The Sociology of Health and Illness

Gower College Swansea

This reader provides a comprehensive collection of classic writings and more recent articles in the sociology of health and illness. It is organised into the following Parts:

- health beliefs and knowledge
- inequalities and patterning of health and illness
- professional and patient interaction
- chronic illness and disability
- evaluation and politics of health care

Each Part has an introduction, summarising the content and argument of each article in turn. The reader also has a general introduction which sets the scene for the field as a whole, contextualises each Part and provides additional reading. The reader includes a number of different perspectives on health and illness, it is international in scope and will provide an invaluable resource to students across a wide range of courses in sociology and the social sciences.

Michael Bury is Emeritus Professor of Sociology at Royal Holloway, University of London.

Jonathan Gabe is Reader in Sociology at Royal Holloway, University of London.

Routledge Student Readers

Series Editor: Chris Jenks, Professor of Sociology,
Goldsmiths College, University of London

Already in this series:

The Sociology of Health and Illness

A reader

Edited by

Michael Bury and Jonathan Gabe

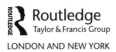

Routledge
Taylor & Francis Group

LONDON AND NEW YORK

First published 2004
by Routledge
11 New Fetter Lane, London EC4P 4EE

Simultaneously published in the USA and Canada
by Routledge
29 West 35th Street, New York, NY 10001

Routledge is an imprint of the Taylor & Francis Group

Typeset in Perpetua and Bell Gothic by RefineCatch Limited, Bungay, Suffolk
Printed and bound in Great Britain by TJ International Ltd, Padstow, Cornwall

British Library Cataloguing in Publication Data
A catalogue record for this book is available from the British Library

Library of Congress Cataloging in Publication Data
The sociology of health and illness: a reader/edited by Mike Bury and
Jonathan Gabe. – 1st ed.
p. cm. – (Routledge student readers)
Includes bibliographical references and index.
1. Social medicine. I. Bury, Michael, 1945–II. Gabe, Jonathan. III. Series.
RA418.S67384 2003
306.4′ 61 – dc21   2003006786

ISBN 0–415–25755–7 (hbk)
ISBN 0–415–25756–5 (pbk)

Contents

Illustrations

Tables

Figures

Boxes

Contributors

Ellen Annandale   Senior Lecturer, Department of Sociology, University of Leicester, UK

David Armstrong   Reader in Sociology as Applied to Medicine, Department of General Practice, Guy's, King's and St Thomas's School of Medicine, London, UK

Paul Atkinson   Professor of Sociology, School of Social Sciences, University of Cardiff, UK

Lisa F. Berkman   Professor, Harvard School of Public Health, Boston, USA

Mildred Blaxter   Professor Emerita, School of Medicine, Health Policy and Practice, University of East Anglia, UK

Mary Boulton   Professor of Sociology, School of Social Sciences and Law, Oxford Brookes University, Oxford, UK

Ian Brissette   Department of Psychology, Carnegie Mellon University, Pittsburgh, USA

Phil Brown   Professor of Sociology, Brown University, Rhode Island, USA

Michael Bury   Emeritus Professor of Sociology, Royal Holloway, University of London, UK

Michael Calnan   Professor of Medical Sociology. MRC Health Services Collaboration, Department of Social Medicine, University of Bristol, UK

Sarah Cant   Senior Lecturer in Sociology, Canterbury, Christchurch University College, UK

Danièle Carricaburu   Centre de Recherche Médecine, Sciences, Santé et Société (Cermes) Paris, France

Cathy Charles   Associate Professor, Department of Clinical Epidemiology and Biostatistics, McMaster University, Hamilton, Ontario, Canada

George Davey Smith   Professor of Social Medicine, Department of Social Medicine, University of Bristol, UK

Charlie Davison   Fellow of the Health and Social Services Institute, University of Essex, UK

Jenny L. Donovan   Professor of Social Medicine, Head of Health Services Research Division, Department of Social Medicine, University of Bristol, UK

Katie Featherstone   School of Social Science, Cardiff University, UK

David Field   Professor of Sociology, Department of Epidemiology and Public Health, University of Leicester, UK

Ray Fitzpatrick   Professor of Public Health and Primary Care and Fellow of Nuffield College, University of Oxford, UK

Arthur Frank   Professor, Department of Sociology, University of Calgary, Alberta, Canada

Stephen Frankel   Professor of Epidemiology and Public Health Medicine, Department of Social Medicine, University of Bristol, UK

Eliot Freidson   Professor Emeritus, Department of Sociology, New York University, USA

Jonathan Gabe   Reader in Sociology, Royal Holloway, University of London, UK

Amiram Gafni   Professor, Department of Clinical Epidemiology and Biostatistics, McMaster University, Hamilton, Ontario, Canada

Thomas Glass   Centre of Aging and Health, Johns Hopkins Medical Institutions, Baltimore, USA

Stephen Harrison   Professor of Social Policy, Department of Applied Social Science, University of Manchester, UK

Claudine Herzlich   Professor, Centre de Recherche Médecine, Sciences, Santé et Société (Cermes) Paris, France

Alistair Howitt   Principal in General Practice, Warders Medical Centre, Tonbridge, Kent, UK

David Hughes   Professor of Health Policy, School of Health Sciences, University of Wales, Swansea, UK

Kate Hunt   MRC Social and Public Health Sciences Unit, University of Glasgow, UK

Raymond Illsley   Visiting Professor, Department of Social and Policy Sciences, University of Bath, UK

Michael P. Kelly   Director of Research, Health Development Agency, London, UK

Donald W. Light   Professor of Comparative Health Care Systems, University of Medicine and Dentistry, New Jersey and Fellow of the Centre for Bioethics, University of Pennsylvania, USA

Deborah Lupton   Professor in Sociology and Cultural Studies, School of Social Sciences and Liberal Studies, Charles Sturt University, Bathurst, Australia

Sally Macintyre   Professor and Director of the MRC Social and Public Health Sciences Unit, University of Glasgow, UK

James Y. Nazroo   Senior Lecturer in Sociology, Department of Epidemiology and Public Health, University College, University of London, UK

Mike Oliver   Professor of Disability Studies, University of Greenwich, London, UK

Evelyn Parsons   Reader and Senior Research Fellow, University of Wales College of Medicine, Cardiff, UK

Janine Pierret   Centre de Recherche Médecine, Sciences, Santé et Société (Cermes) Paris, France

Teresa E. Seeman   Division of Geriatrics, School of Medicine, University of California, Los Angeles, USA

Ursula Sharma   Professor of Comparative Sociology, University of Derby, UK

David Silverman   Professor Emeritus, Department of Sociology, Goldsmiths College, University of London, UK

Helen Sweeting   MRC Social and Public Health Sciences Unit, University of Glasgow, UK

Denny Vågerö   Professor of Medical Sociology, Stockholm Centre on Health in Societies in Transition, University of Stockholm, Sweden

M. E. J. Wadsworth   Professor and Director, MRC National Survey of Health and Development, Department of Epidemiology and Public Health, University College, University of London, UK

Tim Whelan   Department of Sociology, McMaster University, Hamilton, Ontario, Canada

Richard G. Wilkinson   Professor of Social Epidemiology, Division of Public Health Sciences, School of Community Health Sciences, University of Nottingham, UK

Gareth Williams   Research Professor, School of Social Sciences, Cardiff University, UK

Series Editor's Preface

THIS VOLUME ENTITLED *The Sociology of Health and Illness* is the third major contribution to our highly successful series of Routledge Student Readers in Sociology and it promises to maintain the quality that we have become accustomed to. The editors are both well-respected figures from within this specialist field, Michael Bury having been one of the founding fathers of the subdiscipline in the UK.

It is interesting that although issues of health and illness inevitably and fatefully touch us all in our everyday lives it is nevertheless an area of understanding that for decades was 'left to the professionals'. People have always, of course, been concerned if something was wrong with them yet for generations they presented themselves as cases to be assumed or taken over by medicine. Doctors diagnosed, absorbed and processed people as instances of disease and their abstract skills remained removed from and impenetrable by the laity, even to the point of Latin providing the vocabulary of both complaint and medication. In a peculiar way, then, one of the most advanced elements of Western reason became shrouded in mystification and preserved as if a form of magic. Perhaps as embodiment and social identity became more closely aligned through late-modernity people began to redefine their relationship with medicine in terms of health rather than just illness. Self-care, pro-active health pro-motion and maintenance and positive self-regard became markers of identity in the late twentieth century. This sudden insurgence of agency in the populace's interaction with the professions led to an increasing democratisation of medicine and the *citadel* of privacy, insulated from the contamination of everyday concern, that its knowledge base had become. The sociology of medicine, as it was originally designated, played no small part in this transition. These sociologists were making such heretical announce-ments as the fact that people were suffering from and dying from diseases at different rates according to their position within the system of social stratification. Through the same period sociologists of education were similarly noting that ability was socially rather than bio-genetically distributed. These inequalities, and inequities, were intolerable within advanced, democratic societies and as a consequence such areas of social theorising began to impact significantly on social policy. The fact that social class, gender and ethnicity are still significant variables in the distribution of health and illness attests to the fact that there is still a gradient to be climbed and that this field of study is of critical concern to modern sociologists.

Interestingly enough, part of this process of democratisation and demystification has been the mainstreaming of the sociology of medicine and its re-designation as 'health and illness'. Previously such researchers were most likely attached to specialist medical units and continuing the epidemiological tradition of work started by the nineteenth-century philanthropists. Increasingly sociology integrated these colleagues as it became apparent that their work contributed centrally to our concerns with both theory and methodology, as well as their substantive focus. And the more recent title of 'health and illness' reflected the broadening of concerns into the areas of knowledge and belief; doctor–patient interaction and professional process; chronic illness, disability and dying; assessment, evaluation and health care; as well as inequality and patterns of health – all areas that are highlighted in this volume.

Today the sociology of health and illness is an important and influential field within our discipline. It has influenced and continues to influence both social policy and medical practice. It now constitutes a voice loud enough to contribute to the multi-disciplinary explanations of the determinants of health and illness. The burgeoning paradigm of this work has a forceful empirical base, which contributes to its legitimation, yet it also routinely contributes to current theoretical debates about issues as divergent as inclusion, exclusion, marginalisation, identity formation, risk, discourse and surveillance. This is clearly a fecund zone especially when one understands that none of these topics can be addressed independent of considerations of politics, ethics and the law. A positive playground for the young imaginative sociologist then – welcome to the text!

Chris Jenks, Professor of Sociology
Goldsmiths College, University of London

Acknowledgements

The publishers would like to thank the following for permission to reprint their material:

Blackwell Publishing for permission to reprint Annandale, 'Working on the front line: risk culture and nursing in the new NHS', from *Sociological Review* 44, 1996; Davison, Davey Smith and Frankel, 'Lay epidemiology and the prevention paradox: the implications of coronary candidacy for health education', from *Sociology of Health and Illness* 13, 1991; Nazroo 'Genetic, cultural or socio-economic vulnerability? Explaining ethnic inequalities in health', from *Sociology of Health and Illness* 20, 1998; Light and Hughes 'A sociological perspective on rationing: power, rhetoric and situated practices' in Hughes and Light (eds), *Rationing: Constructed Realities and Professional Practice*, 2002; Brown 'Popular epidemiology, toxic waste and social movements' from Gabe (ed.) *Medicine, Health and Risk: Sociological Approaches*, 1995; Williams 'The genesis of chronic illness: narrative reconstruction', from *Sociology of Health and Illness* 6, 1984; Kelly and Field 'Medical sociology, chronic illness and the body' from *Sociology of Health and Illness* 18, 1996; Carricaburu and Pierret 'From biographical disruption to biographical reinforcement: the case of HIV-positive men', from *Sociology of Health and Illness* 17, 1995; and Parsons and Atkinson 'Lay constructions of genetic risk' from *Sociology of Health and Illness* 14, 1992.

The BMJ publishing group for permission to reprint Fitzpatrick and Boulton 'Qualitative methods for assessing health care' from *Quality in Health Care* 3, 1994; Howitt and Armstrong 'Implementing evidence-based medicine in general practice' from the *British Medical Journal* 318, 1999; and Featherstone and Donovan 'Random allocation or allocation at random? Patients' perspectives of participation in a randomised control led trial' from the *British Medical Journal* 317, 1998.

Michael Calnan for permission to reprint his article 'Lifestyle and its social meaning', originally published in Albrecht (ed.) *Advances in Medical Sociology, volume 4*, JAI Press, 1994.

Daedalus for permission to reprint Wilkinson 'The epidemiological transition: from material scarcity to social disadvantage?' from *Daedalus* (Journal of the American Academy of Arts and Sciences) 123, 1994.

The Disability Press for permission to reprint Bury 'Defining and researching disability: challenges and responses' in Barnes and Mercer (eds) *Exploring the Divide: Illness and Disability*, 1996; and Oliver 'Defining impairment and disability: the issues at stake' in Barnes and Mercer (eds) *Exploring the Divide: Illness and Disability*, 1996.

Elsevier Science for permission to reprint Berkman, Glass, Brissette and Seeman 'From social integration to health: Durkheim in the new millennium' from *Social Science and Medicine* 51, 2000; Wadsworth 'Health inequalities in the lifecourse perspective' from *Social Science and Medicine* 44, 1997; Macintyre, Hunt and Sweeting 'Gender differences in health: are things really as simple as they seem?' from *Social Science and Medicine* 42, 1996; Lupton 'Consumerism, reflexivity and the medical encounter' from *Social Science and Medicine* 45, 1997; and Charles, Gafni and Whelan 'Decision-making in the physician–patient encounter: revisiting the shared treatment decision-making model' from *Social Science and Medicine* 49, 1999.

Oxford University Press for permission to reprint Vågerö and Illsley 'Explaining health inequalities: beyond Black and Barker', from *European Sociological Review* 11, 1995.

The Policy Press for permission to reprint Harrison 'The politics of evidence-based medicine in the United Kingdom' from *Policy and Politics* 26, 1998.

Sage Publications for permission to reprint material from Silverman *Communication and Medical Practice: Social Relations in the Clinic*, 1987.

The University of Chicago Press for permission to reprint material from Frank *The Wounded Story Teller: Body, Illness and Ethics*, 1997; and material from Freidson *Profession of Medicine: A Study of the Sociology of Applied Knowledge*, 1970.

The Publishers have made every effort to contact authors and copyright holders of works reprinted in *The Sociology of Health and Illness: A Reader*. It has not been possible in every case, however, and we would welcome correspondence from individuals or companies we have been unable to trace.

General introduction

■   Michael Bury and Jonathan Gabe

Background

IT IS ONLY IN RECENT YEARS that the idea of putting together a Reader on the sociology of health and illness has seemed a possibility in the UK. Though medical sociology has been established and active for the last thirty years, it has not always been part of the sociological mainstream. While UK medical sociology has been very successful in research and teaching this has mainly developed in medical settings. For many years, and still today, sociologists with an interest in health and illness have worked in academic departments of public health, general practice and psychiatry. In university sociology departments the attitude towards health and illness as substantive topics was often lukewarm. Health, illness and health care were not regarded as a main area of enquiry, in comparison with labour markets, social divisions and even religion.

All this has changed dramatically in recent years, to the point where few under-graduate programmes today in the social sciences, and in sociology in particular, are without a course on health and illness. Most, if not all, general textbooks in sociology have a section on the topic. Far from being seen as a peripheral area of social life, health and illness are now rightly regarded as being at the centre of the study of 'private troubles and public issues'. More than this, much that is exciting in con-temporary sociology is gaining from, and contributing to, the field of health and illness. This is true for both theory and empirical research, both of which are reflected in the current collection. A Reader that is explicitly sociological can also supplement other texts concerned with health and illness. The work of the current editors (Bury 1997, Gabe 1995, Williams *et al.* 2000) has dealt with a number of contemporary issues in health and illness and some of these have guided our selection for the Reader, but we have taken a broad view of its scope.

In this General Introduction we intend to provide a guide to some of the most important developments in the sociology of health and illness over the last thirty years. These developments are discussed thematically and provide the rationale for the different sections that make up the Reader. Specific commentary on the themes and arguments of individual articles or extracts is left to the shorter introductions given at the beginning of each Part.

The sociology of health and illness

We have organised the Reader round the following topics:

- health beliefs and knowledge;
- inequalities and patterning of health and illness;
- professional and patient interaction;
- chronic illness and disability;
- evaluation and politics in health care.

Although any exercise in dividing up a field of study is to some extent arbitrary, the above topics seem to us to cover the most important areas of work undertaken over the last ten years or so. Though we have included some 'classic' pieces (e.g. those from Herzlich and Freidson) we have concentrated on selecting pieces that best illustrate recent work, and that we believe deal with a range of topics that will continue to influence the field in the years to come. We have, of course, been forced to leave out or under-represent areas where more could easily have been included, such as the relationship between age and health, including research on children that in recent years has been gaining momentum (Mayall 1996). We have also had to leave out some topics such as the link between place and health, where current research is attempting to shift attention away from individuals alone and on to wider community structures and processes (Macintyre *et al.* 2002). Nonetheless, many of the readings in the book touch on issues such as these, and can be followed up elsewhere. The references at the end of this Introduction provide a starting point for such an exercise, and can act as a guide to further reading.

At the end of the Introduction we also provide a brief guide to the use of the Reader. First, however, we introduce the main themes of the sections of the book and the background to the issues that are currently the focus of medical sociology research and writing.

Knowledge and beliefs in the sociology of health and illness

An important starting point concerns beliefs and knowledge about health and illness, both in the clinic and in everyday settings. Until the 1980s sociological writing tended to focus on the enormous influence of the medical model of illness in modern society, and its employment in medical settings (Freidson 1970). This was occasioned in part by the rapid expansion of biomedical research, which, of course, has continued unabated. The sociological preoccupation with 'medicalisation' and 'medical dominance' helped to establish an independent and critical approach both to medical knowledge and to medical practice. The tendency for more and more problems (social as well as strictly disease-related) to be regarded and treated as medical ones led sociologists also to examine deviance in a new light: the impact of medical knowledge in transforming 'badness' into 'sickness' (Conrad and Schneider 1980). This more critical approach also led to the analysis of the medical profession not simply as providing 'neutral' technical services, but as carriers of a culture where scientific expertise and professionally based authority could overshadow lay understandings and action. Moral and political issues were seen in these critiques to be transformed into medical ones.

Studies of the way in which the lay experience of illness was excluded from medical practice, and the mechanisms that turned people into patients (Robinson 1973, Zola 1973) were related popular topics. Once in the clinic the lay voice was seen to be effectively silenced, under the impact of medical authority, a rationalising technology and an oppressive bureaucracy (Strong 1979). The patient was offered little more than a passive role in proceedings, with strong expectations of unquestioning compliance with treatment decisions. The dominance of a disease model was thus seen to serve the power of medical interests, rather than the needs of a populace in a modern democratic society.

In the 1980s, however, the examination of medical power began to be balanced by studies that moved out of the clinic and into the community, where the beliefs of people outside of the medical arena could be studied (Calnan 1987). In so far as professional expertise was the focus of attention it was the activities of those engaged in health promotion, rather than those delivering clinical services, that now came under the spotlight, and in relation to the assimilation or resistance of their advice in lay settings (Pill and Stott 1982, 1985). It is not difficult to see why, from this viewpoint, the idea of researching lay people's views outside of the clinic began to hold attractions for sociologists, or can still do so today. Although, for example, warnings of the effects of smoking have long been a feature of health education and health promotion aimed at the whole population, it is only in recent years that attempts have been made to understand how this has led to a pattern of consumption where some 45 per cent of adult male unskilled manual workers smoke while only 15 per cent of professionals do so (*Social Trends* 2000).

Clearly, the study of health and illness could not be left at the door of the clinic or in relation to the exercise of medical power. Many more influences, and of a complex kind, were at work in modern communities. Several studies in the developed world, including the UK, began to examine the factors that might lead to patterning of behaviours and lay beliefs about health and illness, together with their determinants (Blaxter 1990, Calnan 1987). These studies have produced a much more nuanced picture of everyday understandings and actions, which have thrown important light on health promotion activities as well as on wider processes. To stay with smoking for a moment, it is clear that a number of social structural and cultural factors interact to produce the observed pattern of consumption, including levels of stress experienced by social groups, the interaction of health behaviours and work, and the differential experiences of men and women in these regards (Blaxter 1990, Graham 1993). But consumption also reflects the active choices people make in different social circumstances. After all, even in the figures given above, the majority of unskilled manual workers do not smoke.

At the same time research on lay beliefs in such areas has revealed important dynamics of modern cultures; differing lay views of personal responsibility and social determinants of behaviour, the continuing influences of ideas about fate and luck alongside more rational influences, and lay perceptions of risk (Davison *et al.* 1992). The latter issue is of particular note, especially as the results of modern laboratory-based medical science have fed into the wider society. Comparing lay perceptions of health and risk, including genetic risk, with the assumptions made by medical experts has added a further dimension to earlier studies of health behaviours and health promotion (Gabe 1995). Not infrequently, sociological work has exposed misperceptions among experts, who too often expect scientific knowledge to 'trickle down' and be assimilated in lay populations, and become frustrated when it does not, or when is assimilated in ways that the experts find difficult to understand. Sociological work has provided a number of important clues to why and how these 'mismatches' occur.

Exploring these issues has led some writers to question the whole notion of 'belief' as it has developed in the sociological and anthropological literature (e.g. Good 1994) and in its application to areas such as health. Part of the problem lies in the implicit, if not explicit, contrast between 'belief' and 'knowledge', which sociological work may unwittingly convey. It is as if lay people are restricted to holding beliefs while experts are able to produce knowledge. Yet it is clear that expert opinion is itself a carrier of a wide range of beliefs, and everyday 'lay' behaviours may often be based on a knowledgeable and rational assimilation of expertise, and on an understanding of its limitations and contradictions.

Of course, it is important not to press this argument too far. The study of lay experiences of health and illness contains considerable evidence of admitted ignorance and an understandable belief that the expert knows best. Such responses in themselves need to be taken seriously by sociologists. However, it is also clear that lay people can and do become knowledgeable about health matters, and can develop sophisticated models that reconcile or challenge what is offered by medical science and health promotion. Moreover, this is not simply a matter of individual reflection, but can take on collective dimensions as people campaign over health issues in their local communities or even in national and international contexts (Williams and Popay 1994, Brown 1995). In such circumstances the line between belief and knowledge becomes blurred, as does the role of the expert and the lay person. In many campaigns today (medical) scientific experts work closely with lay groups. In others, experts and lay people may come into conflict when the evidence does not provide an unequivocal answer. Freidson's 'clash of perspectives' can now take on more collective dimensions outside of the clinic. Through the study of health beliefs we are able to see, therefore, some of the larger contours of late modern societies, and not just those of medicine. These contours are illustrated in the readings chosen to illustrate work on health beliefs and knowledge.

Inequalities and the patterning of health and illness

Of all the 'public issues' that medical sociology has tackled, inequalities in health are among the most important. It has long been observed that mortality varies by social class, producing a picture where the better off have lower mortality than those living in more straitened circumstances. The publication of the 'Black Report' in the UK in 1980 (Townsend and Davison 1990) marked a renewed interest in the subject, and immediately became the focus of intense debate. Among (conservative) critics the Report's recommendations seemed to amount to little more than a call for the abolition of relative poverty. Government ministers of the time regarded the science as flawed and the recommendations as outrageously expensive. At the same time, debate inside medical sociology and health policy circles was no less intense. While some researchers added further evidence to that produced by the Black Report, especially on measures of morbidity (self-reported illness and disability, e.g. Blaxter 1990), others questioned the validity of the whole approach and the assumption that all inequalities were 'unacceptable' (see Bury 1997: 66–72 for a review).

In looking back over this period of discussion and argument, two themes are worthy of note in relation to the selection of material in the Reader, and may help explain some of the heat if not the light generated in the area. First, on an inter-national scale, the inequalities observed in highly developed countries such as the UK or the US pale in comparison with the health status of populations in developing countries. Take, for example, the situation with infant mortality rates (IMR) expressed as the number of deaths in the first year of life per thousand live births. This measure has been universally regarded as one of the most important indicators of both the health of populations and economic and social development. Today, Bangladesh has an IMR of 70 per thousand live births and Mali, in sub-Saharan Africa, 121. In the UK the figure is 5.5 and in the US 6.5. The magnitude of these differences helps explain, perhaps, the reluctance of some in the developed world to accord health inequalities of the kind discussed in developed countries the highest of priorities. Even the poorest people in developed countries experience a level of health only dreamt about in many parts of the world (Gray 2001).

Second, the emphasis on mortality data in much of the health inequalities literature has seemed to miss the point that longevity in the developed (and now in many developing) countries has been steadily increasing. Indeed, recent evidence on average life expectancy in the UK shows that when survival is the focus of attention rather than mortality, the picture emerging on inequalities is somewhat less dramatic than the Black Report seemed to show. The difference in life expectancy between unskilled manual workers and professional groups is about five years, which, while significant, is less dramatic than the very wide differences seen in mortality data, especially when expressed as ratios (Drever and Whitehead 1997). As people from all social groups live longer, early mortality (deaths in infancy and adult life before retirement) has, accordingly, become a less sensitive indicator of the public health, HIV/AIDS notwithstanding. Today the issues associated with disability and health in later life are as important as those of premature mortality. Moreover, studies of gender and ethnic inequalities in health have taken on greater salience, in comparison with the emphasis on occupational social class, as sociology has re-orientated much of its work on inequalities in the face of economic and social restructuring and the increasing significance of new forms of social division. The availability of new data such as those stemming from the combination of 'ethnic questions' and measures of long-term illness since the 1991 UK census has also been significant. Research is now exploring the role of racism in health inequalities and disentangling the relationship between gender, culture, context and class and their influence on health.

In addition to these considerations, two further theoretical issues have influenced developments in the field, and, again, the readings included in this Part of the book. The first is that much of the literature calls on and contributes to two different sociological traditions. On the one hand there is a structural or materialist tradition, emphasising economic relations and the effects of deprivation and poverty. The Black Report drew heavily on this approach to health inequalities and in its anti-poverty recommendations. Culture and individual behaviour were effectively sidelined in favour of emphasising the effects of occupational social class. On the other hand there is a more Durkheimian tradition, which emphasises social solidarity, social networks and the need for social support as the key determinants of good health. The absence of the same factors is seen to produce the conditions that may predispose towards poor health. Social dislocation, disorientation, insecurity and poor social support have significant health implications in this view. While these may be related to deprivation, they can be found in, and may be typical of, social circumstances where inequalities are marked but where absolute material hardship is less evident. Wide variations in circumstance rather than absolute poverty are the issues here. Anomie rather than alienation predominates. In this Durkheimian approach material forces are seen to play less of a role in determining health (at least, in developed countries) and social cohesion or its absence more so (Wilkinson 1996).

The second theoretical issue concerns biography and history. Modern societies are not static and this has important implications for the sociological study of inequalities in health. At the very least, the presence of at least a degree of social mobility produces a situation where good health along with other factors favours upward movement in the system and poor health downward movement. This issue of 'health selection' has been widely debated in the health inequalities literature, but in recent years research has re-focused its efforts to concentrate on the nature of 'lifecourse' influences on health in order to unravel such processes more fully (Bartley et al. 1999). 'Lifecourse' approaches mean that rather than rely on cross-sectional data gathered at one point in time (say, mortality data for 1990/1991) researchers focus instead on data which captures influences on samples of people over periods of their lifetime, preferably beginning with data collected at their birth. Data on the biological and social characteristics of both mothers and their infants born within a specified time period can be compared with data collected periodically at later points. Even if the starting point is later than birth, longitudinal studies can examine changes over subsequent periods of the lifecourse. The interaction of social selection and health status can then be documented as people move through their lives, and up or down the social system.

By studying the health of groups of people over time it is possible to chart the influences on health of particular historical circumstances and the biographies of individuals (Blaxter 2000). Such longitudinal research has begun to reshape the field of health inequalities by showing how the risks of poor health may build up over time and how they may be avoided. Pathways to poor health and, perhaps more significantly, pathways to good health can then be described. The processes that drive good health can be more easily identified than is possible from 'snapshot' cross-sectional data. Importantly, such studies may be able to examine biological as well as social factors present at birth and the interaction of these with social processes and health-related behaviour as time unfolds. Work along these lines has provided the opportunity to examine the influence of such factors as education and social networks, as well as early exposure to material hardship and deprivation, helping to bridge the materialist and Durkheimian perspectives (Wadsworth 1991).

More recently attention has turned to the health of older age groups, as the cohorts being studied enter retirement. In this context it has been shown in one study, for example, that those from poorer backgrounds and who had poorer health at birth are more likely to have raised blood pressure in later life if they are overweight or obese. Those from equally poor backgrounds, in both biological and social terms, but who are not overweight or obese in later life have reduced risk of high blood pressure (Bury and Wadsworth 2003). Thus, factors operating across the lifecourse can either protect or increase health risks conferred on individuals at birth or in infancy. Work on health inequalities of this kind points to the protective potential of favourable health behaviours or circumstances in adult life and thus of the need to encourage policies which help develop them. The tendency for health inequalities work to either be pessimistic about effective social change or passive in the face of risks present at birth can thus be challenged. Research on health pathways across the lifecourse is therefore taking on renewed intellectual and practical significance.

Professional and patient interactions

While work on health inequalities has focused on the nature of material and social determinants of health, the role of health services has been somewhat downplayed. This has partly stemmed from the observation made by McKeown (1976) and others in the 1970s that, historically, health services have played little role in the improvement of the health of the public. Most improvements in health status in the last 150 years, up to the post Second World War period, occurred before medical science formulated a clear understanding of the mechanisms at work (e.g. regarding infections) and thus before effective treatments became available. Social factors such as clean air, clean water and improved diet, rather than modern medical knowledge and practice, have been the most important. It is doubtful, however, whether such a clear-cut division between 'external' influences on health and those of health services could be made with respect to any similar assessment covering the last twenty years. It has been estimated that significant improvements in population health during this period may be the result of medical intervention, most notably more successful surgery and

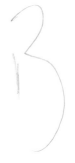

effective pharmacological treatments (Bunker *et al.* 1994). For this reason alone the issue of people's experience of health services and their organisation must be a central part of medical sociology's remit.

Early work on people's encounters with health care professionals such as that of Parsons (1951, 1978) focused on doctors and stressed the shared values and consensus between doctors and patients. Subsequently, in the 1970s and 1980s, conflict and professional power, if not class interests, were given centre stage. For instance, in Freidson's (1970) view, conflict was endemic if muted in medical practice, and the worlds of lay and professional existed in parallel rather than harmony. Others, as noted earlier, focused on how doctors medicalised everyday life by defining patients' problems that had a social origin in terms of a medical model and individualised aetiology (Zola 1975), and legitimised and reinforced existing hierarchical social relations by their attitudes and behaviour towards patients, especially female patients (Barrett and Roberts 1978, Oakley 1981). However, a problem existed at the heart of this conceptualisation. The picture created of the 'lay world' in this more critical sociology was largely one of the passive citizen or patient. Medical dominance ruled, and there seemed little scope for patients or lay people to do much about it. A few sociologists took pains to examine the 'countervailing power' that patients might exert (Stimson and Webb 1975) as well as the processes of 'demedicalisation' that were occurring alongside 'medicalisation' (Conrad 1992). Despite this, most medical sociology in the 1970s and 1980s was characterised by a tendency to see the medical profession, if not all practitioners, in a largely negative light. Part of the justification for this lay in the fact, as we have noted, that medicine had come to occupy a strategic place in modern society, embodying an ever expanding role for science and technology, and epitomising the growing ascendance of 'expertise' in tackling a wide range of social issues. Medical sociology's preoccupation with medicine as an institution can be seen, therefore, as a major contribution to the sociology of the professions and the study of modernity more broadly.

These earlier concerns with the medicalisation of society remain relevant to the sociological enterprise, if only because continuing large-scale consumption of medical treatments brings with it the possibility of deleterious side effects for individuals and a growing culture reliant on expertise and technical 'fixes', along demonstrable benefits (*British Medical Journal* 13 April 2002). Moreover, though sociologists have argued that the medical profession is going through a major transition away from its pre-eminent position of power in the health care sector, to a position where it has become 'corporatised' if not 'proletarianised' – what McKinlay and Marceau (2002) have recently called the 'end of the golden age of doctoring' – the jury remains out concerning the extent of this transition. Medical authority still holds great sway over the public imagination, despite high-profile and damaging scandals, the advent of greater regulation by governments and corporations, and the growth of a more assertive, litigious and critical public. Medical science continues to grow apace, especially in the field of post genome research, and still receives strong governmental backing and large-scale research funding. In many day-to-day interactions, patients may still be cast in a passive and deferential role, or may indeed actively seek it. But having said this, it needs to be recognised that medical practice covers a very wide range of activities, from dealing with the most frightening life-threatening effects of disease, through the treatment of trauma and diffuse forms of physical illness, to the treatment of chronic physical or mental illness. It would be surprising if this huge range of activity could adequately be characterised by one overriding form of interactional style or display of power and authority.

It is for this reason that the nature of the doctor–patient relationship as an instance of 'negotiated order' retains its attractions, if only because such a perspective points to the contingencies that surround the many different forms of medical encounter. Even here, though, the changing nature of medical practice needs to be recognised. A number of important developments have suggested themselves for consideration and have influenced our choice of extracts for the Reader. The first of these is the question of health care professions other than medicine. It is possible to argue that initial interest in 'medical dominance' among medical sociologists gave too much attention to doctors and not enough to other significant groups such as nurses. Much of the everyday practice of medicine is carried out by nurses (and other professional groups) and much of the mediation of medical knowledge and communication about health and health care risks, including such matters as genetic risk, is carried through by them.

In a similar vein it is also possible to see more clearly from today's perspective that much of the focus of medical sociology in the UK (with notable exceptions, e.g. Silverman 1987, Calnan *et al.* 1993) was overly concerned with interactions in the National Health Service (NHS). While this was understandable during a period when the NHS represented virtually the only point of contact with health care professionals, this has increasingly become less true. The expansion of the private sector, especially for non-urgent treatments, and the growth of complementary or 'alternative' forms of medicine for a large number of medical conditions has led to an even greater range of professional–client interactions than before. Not surprisingly, medical sociology has therefore begun to take these forms of 'plural' medical consumption into account in its research activity (Cant and Sharma 1996).

The issue of 'consumerism' in health care is of note in this changing picture. In the mid 1970s medical sociologists such as Stacey (1976) were able to argue that the idea of patients as consumers was a basic misconception. The social relations of health care – or at least those of the dominant NHS – were anathema to such a formulation. Patients simply could not be consumers because they lacked the ability to choose, were deficient in knowledge and power compared with their doctors, and could not exercise the right to return or effectively complain about the 'product', so often the hallmarks of consumerism. At the most basic level this argument seemed to be self-evident – it is difficult to imagine returning to a surgeon and demanding another type of operation because the one that has been given has not worked properly.

Yet, despite these obvious limitations, consumerism has come to play a greater role in professional–patient interactions than had been thought possible. Changes in the organisation of care, including a more 'businesslike' orientation in health care delivery based on the patient rather than the provider, greater lay knowledge of medicine especially among those living with and managing chronic disorders, and at least some reduction in hierarchical relationships in health care have helped to create a more consumerist approach. As important has been the increase in litigation in countries such as the UK, where until recently patients have rarely challenged their doctors' judgement or behaviour in the courts. In addition, as well as greater regulation by governments through formal procedures such as audit and clinical governance, there have been more subtle assaults on medical autonomy such as the development of evidence-based practice (Armstrong 2002). Clinical governance and evidence-based practice (where guidelines based on research findings are supposed to inform clinical judgement) constrain doctors' autonomy, and limit their freedom to practise as they choose. If we then add to this the role of the media, which no longer treats the medical profession as a 'protected species' (Bury and Gabe 1994), then a very different picture of medical practice emerges for sociological attention.

To this heady brew we should also mix in one last ingredient that has arguably both reinforced and altered the view of the patient as consumer, namely the rhetoric surrounding 'partnership' (Calnan and Gabe 2001). In many developed countries, but most notably in the UK, government policies on many fronts, and especially in the health sector, now emphasise 'partnership' as a key element of policy development. Government departments in the UK have issued a number of important statements on the subject, and, through a variety of initiatives, the view that patients (indeed, lay people in general) should be involved in the development of services as well as their delivery has been reinforced. At the point of contact, shared decision making is to be the watchword of professional–client relationships. Within the social scientific and medical press a number of programmatic statements on partnership have reinforced this view (Coulter 1999, Charles *et al.* 2000). The scene is set therefore for sociological research on professional–patient interactions to enter a new phase, if only in analysing and assessing the realities and rhetorical uses of partnership in health care.

Chronic illness and disability

The overarching theme of this Introduction is to emphasise the changes in health and society that have influenced the medical sociology agenda in the last ten years or so, and thus the selection of readings for this volume. As far as health itself is concerned the most important change in countries such as the UK, which we have already touched on in the inequalities Part, is what has been referred to as the 'epidemiological and health transition' (Gray 2001: 127). This refers to a situation where infectious diseases and those resulting from food shortages give way to conditions associated with later life such as heart disease and cancer. These 'degenerative' diseases pose new problems of living for those affected, and demand new forms of health care. As the latter become more effective, so people may live longer with their symptoms, or in a 'post recovery' situation.

Just as important is a wider range of non-life-threatening but disabling disorders, which, though containing many which have early onset such as cystic fibrosis and trauma from accidents, are typically characterised by late onset and long duration in the later years of life. These chronic disabling illnesses have been the focus of considerable sociological research. In recent years, work in this area by medical sociologists has also provoked a growing and sometimes heated debate with some sections of the disability movement.

The early study of chronic illness, like that of the doctor–patient relationship, was strongly influenced by interactionist perspectives, emphasising the contingencies surrounding diagnosis, treatment and everyday actions in living with a disorder (Gerhardt 1989). While research on health inequalities was preoccupied with factors that might predispose or play a causal role in disease occurrence, sociological attention in chronic illness focused on the situation of those already living with health problems, and how long-term experiences were shaped by social actions – both of self and others in the face of symptoms. While initial research centred on the behavioural patterns in everyday life (Strauss and Glaser 1975) other studies, especially in the UK, increasingly examined links between illness, the body, self and society (e.g. Kelly and Field 1996). Research also focused on the effects of chronic illness on significant others, particularly in the context of the family (Anderson and Bury 1988).

As work on chronic illness has grown a number of issues have emerged of wider relevance to sociology as a whole. In order to contextualise the readings included in this volume we would mention three issues in particular. The first concerns postmodernism and the sociology of the body. One of the criticisms levelled against earlier work on chronic illness is that although many problems faced by people with such conditions relate to the 'embodied' character of social life, an explicit exploration of the issue was noticeable by its absence. Since the 1980s considerable debate has ensued concerning the role of the body in social action and in sociological theorising (Turner 1984, 1992, Shilling 1993). The study of chronic illness has begun to throw particular light on a number of important issues in this regard.

Take, for example, the issue of 'cultural competence'. It may plausibly be argued that modern societies, especially in their 'late modern' or 'postmodern' form, give particular emphasis to the nature of bodily appearance. Giddens (1991), for example, argues that the body in such societies is less an 'extrinsic given' and more involved in 'internally referential systems' (Giddens 1991: 7). This means that in an increasing number of areas of life, whether to do with the consumption of food, body maintenance, leisure and sport, or even medical and reproductive interventions, strategic sites develop where cultural competence can be displayed, consumerism pursued, and, indeed, where there is pressure to do both. Postmodern cultures set up tensions between strongly normative images of cultural propriety (for example, a slim body image) and at the same time emphasise diversity in lifestyle, appearance and the pursuit of consumer freedom.

Against such an ambiguous backcloth, those suffering from the disruption that chronic illness brings find themselves creating a number of different responses. Studies have shown how disruptive lives may be repaired or at least mitigated to meet social and cultural demands, providing at least a degree of continuity (Charmaz 2001). It is important to note, however, that active and positive responses to these pressures are not ubiquitous. The sociological literature shows also that some can be overwhelmed by their illness and by the demands placed upon them, especially in situations where competence in bodily display and emotional control is required but where 'failure' is inevitable, or where feelings of chaos dominate (Becker 1997). However, the pressure from a culture that at many points seems strongly conformist in terms of its view of the body is counterbalanced by a postmodern display of such matters as disfigurement or physical disability which would earlier have been at least partly hidden from view. In medical sociology, an emphasis on illness narratives has illustrated this more expressive form of postmodern culture (Bury 2001, Morris 1998). For some sociologists the emphasis on a more diverse and expressive culture is to be welcomed, as providing a more conducive and supportive environment for living with illness. For others, a postmodern culture is seen to bring about a hazardous situation for the chronically ill, in insisting on making public what would otherwise be dealt with in private.

The second issue of note concerns the place of material factors alongside inter-actional ones. One of the common criticisms of interactionist sociology has been that it has underplayed, either wittingly or otherwise, the role of material forces on people's lives. In the study of chronic illness similar criticisms have been made. Links between the sociology of illness experience, especially its biographical dimensions, and that of epidemiological work on chronic disease (Kuh and Ben-Shlomo 1997) has not been much in evidence. Thus the contextualising of the disruption of chronic illness, whether in terms of its place in the lifecourse, or in terms of the material factors that may significantly influence its course, has still to be examined more systematically (Williams 2000).

One of the key issues here is that of age. As with work on the body, much of the chronic illness literature has taken age as a given, referred to often only in passing. Much research has been on young or middle-aged adults but with little reference to ageing as a process or as a major contextual factor. Though writers in the US (Zola 1991) and in the UK (Arber and Ginn 1991) have drawn attention in different ways to the links between age, material factors and chronic illness and disability, more work needs to be done in better understanding those links. There is some evidence to suggest that ideas concerning the 'disruptive' nature of chronic illness, let alone pre-occupations with late modern cultural motifs concerning the body, are less in evidence among older age groups (Pound et al. 1998, Sanders et al. 2002). However, given that later life itself covers substantial periods of biographical time and is characterised by wide variations in material circumstances, generalisations should be expressed with caution.

The last issue under this heading, important to an understanding of contemporary work on chronic illness, concerns that of its relationship to disability. Up to this point we have used the terms 'chronic illness' and 'disability' in an interchangeable way. As indicated above, however, considerable controversy has grown, in the UK especially, between medical sociologists and disability activists about the nature of disability and its portrayal in the medical sociological literature. In part this stems from the criticisms of interactionism already mentioned, namely that it concentrates overly on day-to-day experiences and not enough on the material context in which these experi-ences take place. While it is overstating the argument to claim that, whatever the circumstances, daily interactions are central to those living with long-standing illness, the force of this argument is difficult to resist entirely, as some disability activists seem to do.

However, the disability movement has levelled a stronger charge against medical sociology. In brief, this has been that disability is essentially a social product, and should be separated off from issues to do with chronic illness or the body. While people may suffer from impairments (symptoms, altered bodies) the disability they experience is best conceived of in strictly social terms, indeed in terms of discrimination and rights. Barnes (1991) and Oliver (1996) among others have argued that such a view allows attention to focus on the real causes of disability, namely the oppressive and discriminatory practices that have excluded those with certain impairments from mainstream social life. From this viewpoint, attention to bodily symptoms and illness distracts the analyst from attending to the need to oppose the oppressive character of social structures and of medicine's involvement in managing disability.

There is not space here to enter into a full discussion of the 'social model' of disability that underpins such critiques. There is now an extensive literature on 'disability studies' that tackles many of the arguments to which it refers (e.g. Barnes *et al.* 1999, Albrecht *et al.* 2001, Williams 2001). Suffice it to say for the present purposes that the relationship between chronic illness and disability remains a complex one. While some forms of impairment and disability are not caused or immediately related to illness (for example, those related to accidents) many are, especially in later life.

Empirical evidence suggests that while the 'social model' may have attractions for some disabled people and be relevant to some aspects of disability in terms of discrimination (for example, in the workplace and in education) many chronic disorders are still widely regarded in lay circles as disabling, in the sense of restricting activity and reducing quality of life. Research on older age groups suffering from disabling conditions such as arthritis has found radical ideas about disability to be of little relevance (Sanders *et al.* 2002). Not only does it prove difficult to maintain a strict separation of illness and impairment from disability (however defined) but disability activism, important though it undoubtedly is in some quarters, can be no substitute for good medical care where it is proven to be beneficial. At the least, the study of chronic illness looks set to continue to touch on significant sociological issues, and on continuing debates.

Sociology and the evaluation of health services

Until recently the involvement of medical sociology in the evaluation of health services has been restricted to its more 'applied' wing in the guise of health services research or health policy analysis. Enough has been said so far in this Introduction, however, to underline how important health care is to modern social systems. Health care not only acts as a major 'carrier' of a culture in which professional expertise is central (if not longer entirely dominant and unchallenged) but also bears witness to the way in which health and illness have taken on ever greater significance in daily life. The health risks of food, the environment, drugs both licit and illicit, genetic endowment and a variety of psychosocial stresses have all acted to bring people into regular contact with health care agencies and those concerned with health promotion.

Late modern cultures are shot through with the motifs of health and illness, to the extent that it is difficult sometimes to imagine a medically free or truly healthy existence. It has recently been pointed out that self-reported illness in the US, for example, is over three times higher than in India, suggesting that North Americans are experiencing much worse health than those in a much poorer country (Sen 2002). This, of course, is difficult to reconcile with health status measures of a more traditional public health kind. In 2001 life expectancy in the United States was 77 years and infant mortality 7 per thousand live births. In India life expectancy was 63 years and infant mortality 63 per thousand live births. Clearly, the dynamics affecting perceptions of health and the role of health services in meeting expressed 'needs' in the developed world require careful study. We should also note in this connection that the use of prescribed drugs in the developed countries has also increased enormously. In England alone, prescriptions for just one class of drugs – anti-depressants – have risen from some 8 million in 1991 to 22 million in the year 2000 (Double 2002).

For these reasons it is important that medical sociology continues to be involved in the evaluation of health services and to provide a critical perspective on the politics of health care. Our selection of readings under this heading attempts to reflect this growing field. As far as the politics of health care is concerned, two broad themes emerge from the literature. The first concerns the continuing crisis with respect to the public funding of health care. The apparent shortfall of provision against demand, as witnessed in the UK at least by continuing controversies surrounding waiting times for common procedures, has led to a call for the raising of levels of expenditure in the UK to those in the rest of Europe, that is to about 8 per cent of GDP. Yet given the level of demand, illustrated by Sen's data on self-reported illness, it seems unlikely that increases in expenditure will by themselves help to meet demand in any absolute sense. Like motorways, the more health services that are provided the more seem to be needed. There are good reasons to argue that some groups in modern society have been undertreated in the health care system, for example the elderly who have frequently been denied acute care by virtue of age alone (Ebrahim 2002). However, the tendency to treat old age as if it were a disease (senescence) has also been a feature of a critical sociology of ageing (Katz 1996), stressing the negative as well as the positive effects of developments such as geriatric medicine. Sociological analysis needs to tackle the contradictions that these kinds of observation produce. Notions such as the medicalisation of society need to be revisited in the light of these tensions, and in the light of both explicit and hidden forms of rationing which attempt to manage demand.

Linked to this is the theme of clinical governance and evidence-based practice. As we have noted above, most developed countries have taken steps to control medicine by controlling medical activities and their costs, and by encouraging, and in some cases demanding, better evidence of effectiveness of treatments. The observations made by the epidemiologist Archie Cochrane (1972) some thirty years ago that most routine procedures in the health services have never been evaluated, chimed in with critiques that others in the public health movement had made concerning the limited effectiveness of health care. Mention has already been made of McKeown's historical thesis that health care has played only a minor role in the improvement of the population's health. These public health broadsides against clinical medicine met with considerable sympathy in some policy circles (including some in government who were keen to limit health service expansion) and among other groups with a history of scepticism towards the medical profession, including sociologists.

Today, however, the agenda concerning evaluation is arguably very different. The presence of large-scale research activity in assessing outcomes of medical treat-ments poses new and important sociological and political issues. The very existence of organisations such as the Cochrane Collaboration is of great significance. This collaboration is an international network of researchers working on the evaluation of health care effectiveness (often through the use of randomised controlled trials, strongly advocated by Cochrane himself) and is testament to the rapidity of change. A search on any internet search engine can produce up to 35,000 links around the world, under the Collaboration heading alone. Though some sociologists of an applied nature may be interested in participating in the carrying out of such evaluations, for example, through collecting different kinds of data, including qualitative data (Dixon-Woods and Fitzpatrick 2001) there are also important questions about their political impact. It is clear, for example, that the idea of developing 'evidence-based medicine' is attractive not only to managers trying to reduce costs and ration services, but also to professional elites who wish to exercise greater control over the medical profession and indicate to governments their willingness to undertake 'internal' regulation and develop tighter clinical governance mechanisms (Armstrong 2002). Developing a pro-fessional ideology based on evaluation chimes in with 'modernisation' agendas and shows a willingness to limit professional autonomy. The sociological consequences of this for the doctor–patient relationship require careful study, as doctors attempt to use research evidence more directly in their dealings with patients.

This brings us to the wider issues of evaluation, aside from its political dimensions. Within medicine it is often assumed that the mechanisms and methodologies of evaluation are largely neutral in their social effects. Yet a growing body of sociological work indicates otherwise. Two points can illustrate what is at stake here. The first brings us back to the issues of lay views and beliefs versus expert opinion. Evaluation research makes the assumption that its procedures are scientific and rational and that, therefore, implementation should be relatively straightforward. With goodwill both doctors and patients should be able to implement the findings of trials or other systematic evaluation procedures. No reasonable person would do otherwise. However, there is much to indicate that health care delivery, like health and illness themselves, is a complex phenomenon, open to a number of different kinds of rationality. It may well be the case that science offers a form of rationality that is more rational than others, to borrow a phrase from Gellner (1992), but everyday practice suggests that interactional contingencies and lay views often introduce other, no less compelling forms of behaviour and assessment into the medical arena. The pattern of health care consumption may be less amenable to rational change than the advocates of scientific evaluation allow.

Second, the introduction of large-scale evaluation into the health services brings with it major new issues to do with consent and the ethics of health care. Cochrane took the view that it was unethical to offer treatment that had not been properly evaluated by randomised controlled trials, but the circumstances where this meets sociological limits is, again, more frequent than is often recognised in medical circles. These limits may refer to types of treatment or types of patient. Potentially life-saving procedures, for which there are no proven alternatives, present acute problems for evaluation. Despite many improvements in health care some areas remain frustratingly intractable. For example, the outlook for people diagnosed with lung cancer (the largest cause of cancer deaths) remains poor, and surgery may well be the only option available. It is difficult to imagine in such circumstance randomly allocating some patients to surgery and others to alternative treatments, in order to assess which fares better. Indeed, it is arguable that it would be quite unethical to evaluate treatment by such means, if randomisation means death for some patients. The only chance of survival may lie in surgical intervention, and thus the denial of treatment, even for the 'higher' goal of assessing its effectiveness, may not be possible. Wanting to meet the immediate needs of the individual patient is no less rational than the desire to evaluate the treatment being offered by studying patients in aggregate.

Moreover, many groups of patients face difficulty in participating in evaluation exercises, or indeed treatment itself, by virtue of such factors as their age, their cognitive status or their social relationships. Research on treatments among babies and children, for example, requires the involvement (we might say 'partnership') of at least one adult, and often two, with the professionals involved. At the other end of the lifecourse research on the treatment of older people may present similar difficulties. Evaluating the treatment of Alzheimer's disease is an obvious case in point, though it is but one of many disorders that limit the ability to make rational judgements or to set up randomised trials.

Sociological research is also showing that 'informed consent' is sometimes more apparent than real in evaluative research, even where cognitive abilities are not compromised. It has been shown that the ability of lay people fully to understand the nature of scientific procedures, in which they may be involved by agreeing to participate in evaluative research, is less than adequate (Featherstone and Donovan 2002). Such difficulties are also unlikely to be overcome easily by the researching clinician. Indeed, recent evidence from Australia has shown that family practitioners themselves admit that they neither understand many of the terms and procedures involved in evaluation research, nor have confidence in their ability to explain the procedures to their patients (Young *et al.* 2002). Here, as elsewhere in the health and health care field, sociological research is urgently needed, to understand what is going on in such circumstances and the wider social and cultural implications of the major developments that are underway.

The medical sociology agenda

As we hope we have been able to show above, the field of medical sociology has strands of continuity and innovation in research stretching back over thirty years or more. Part of its strength lies in the fact that it operates on two levels. On one level a sociological perspective contributes to the study of health, illness and medicine by showing how they are influenced and shaped by social factors and processes. On the other level, the sociological study of health, illness and medicine illustrates how these phenomena have become major features of contemporary structures, cultures and social interaction. These two levels allow for a rich empirical base to develop and for theoretical issues to be explored. As we have said, the Reader aims to provide examples of some of the most important work in the field, particularly over the last ten years or so, which can be used in their own right and followed up in further study. The extended extracts, and in some cases the whole articles we have selected, are designed to provide a resource for those interested in substantive and critical topics.

In summary, we can identify the following themes and objectives that run throughout the body of work included here that may be of help to those using the Reader:

* Research in medical sociology aims to throw new light on the determinants of health and illness alongside other perspectives, including those of medicine.
* The topics dealt with in medical sociology illustrate key mainstream issues in sociology, and deal with major political and policy matters.
* Medical sociology has a strong empirical base, but also contributes to theoretical developments.
* Earlier preoccupations with such matters as medical autonomy, medical dominance and medicalisation are now being explored in new contexts.
* Research in areas such as health inequalities and the experience of illness, especially chronic illness, have been refocused to take account of new conceptualisations and debates.
* The evaluation of health care offers opportunities for the exploration of critical social and ethical issues as well as for sociology to participate in the process of evaluation itself.

While the methodologies and topics grouped together under the rubric of the Sociology of Health and Illness are many and various, we have aimed in the Reader, and in this Introduction, to show that the field is both coherent and exciting. It is our belief that the key areas of study, which form the main structure of the Reader, deal with some of the most pressing problems facing both individuals and groups in late modern societies. The health and illness field is constantly changing, as patterns of health and health care themselves change, and as society attempts to respond to new challenges and difficulties. Medicine, conceptualised in terms of its scientific and technical base as well as its professional organisation, is likewise going through major restructuring as it comes under pressure from a more assertive patient body and regulatory government pressure. The traditions of sociological enquiry into the medical profession, as into other matters medical, provide a number of important conceptual frameworks for analysis. We hope that those using the Reader will be enthused to follow up the issues dealt with here.

References

Albrecht, G., Seelman, K.D. and Bury, M. (eds) (2001) *Handbook of Disability Studies*, Thousand Oaks: Sage.

Anderson, R. and Bury, M. (eds) (1988) *Living with Chronic Illness: The Experience of Patients and Their Families*, London: Unwin Hyman.

Arber, S. and Ginn, J. (1991) *Gender and Later Life: A Sociological Analysis of Resources and Constraints*, London: Sage.

Armstrong, D. (2002) 'Clinical autonomy, individual and collective: the problem of changing doctors' behaviour', *Social Science and Medicine*. 55, 10: 1771–7.

Barnes, C. (1991) *Disabled People in Britain and Discrimination*, London: Hurst.

Barnes, C., Mercer, G. and Shakespeare, T. (1999) *Exploring Disability: A Sociological Introduction*, Cambridge: Polity Press.

Barrett, M. and Roberts, H. (1978) 'Doctors and their patients: the social control of women in general practice', in C. Smart and B. Smart (eds) *Women, Sexuality and Social Control*, London: Routledge and Kegan Paul.

Bartley, M., Ferrie, J. and Montgomery, S. (1999) 'Living in a high unemployment economy: understanding the health consequences', in M. Marmot and R.G. Wilkinson (eds) *Social Determinants of Health*, Oxford: Oxford University Press.

Becker, G. (1997) *Disrupted Lives: How People Create Meaning in a Chaotic World*, Berkeley: University of California Press.

Blaxter, M. (1990) *Health and Lifestyles*, London: Routledge.

Blaxter, M. (2000) 'Class, time and biography', in S.J. Williams, J. Gabe and M. Calnan (eds) *Health, Medicine and Society. Key Theories, Future Agendas*, London: Routledge.

Brown, P. (1995) 'Popular epidemiology, toxic waste and social movements', in J. Gabe (ed.) *Medicine, Health and Risk*, Oxford: Blackwell.

Bunker, J.P., Frazier, H.S. and Mosteller, F. (1994) 'Improving health: measuring effects of medical care', *Milbank Quarterly* 72: 225–58.

Bury, M. (1997) *Health and Illness in a Changing Society*, London: Routledge.

Bury, M. (2001) 'Illness narratives: fact or fiction?' *Sociology of Health and Illness* 23, 3: 263–85.

Bury, M. and Gabe, J. (1994) 'Television and medicine: medical dominance or trial by media', in J. Gabe, D. Kelleher and G. Williams (eds) *Challenging Medicine*, London: Routledge.

Bury, M. and Wadsworth, M. (2003) 'The "biological clock"? Ageing, health and the body across the lifecourse' in, S.L. Williams, L. Birke and G. Bendelow (eds) *Debating Biology: Sociological Reflections on Health, Medicine and Society*. London: Routledge.

Calnan, M. (1987) *Health and Illness: The Lay Perspective*, London: Tavistock.

Calnan, M. and Gabe, J. (2001) 'From consumerism to partnership? Britain's National Health Service at the turn of the century', *International Journal of Health Services* 31, 1: 119–31.

Calnan, M., Cant, S. and Gabe, J. (1993) *Going Private: Why People Pay for Their Health Care*. Buckingham: Open University Press.

Cant, S. and Sharma, U. (eds) (1994) *Complementary and Alternative Medicines: Knowledge in Practice*, London: Free Association Books.

Charles, C., Gafni, A. and Whelan, T. (2000) 'How to improve communication between doctors and patients', *British Medical Journal* 320: 1220–1.

Charmaz, K. (2000) 'Experiencing chronic illness', in, G.L. Albrecht, R. Fitzpatrick and S.C. Scrimshaw (eds) *The Handbook of Social Studies in Health and Medicine*, London: Sage.

Cochrane, A. (1972) *Effectiveness and Efficiency: Random Reflections on the Health Service*, London: Nuffield Provincial Hospital Trust.

Conrad, P. (1992) 'Medicalisation and social control', *Annual Review of Sociology* 18: 209–32.

Conrad, P. and Schneider, J.W. (1980/1992) *Deviance and Medicalisation: From Badness to Sickness*, Philadelphia: Temple University Press.

Coulter, A. (1999) 'Paternalism or partnership?' *British Medical Journal* 314: 719–20.

Davison, C., Frankel, S. and Davey Smith, G. (1992) 'The limits of popular lifestyle: re-assessing "fatalism" in the popular culture of illness prevention', *Social Science and Medicine* 34, 6: 67–85.

Dixon-Woods, M. and Fitzpatrick, R. (2001) 'Qualitative research in systematic reviews', *British Medical Journal* 323: 765–6.

Double, D. (2002) 'The limits of psychiatry', *British Medical Journal* 324: 900–4.

Drever, F. and Whitehead, M (eds) (1997) *Health Inequalities: Decennial Supplement*, Government Statistical Service, Series DS No. 15, London: The Stationery Office.

Ebrahim, S. (2002) 'The medicalisation of old age – should be encouraged', *British Medical Journal* 324: 861–3.

Featherstone, K. and Donovan, J.L. (2002) ' "Why don't they just tell me straight, why allocate it?" The struggle to make sense of participating in a randomised controlled trial', *Social Science and Medicine* 55, 5: 709–719.

Freidson, E. (1970/1988) *Profession of Medicine: A Study of the Sociology of Applied Knowledge*, Chicago: University of Chicago Press.

Gabe, J. (ed.) (1995) *Medicine, Health and Risk: Sociological Approaches*, London: Routledge.

Gellner, E. (1992) *Reason and Culture: The Historic Role of Rationality and Rationalism*, Oxford: Blackwell.

Gerhardt, U. (1989) *Ideas about Illness: An Intellectual and Political History of Medical Sociology*, London: Macmillan.

Giddens, A. (1991) *Modernity and Self Identity*, Cambridge: Polity Press.

Good, Byron J. (1994) *Medicine, Rationality and Experience: An Anthropological Perspective*, Cambridge: Cambridge University Press.

Graham, H. (1993) *When Life's a Drag: Women, Smoking and Disadvantage*, London: HMSO.

Gray, A. (ed.) (2001) *World Health and Disease*, Buckingham: Open University Press.

Katz, S. (1996) *Disciplining Old Age: The Formation of Gerontological Knowledge*, Charlottesville: University of Virginia.

Kelly, M. and Field, D. (1996) 'Medical sociology, chronic illness and the body', *Sociology of Health and Illness* 18, 2: 241–57.

Kuh, D. and Ben-Shlomo, Y. (1997) *A Lifecourse Approach to Chronic Disease Epidemiology*, Oxford: Oxford University Press.

Macintyre, S., Ellaway, A. and S. Cummins (2002) 'Place effects on health; how can we conceptualise, operationalise and measure them'? *Social Science and Medicine* 55: 125–39.

McKeown, T. (1976) *The Role of Medicine: Dream, Mirage or Nemesis*? London: Nuffield Provincial Hospitals Trust.

McKinlay, J.B. and Marceau, L.D. (2002) 'The end of the golden age of doctoring', *International Journal of Health Services* 32, 2: 379–416.

Mayall, B. (1996) *Children, Health and the Social Order*, Buckingham: Open University Press.

Morris, D. (1998) *Illness and Culture in the Postmodern Era*, Berkeley: University of California Press.

Oakley, A. (1981) 'Normal motherhood: an exercise in self control?' in B. Hutter and G. Williams (eds) *Controlling Women: The Normal and the Deviant*, London: Croom Helm.

Oliver, M. (1996) *Understanding Disability: From Theory to Practice*, Basingstoke: Macmillan.

Parsons, T. (1951) *The Social System*, New York: Free Press.

Parsons, T. (1978) 'The sick role and the role of the physician reconsidered', in *Action Theory and the Human Condition*, New York: Free Press.

Pill, R. and Stott, M. (1982) 'Concepts of illness causation and responsibility: some preliminary data from a sample of working class mothers', *Social Science and Medicine* 16: 43–52.

Pill, R. and Stott, M. (1985) 'Preventive procedures and practices among working class women: new data and fresh insights', *Social Science and Medicine* 21: 975–93.

Pound, P., Gompertz, P. and Ebrahim, S. (1998) 'Illness in the context of older age: the case of stroke', *Sociology of Health and Illness* 20: 489–506.

Robinson, D. (1973) *Patients, Practitioners and Medical Care*, London: Heinemann.

Sanders, C., Donovan, J. and Dieppe, P. (2002) 'The significance and consequences of having painful and disabled joints in older age: co-existing accounts of normal and disrupted biographies', *Sociology of Health and Illness* 24, 2: 227–53.

Sen, A. (2002) 'Health: perception versus observation. Self reported morbidity has severe limitations and can be extremely misleading', *British Medical Journal* 324: 860–1.

Shilling, C. (1993) *The Body and Social Theory*, London: Sage.

Silverman, D. (1987) *Communication and Medical Practice: Social Relations in the Clinic*, London: Sage.

Social Trends (2000) London: The Stationery Office.

Stacey, M. (1976) 'The health service consumer: a sociological misconception', in *The Sociology of the NHS*, Sociological Review Monograph No. 22, Keele: University of Keele.

Stimson, G. and Webb, B. (1975) *Going to See the Doctor: The Consultation Process in General Practice*, London: Routledge and Kegan Paul.

Strauss, A. and Glaser, B. (eds) (1975) *Chronic Illness and the Quality of Life*, St Louis: Mosby.

Strong, P.M. (1979) *The Ceremonial Order of the Clinic: Parents, Doctors and Medical Bureaucracies*, London: Routledge.

Townsend, P. and Davison, N. (1990) *Inequalities in Health: The Black Report*, Harmondsworth: Penguin Books.

Turner, B. (1984) *The Body and Society: Explorations in Social Theory*, Oxford: Basil Blackwell.

Turner, B. (1992) *Regulating Bodies: Essays in Medical Sociology*. London: Routledge.

Wadsworth, M. (1991) *The Imprint of Time: Childhood, History and Adult Life*, Oxford: Oxford University Press.

Wilkinson, R.G. (1996) *Unhealthy Societies: The Afflictions of Inequality*, London: Routledge.

Williams, G. (2001) 'Theorising disability', in, G. Albrecht, K.D. Seelman and M. Bury (eds) *Handbook of Disability Studies*, Thousand Oaks: Sage.

Williams, G. and Popay, J. (1994) 'Lay knowledge and the privilege of experience', in J. Gabe, D. Kelleher and G. Williams (eds) *Challenging Medicine*, London: Routledge.

Williams, R. (1990) *A Protestant Legacy: Attitudes to Death and Illness among Older Aberdonians*, Oxford: Clarendon Press.

Williams, S. (2000) 'Chronic illness as biographical disruption or biographical disruption as chronic illness? Reflections on a core concept', *Sociology of Health and Illness* 22, 1: 40–67.

Williams, S.J, Gabe, J. and Calnan, M. (eds) (2000) *Health, Medicine and Society: Key Theories, Future Agendas*, London: Routledge.

Young, J.M., Glasziou, P. and Ward, J.E. (2002) 'General practitioners' self ratings of skills in evidence-based medicine: validation study', *British Medical Journal* 324: 950–1.

Zola, I. (1973) 'Pathways to the doctor, from person to patient', *Social Science and Medicine* 7: 677–89.

Zola, I. (1975) 'In the name of health and illness: on some socio-political consequences of medical influence', *Social Science and Medicine* 9, 2: 83–7.

Zola, I. (1991) 'Medicalisation of aging and disability', in G. Albrecht and J.A. Levy (eds) *Advances in Medical Sociology Vol. 2*, Greenwich, Conn.: JAI Press.

PART ONE

Health beliefs and knowledge

IN THIS FIRST PART of the Reader we provide a selection of articles that will help orientate those approaching the field of medical sociology for the first time, as well as those already familiar with some of its preoccupations. These articles cover two of the basic issues confronting a sociological view of medicine, namely how lay people conceptualise health and illness, and how far these views differ from those of doctors and other experts. One of the ways this is often conceptualised is to say that lay people are concerned with illness, and doctors with disease. While this may often be the case, research on lay beliefs and knowledge, in modern societies at least, shows that there is not a clear-cut set of 'folk beliefs' separate from medical ideas, and that there are complex interactions between the two operating in different contexts. Research in this area provides an important window on lay ideas and actions in their own right, but also informs research covered elsewhere in this volume.

In the first extract by Herzlich, accounts of lay views of the origins of disease are taken from a study of middle-class French respondents. In these accounts – for Herzlich, 'representations' – of disease, the 'way of life' predominates, especially that linked to urban living. Stress, fatigue and exhaustion can all exacerbate underlying problems, or be the source of new disorders, and are seen to upset the balance between the individual and his or her environment. This lay 'equilibrium' model of illness resonates with long-standing views of illness among both lay and expert opinion dating back many centuries. In modern settings, however, issues such as environmental pollution or road traffic accidents come into the picture. On the other hand Herzlich demonstrates that lay thought also emphasises the constitution, temperament and heredity of individuals and how these interact with the environment. The value of Herzlich's work is that it shows how complex and important beliefs about illness are to lay people in modern societies and how they touch on matters fundamental to the organisation of modern life.

In the next extract by Blaxter, this time based on a study of Scottish working-class women, a different emphasis emerges. While in Herzlich's work lay people can be heard speaking in detail about the impact of the environment on health, here the responsibility of the individual is more in evidence. This, for Blaxter, is something of a paradox, given that public health and epidemiological research has emphasised that it is structural factors that explain poorer health among working-class groups. Little of this was in evidence in Blaxter's study of lay views. Rather than blame the environment, urban or otherwise, the women here emphasised their own responsibility. Deprivation and poor environments in the past were recognised, but responsibility for 'who they were' in the present was equally strong, if not stronger. Through this qualitative study, Blaxter calls on both sociological and epidemiological research not to overestimate the relevance of structural explanations for people in everyday settings.

If Blaxter's findings seem to reinforce individual responsibility for health (and indeed, the wider individualism of the 'Protestant Ethic') and Herzlich's the role of the environment, the next extract by Davison et al. provides an anthropological view of some of the complexities at work. In this study, set in South Wales, interviews and observations of lay responses to health focused on one disorder, namely heart disease. Davison et al. show that the lay idea of the 'coronary candidate' confounds medical opinion. While it is clear from the study that lay populations have assimilated many of the medical and health promotion messages about heart disease – essentially those about individual risk behaviours such as fatty diets, smoking and alcohol consumption – they are combined with other equally important observations. In lay settings, the coronary candidate appears to be almost anyone, given the widespread nature of risk behaviours and such factors as being overweight. This allows for ideas of chance and fate to retain their explanatory power, and their rationality. Davison et al.'s respondents drew attention to the exceptions to the rule concerning risk behaviours. The 'Uncle Norman' figure was frequently cited, who, though obviously at risk, lives his life without dying from heart disease. These lay views also revealed a critical feature of the population approach to health risks and a dilemma in health promotion: the so-called 'prevention paradox'. This refers to the situation where whole populations are persuaded to change their behaviour (e.g. consume less fat) but with no personal benefit to many of the individuals involved – for the simple reason that they would not have had a heart attack anyway. Davison et al.'s study reveals important features of expert as well as lay opinion concerning individual risk and the health of populations.

The next two contributions move the analysis of lay beliefs even more sharply away from a focus only on individuals. In Calnan's extract on lifestyle a contrast is made between individual psychological models of health beliefs, based on ideas such as the 'locus of control' which emphasise feelings of control or powerlessness over behaviour, with a sociological perspective which connects beliefs with wider contextual processes. For example, Calnan emphasises that health is not always the most important aspect of daily life, and beliefs about health may only surface during times of crisis. Moreover, social and economic circumstances, rather than individually held beliefs, may constrain or facilitate certain health behaviours. As we have seen with Herzlich's and Blaxter's articles, social class differences may be strongly related to differences in health beliefs and behaviours, though not always in the predicted direction. Calnan attempts to reconcile work on individual beliefs and on social circumstances, by proposing a sociological approach that emphasises the meanings attached to health beliefs and behaviour and how these might be linked with key aspects of daily life, such as work.

Brown's article on 'popular epidemiology' takes research on social contexts and lay beliefs one step further, to document their relationship to the emergence of collective actions. In the case of occupational or environmental causes of disease, Brown argues that lay groups are increasingly playing a key role in the shaping of both public debate and political responses. Taking the example of toxic waste contamination in the US, Brown shows how lay beliefs about deleterious effects can become the source of important campaigns to persuade governments or sue companies they believe to be responsible. Such lay involvement erodes the clear distinction between belief and scientific knowledge, which we discussed in the General Introduction to this volume. Lay campaigns over health hazards will typically involve collaboration with sympathetic doctors, scientists and epidemiologists, or challenging the science of opponents. Thus, relays between knowledge and belief occur across the lay–expert line. Brown shows how such 'popular epidemiology' is helping to constitute new social movements around health issues, and provides a new terrain for the study of 'claims making' activity in modern society.

Finally, in this first Part of the Reader, we include an extract from Parsons and Atkinson dealing with an equally important development in lay understandings of health, namely those concerning genetic risk. The focus of the study presented is on the beliefs of those affected by a particular genetic disorder, Duchenne Muscular Dystrophy. In the article the authors attempt to understand the outlook of a group of Welsh women who have been defined as having a specific level of risk in relation to this disorder. Through detailed interviews with 22 mothers and 32 daughters, Parsons and Atkinson found significant discrepancies between lay understanding of such risks and those of medical experts. Calculating risk in this disorder is complex, but the process results in a statistic for each individual, summarising her carrier status and reproductive risk. However, Parsons and Atkinson found that many of the women in the study translated their 'risk statistic' into descriptive statements that provided a more certain foundation for decision making about reproduction. Rather than seeing health beliefs as fixed, these authors show that health beliefs are defined and redefined on a continuous basis. However, as with other studies discussed above, the overriding concern is to maintain a sense of identity and provide 'everyday recipes' that can inform action in a way that medically derived expertise cannot. The need for forms of knowledge that address existential as well as scientific issues is a thread running though much of the sociological research on lay health beliefs.

Chapter 1

Claudine Herzlich

THE INDIVIDUAL, THE WAY OF LIFE
AND THE GENESIS OF ILLNESS

From *Health and Illness: A Social Psychological Perspective*, London and New York: Academic Press, in cooperation with the European Association of Experimental Social Psychology (1973).

WHERE DO DISEASES COME FROM? How do they originate? What is involved in illness and what is involved in health? These questions arise immediately in conversations with subjects and our first task will be to analyse the answers which they give.

Anthropologists and historians of medicine are in general agreement that causal conceptions of illness – whether popular notions or medical theories – range between two extremes. On the one hand, illness is endogenous in man, and the individual carries it in embryo; the ideas of resistance to disease, heredity and predisposition are here the key concepts. On the other hand, illness is thought of as exogenous; man is naturally healthy and illness is due to the action of an evil will, a demon or sorcerer, noxious elements, emanations from the earth or microbes, for example. Medical theories can also be classified according to their view of the relations between normal and pathological phenomena. Health and illness may be considered as radically heterogeneous, like two conflicting factors within the individual, or, on the other hand, as relatively homogeneous, like two modes of vital phenomena differing only in degree.

At various periods, in different societies and in various guises, we can see the persistence of these broad currents of thought, and often their alternation. In this respect, scientific thinking, like popular thinking, seems to consist of an infinite number of variations on the same themes.

We have also found these two themes in the thinking of the subjects we interviewed, expressed in their own words. The endogenous theme is represented by the individual and his part in the genesis of his condition. The exogenous theme is the way of life of each person. We shall examine in turn the relations of each of these factors – the individual and his way of life – with health and illness, starting with the way of life, which would appear to play the more important part.

Actually, the picture which is obtained in this way corresponds to a kind of selective perception or schema of reality. In the complex world of health and illness, the subjects choose certain aspects at the expense of others, from among the variety of factors which they learn about by experience or from other sources. The relations among the elements chosen can then be classified under a few simple headings.

Way of life

The way of life to which such a preponderant role is assigned, it must be noted, is life in towns. In fact, it is life in Paris that its citizens without exception refer to.[1] When some of them describe life in the country, it is to contrast it with their habitual way of life; the country dwellers delineate the encroachment of urban aspects on country life. In this sense the two attitudes can be regarded as similar.

In both cases, the urban way of life is always associated with illness, and its influence always undesirable. Its effect can, however, be viewed in several ways; it varies in degree from simple 'harmful effects' to 'appearance of an illness'. The decline in health can have various starting points. The way of life creates in the individual, or makes use of, 'weak points'; its effects will be felt especially where resistance is least. 'You can have a mild intestinal infection, the first signs of a stomach ulcer, slight irritation following certain food, discomfort, early symptoms resulting from a faulty way of living . . . your organism being less ready to resist, these minor signs grow into illness.'

Most frequently, however, the attack is a general one. The perceptible symptoms of it are fatigue, 'nerves' and premature ageing, which all indicate weakness and physical wear and tear. For the individual, they represent entry into an 'intermediate state'. . . . which is neither illness nor health. Subjects almost unanimously describe, often vehemently, how city life produces a world of fatigue and nervous tension. Way of life and fatigue and disturbance of nervous equilibrium are, in the last resort, synonymous for the individual. 'Paris is fatigue and nervous tension, with this exhausting and rather unhealthy life.' 'The constant commotion isn't made to make people ordinary, they are difficult, nervous, tired; that's the truth about modern life.'

The importance of notions of nervous tension and the frequent mention of feelings of anxiety indicate that the decline concerns psychic as well as organic potential, just as the intermediate state is characterized by both physical fatigue and nervousness.

Declining health and getting into the intermediate state are two aspects of a single process. They subject the individual to the same risk – they reduce his capacity for resistance and bring increased vulnerability to illness. 'You could say that now, with the life we lead, certain diseases are increasing because our body no

[1] Of a total of 80 subjects interviewed, 68 lived in Paris and 12 in a little village in Normandy.

longer reacts because it no longer has enough resistance . . .' 'Modern life induces a kind of fatigue which makes us ill . . . everything to do with modern work and its conditions makes us more vulnerable to most diseases.'

The way of life is thus a contributory factor facilitating attack by a pathological agent. But its effect is not limited to this; the analysis provided by some, of the respective parts and the combination of different pathogenic factors in the genesis of different diseases, indicates that the way of life plays a three-fold role and is of crucial importance in various guises, not only in the development of illness, but at its very origin. Like germs, and factors other than hereditary ones, the way of life is a releaser of illness. Finally, in addition to this releasing effect, and to the facilitating effect already analysed, the way of life is related in another and more complex way to the facts of illness, i.e. it has a role which we shall call 'generating'. The way of life generates the pathological agents themselves. Thus, germs and the phenomena of contagion are related to the way of life. 'I reckon that in life today, the possibilities of infection are too great . . . you're attacked by germs.'

They are, however, sometimes thought to be less frequent or less likely to attack one in the country. 'In the country, there's the air, and so the germs don't have anything like the same effect as here.'

Similarly, accidents are seen as more frequent in contemporary city life. 'Accidents are a disease of our modern society, car accidents and accidents at work, it's due to our mechanized life.'

At a more general level, that of contemporary society, the way of life affects the form and the distribution of illness; it imposes certain particular kinds of illness, diseases of modern life, transforms diseases and creates new ones. 'I have the impression that the diseases of today didn't exist in former times, just as the diseases of former times are no longer with us today. I feel we, well not we but external circumstances and social conditions, create new sources of illness which, while still being called illnesses, take more and more diverse and complicated forms.'

For this subject the association between illness and way of life appears within a bigger time-cycle in which the same process proceeds indefinitely, some diseases characteristic of a way of life becoming rare while others spread. The diseases typical of modern life because more frequent than before are in particular the following.

CANCER   'Cancer I rather associate with current allergies, with very modern allergic diseases, with the physical and nervous strain we undergo in cities, and then in breathing in the present-day atmosphere in cities.'

MENTAL DISORDERS   'Mental illness, that's a disease bound up with modern life . . . You get much more mental wear and tear; the more restless life is, the more people are mad or half mad.'

The notion – if not the expression – of psychosomatic illness appears in this context; the same person in fact carries on: 'I don't know whether it may not have something to do with some other diseases, diseases which might involve a psychic state; it's important in liver disease, when you are very irritated, some people when they are afraid, get jaundice. Jaundice is the beginning of liver disease.'

HEART DISEASE   'Modern life brings too many worries which make people live in a certain state of anxiety, of nervous tension which can have effects on the heart and induce heart trouble.'

The notion of a harmful way of life thus embraces certain particular diseases. Mental disorders, heart disease and, above all, cancer are those most frequently mentioned, but they also have a very special significance. They are, it is said, the diseases that everyone speaks of, and therefore at the heart of the process of social communication; they are the diseases which people themselves fear, and are therefore also at the heart of individual preoccupations. These two facts indicate that the diseases of modern life constitute for the members of our society the most significant picture of illness and represent illness itself for them.

The way of life may have effects in several ways. It may involve intermediate stages (deterioration of health, intermediate state, illness). These may become stabilized; people sometimes live indefinitely in the intermediate state. The logical conclusion, however, is always illness, even if this development does not actually take place. The way of life would appear to be necessarily pathogenic.

Is this strong relation entirely unidirectional? Is there no positive relation between way of life and health? An examination of themes relating to medical progress indicates that there is, and that this takes three forms: triumph over disease by cure or prevention, reduction in the infant mortality rate and increased expectation of life. Only the reduction in infant mortality is mentioned without reservations, and that is emphasized by a few people only. In the other two cases, it is as if there were a tendency to minimize the importance of medical progress which is, in some measure, dissonant with the notion of a harmful way of life. On the factual level, people declare themselves sceptical with regard to the possibilities of prevention or cure of disease. Viewed within the context of the perpetual cycle of new diseases to which we have referred, medical progress loses its absolute quality; its victory over disease is never final. Moreover, with regard to the significance attached to the phenomena concerned, the lengthening of life does not strike everybody as an indisputable gain. To prolong life is to prolong the life of aged invalids and is not, strictly speaking, a matter of bringing or improving health. 'People attach too much importance to longevity . . . why live ten years longer on drugs when you are completely worn out, when you're falling to pieces?'

On the other hand, it is often said that health is necessary to face contemporary life. It is a sort of antidote, a necessary condition for adjustment. 'The rhythm of life isn't adjusted, this rhythm of life is possible for some individuals who are particularly fortunate in the matter of health . . . anyone with good health is better equipped to react to the situation, but the rest . . . they can't get away with it.'

In spite of some slight contributions, the way of life does not make for health, but, on the contrary, basically works against it, while being clearly and strongly related to the incidence of illness.

Individual factors

These constitute the second group of determining factors and are of various kinds. Each of the variables used, predisposition, constitution, temperament, nature of the individual, resistance and self-defensive reaction has a specific meaning. But they are all used for the same purpose: to describe the part played by the individual himself in the genesis of his condition, whether health or illness.

A process analogous to that which we have observed in the case of the way of life is evident; individual factors are regarded in a particular light. In spite of the variety of terms used, none refers to any pathogenic action, but all rather indicate a variable capacity for resistance to disease, and therefore to the inroads of the way of life. The terms involving the idea of resistance often appear alone. They give a sort of significance to individual factors beyond any objective notion. 'There is a kind of resistance in the individual, more or less strong.'

Similarly, for the notions of defence and autodefence of the individual. 'There are individuals who are, so to speak, defenders; there are people whose body defends itself against illness, but there are also others who do not defend themselves and are easy victims. In present-day life everything gets them down, the least thing tires them out, and it doesn't take much for people like that to fall ill.'

Other terms are also used, not to describe pathogenic factors but to refer to the capacity for resistance or defence against illness. This capacity varies according to the individual, and people's constitutions range from strong to weak. 'There are people who are constitutionally more or less all right but who are nevertheless much weaker than others.'

Similarly with the individual's nature. 'There are people who are naturally strong, they are less affected, they put up a better fight than those who are naturally nervous, less resistant.'

Organism and temperament also refer to the capacity for putting up a fight. 'When there is an illness, the organism must react and put up a fight.' 'You have temperaments which react and others which don't.'

The term 'temperament' is sometimes associated with the notion of a qualitative as well as a quantitative difference, i.e. with the notion of a topology. 'People with a sanguine temperament are less affected than people of a nervous type; intelligent people are more affected than less intelligent people.'

Finally, there may be a selective sensitivity to certain kinds of attack, points of minimum resistance. Thus we find the notion of a predisposition towards certain diseases. 'For diseases where you have germs . . . they always say, 'There was a liability to it, the body was vulnerable to just these germs'.'

But if a predisposition is sometimes necessary before an illness can develop, it is never a sufficient condition. Similarly, heredity is not always considered as a pathogenic factor (the notion of hereditary disease or disease due to hereditary factors appears only in some subjects), but as the inheritance of weak or strong points, of fragility or robustness requiring certain precautions of the individual or making certain performances possible for him. We also find references to the inheritance of temperament. In these various cases, hereditary factors will not of themselves bring disease. Impairment by the way of life remains the determining factor. 'I get attacks of anxiety, I can't sleep, I have nervous troubles, it's a matter of one's "climate of life". I have a weak nervous system, which I've certainly inherited, but I might have set up home with a very very placid man, and had a different life, and now . . . I wouldn't have had these troubles.'

Some people also show a tendency to restrict the role of heredity. The implicit question is: Is it really certain? 'We don't really know why some people have abnormal children . . . there's heredity but . . . there are parents who are drunkards and others whose parents aren't drunkards, who are still abnormal.'

Finally, according to some, hereditary diseases are very much rarer than those which are due to the way of life. 'In big cities and certain industrial centres, people are on edge . . . it's legitimate to think that there's a higher incidence of mental disorders than elsewhere where there isn't this restlessness. There's heredity if you like, but it doesn't count for all that much . . . in the cities, you come across so many queer folk in the street you don't really notice them.' We can see that although heredity may be for this man a notion which he knows and uses, it is not really integrated into his thinking or, more generally, into his view of things. He no sooner mentions the case of hereditary diseases than he abandons it to return to what is for him essential and gives him, as it gives many others, a firm basis for his view: the way of life as the cause of our illnesses.

To summarize, the individual does not carry his illness essentially within himself; on the contrary, everything in him resists the encroachments of the way of life which tends to start it off. Internal individual factors play a part in so far as he resists strongly or weakly in the face of attack, but their part appears to be a secondary one compared with that of the way of life which constitutes the principal and active determinant of disease. The individual can only resist; his role, although important, is a secondary and passive one. 'I think the way of life is more important than the actual physical aspect; I don't think the human being is ill as a result of inner factors; it is external conditions which end by making him ill. Nevertheless, there are predispositions . . . . of children who are born less healthy than others, but I think it's much more the environment which creates diseases.'

On the other hand, constitution, temperament and heredity are, in regard to health, determining factors which are both indispensable and sufficient. The order of importance is here reversed. Health comes first and foremost from the individual. 'Health is a very special factor, due first of all to heredity and then to the way of life of each person.'

Thus, if illness is identified unequivocally with the way of life, the individual is conversely described wholly in terms of resistance to disease and, in fact, in terms of health. Generally speaking, then, individual factors, with which we have here been concerned, are assimilated to health.

The outcome of this analysis would appear to be that health and disease must be conceived as the outcome of a struggle between individual equals health and way of life equals disease. In this struggle we have the opposition of an *active* factor, the way of life, which, by its incursions, leads to disease, and a *passive* factor (passive being here synonymous with resistance), the perfect health of the individual (or the perfectly healthy individual). The outcome of the conflict may be either the victory of the individual, resulting in health and adjustment to the way of life, or the invalid way of life with deterioration in health.

The representation thus involves a double opposition. The opposition between health and illness originates in and reflects the opposition between the passive individual and his exacting way of life. There does not seem to be much point in referring again to the selective nature of the schema here developed. If there are other images behind the enveloping images of a harmful way of life and a resistant individual, they are not, as the case of medical progress or of hereditary diseases shows, integrated into a structured conception.

We prefer to draw attention to two other aspects.

1 The rigidly stereotyped nature of the schema immediately strikes one. The notions of way of life as a factor in illness and of diseases of civilization are daily emphasized by the mass media, including the national newspapers and the popular medical press. All the features of stereotypes – frequency and uniformity of expression of content, and the strongly emotional accompanying charge – appear here, and we may well think that subjects are having recourse to a schema which is in daily circulation in society, which is always available to them and which requires neither effort nor original thought.

2 Schematically, such a picture is nevertheless characterized by coherence of content and an organizing role in relation to reality. The struggle between the two opposing elements takes account both of different states (health and illness) and of different stages (in the development of a disease), and also, in this very process, elaborates a view or interpretation of the relations between the individual and his environment. Health and illness are distinguished in terms of the opposition between the individual and his way of life.

Nature, constraint and society

We have shown that there is a coherent representation of the basis of health and illness. This idea, which reflects reality and gives it meaning, would appear to arise because of the attribution of a common significance to the various aspects of the way of life.

Way of life and its meanings

The analysis of the notion of way of life does not consist merely of showing how it works. We must also be concerned with its content, which is made up of distinct elements.

The way of life indicates the spatio-temporal framework of the individual, the space in which he lives and its characteristic features (density of population, atmosphere, etc.), the rhythm of life (time schedules, forms of stimulation) and also the reflections of these in everyday forms of behaviour (eating, activities, sleeping and relaxation, for example). It is therefore in large measure something external to the person, but it also provides the common meaning for all of the conduct of each. Consider the place occupied by work: its setting, its rhythm and its conditions. A person's way of life is determined by his occupation and is subject to the demands of his specific function in society.

Life in cities appears as both *unhealthy* and *constraining*. Its harmful effects are due to these two characteristics. Its effects are channelled through various media

(food, air, noise, rhythm of life and so on), but all of them share these two characteristics. One of the two aspects sometimes predominates. The idea of "unhealthy" is
more important in respect of food, constraint in respect of noise and everything
connected with the rhythm of life. This difference is, however, less important than
what is common to both.

Let us first examine the notion of *constraint*. It comprises the image of a way of
life imposed upon one, of an urban situation as unavoidable as the human situation
itself. Man can neither escape from it nor, in the main, alter it. 'You can't reorganize
your life, you are in a certain situation, it is there; there's a doctor who tells me to
leave my job. That's fine, and I say to him: "You leave *your* job." You'd have to change
your whole life, it isn't possible.'

Confronted with his way of life, the individual thus feels himself passive and
powerless. Constraint excludes any possibility of escaping from harmful conditions
of living. It is also impossible for him, in everyday life, to avoid any of the more
specific attacks on his health. Thus polluted air and noise, both unhealthy, are
described as being imposed on the individual. 'The noise in the street, the fumes in
the air and the dust, how do you think you can move in the direction of health if
technology is attacking you every minute like that?'

Again, every particular aspect appears to the individual as a constraint,
an imperative or a restriction, a noose in which he feels himself strangled
and a prisoner. 'We lead a restricted life, in town you are always shut in . . .
you cross a street, but it seems to me that you are still imprisoned in this same
street.'

Finally, constraint has its effects on conduct. The individual feels himself forced
into certain kinds of behaviour with which he isn't satisfied or which seem quite
wrong to him. The rhythm of life and time schedules are experienced as constraints
which are reflected in the conduct and habits of everyone. As one of the subjects
interviewed said: 'You have to think of everything, you have to think about getting
up, about catching the bus, about getting there in time, about your work . . . you're
always thinking, and that in itself creates a kind of disequilibrium . . . you're in the
street, you aren't free, you have to look out for red lights, you have to pay attention
to this and that, which means you're constantly on the look-out, your body is never
at rest, always on the alert.'

In short, the relation between the individual and his way of life is an externally
imposed relation. The individual does not have the impression that he is creating it
or participating freely in it, or even that he can appreciably modify it; he simply
undergoes it. This leads to antagonism and conflict. A journalist summarizes thus his
view of the contemporary way of life: 'Today, the environment influences man much
more than man influences the environment . . .'

The way of life, the determining factor in illness, is experienced by the individual as something external to him; way of life and illness impose themselves upon
him, attack him and constrain him without, as it seems to him, his having any part in
anything beyond his relatively passive capacity for resistance and adjustment to
conflict.

These constraints and attacks are, in fact, those of social life. It is society, people
think, which finds expression in the way of life, imposing obligations and restrictions
upon us. It is society which brings conflict. 'Very often, in present-day society, you

have to control yourself and this is sometimes quite distressing, for things you can't do anything about anyway . . . You have to give way, society constrains you.'

Similarly, it is because of one's social function, one's position in society that one can't change one's life. 'Our current way of life, it's difficult to change it. If you wanted, as an individual, to live in a more balanced manner, you would be professionally and socially destroyed and that's something which would prevent you from doing it.'

Finally, it is society which, through the way of life, brings illness; at the same time, it is society which demands that the individual should be healthy. 'Good health, I think that in the face of the life you lead today, and the nervous tension you have to maintain, it provides defensive reserves against attack of any kind, whether by illness or by the society in which you live. The individual with good health can rely on himself, so it's a factor which makes for assurance and confidence and that has enormous possibilities for the individual in society . . .'

This man expresses the double role of health in the individual–society conflict. First of all it provides resistance to illness, which is a product of society. It also provides the physical reserve necessary for the effort of social adjustment.

Therein lies the paradox of society: it demands from the individual what it refuses him. We see here a hint of a more complex relation between the two parties to the conflict, which will enrich our initial schema. Society in its double role replaces the way of life – as bringing disease and as requiring health. For the individual, health is both the potential for resistance and the means of solving the conflict. The essential opposition, however, remains – the idea of opposition is even strengthened – between health as a factor internal to the individual, and the external factor of society and the way of life, experienced as threatening. Health is entirely endogenous; what is exogenous comes to stand for illness. . . .

Chapter 2

Mildred Blaxter

WHY DO THE VICTIMS BLAME THEMSELVES?

From A. Radley (ed.) *Worlds of Illness: Biographical and Cultural Perspectives on Health and Disease,* London: Routledge (1993)

T HIS INVESTIGATION OF WHAT it means to say that 'the victims blame themselves' is presented as an example of the interaction of qualitative and quantitative methods. The question, raised by the inevitably superficial results of larger-scale surveys, is: Why do those who are most vulnerable to the environment seem to be most likely to stress self-blame for illness and self-responsibility for health? Can a biographical approach suggest some answers?

There are, of course, two perspectives on the determinants of illness, and especially the cause of social inequality in health: the idea that illhealth is primarily 'self-inflicted', and has behavioural causes, and the view that the major causes are structural and located in the environment. The extent to which people themselves subscribe to one view or the other is a topic which surveys often investigate, and though the alternatives are not necessarily mutually exclusive, the brief questions of surveys ('What is the cause of heart disease?', 'Do you think people are responsible for their own illnesses?'), perhaps with forced-choice answers, tend to create dichotomies. One consistent finding is that although most people, of whatever social group, have learned very well the self-responsible lessons of health promotion, it is those who are most 'unequal' and most exposed to environmental risk who are least likely also to be aware of the structural perspective. Those who are in the lowest social classes, or have the least education, are most likely to confine their explanations to behavioural causes. . . .

The search for explanations

Why should this be so? There are possible explanations of a rather facile nature. It could be argued, for instance, that although this emphasis on the behavioural, as a taught response, has been generally very well learned, alternative or additional modes of explanation are more available to those who are better educated or more exposed to 'scientific' media presentations. The middle class are also more likely to belong to contemporary consumerist and environmentalist movements. It might also be suggested that these findings are no more than an artefact of method: the more articulate are more likely to give elaborate answers in the survey situation, and the less well educated or those without a ready vocabulary of abstract concepts are likely to seek the line of least resistance and give the easiest answers perceived to be the approved ones. Certainly, it was true in the Health and Lifestyle Survey (Blaxter 1990) that education of the respondent was, in general, clearly associated with the length of their open-ended replies or the number of different concepts that an individual expressed.

Are such explanations sufficient? If they are given time to express themselves in a situation less reminiscent of a 'test', is it true that those who are in the poorest social and economic circumstances are still least likely to place the blame for illhealth on their environment? And if it is, how do the disadvantaged, in fact, interpret the relationship between their health and the circumstances of their lives? To answer these questions, ideally, new and clearly focused research should be mounted. In the absence of this ideal, there is the possibility of an alternative strategy: to return to a re-analysis of the qualitative material which initially provided some of the themes guiding the analysis of the Health and Lifestyle Survey.

The qualitative data

The data referred to are long tape-recorded conversations with a group of 47 Scottish women of about 50 years old (Blaxter and Paterson 1982). For other purposes of the study, they had been randomly selected from women who, at the time of their first childbearing 30 or so years before, were in social classes IV or V, and whose adult daughters lived in the same city and were still in the lowest social classes. Thus they belonged to families, neither geographically nor socially mobile, who were likely to have some generations of economic deprivation behind them: a group among whom the relationship between social circumstances and ideas about the cause of illhealth could be clearly tested. The data used here consist of interviews, usually lasting for an hour and often much longer, in which the conversation was guided to cover the woman's health and health history, and her attitudes to illness, doctors and health services.

It must first be noted that the personal and family histories of the women demonstrated not only social deprivation in past generations, in their own childhoods, and at the time of their childbearing (in the early 1950s), but also the very clear association of this deprivation with illhealth. As Herzlich and Pierret (1984) noted of their French respondents, 'the memory of the terrors of the past remained astonishingly vivid'. Diphtheria and scarlet fever had swept through families:

> Because I remember when I was taken away with scarlet fever. I mean, that night is as clear to me as though it happened last week. I wis only four, right enough, but I remember the hospital being packed wi' kids. My husband – there was him and his two brothers – the three of them were taken out o' the house one night and my husband wasnae expected to come back. And after he did come back from the hospital he took it again.
>
> (G37)

Six of the forty-seven women had had TB, and several of their own children: one woman described how her son had caught TB from 'sharing a bed with a lodger, when he came home from sea – we didn't know he had it, you see'. A stark lack of adequate food, clothing and housing was described in the days before the Second World War:

> I always had sore throats, septic throats and that. Before I had diphtheria we stayed in an old house – my mother blamed that. We'd only one room and there was six o' us in one room, two beds in one room at that time. An' your sink was just on the stair an' outside was your toilet.
>
> (G3)

As young women in the 1950s their circumstances had been little better. Many husbands had been working away from home or otherwise absent, and almost all the women began married life either subletting crowded rooms from parents or other relatives, or renting crowded, damp slum property often without running water or inside sanitation. They represented themselves, at that time, as having little control over their fertility. Over half had conceived their first child before marriage, and twenty-nine of the forty-seven women had borne four or more children.

They were very conscious that part of the illhealth of the past had been due to an absence of medical services, and told many stories of not being able to afford or obtain care:

> When you had to pay for a doctor – well, to this day my mother still says that wa the reason I took rheumatic fever. Cos I took scarlet fever – and I was ill for a few days, and my mother took me to the dispensary. Now, I had to walk there, cos my mother didn't have the tramcar fare. With the result – I got my chill – we had to walk to the dispensary because it was free there, we couldn't afford to pull in a doctor. Cos my mother would have had the doctor in her house – well, at least twice a week, because she had eight of us.
>
> (G1)

. . . They were, however, very conscious that 'things had changed'. These family stories were usually told in the context of praise for the National Health Service, universally given credit (together with the 'medical advances' that had provided a cure for TB and, in their eyes, had been responsible for 'conquering' the childhood killers of the past) for major advances in health. [One woman] concluded by saying 'We hinna got that worry nowadays.'

Many of the women were of rural background. This acknowledgement of the effects of poverty produced some conflict with another strong and almost universal theme: the wish to present the days of their youth as in some sense 'healthier', with simple good food, fresh air and sensible living. This was an obvious appeal to a 'golden age' of the past, a response to all they disliked about modern life or all that irritated them about the way in which their grandchildren were brought up; in part, it represented the childhood memories of the rural as opposed to the urban, perhaps typical of a generation experiencing the period of rural depopulation. One woman described a tragic childhood:

> My mother had ten altogether – six of us survived. She died in the April and I was 13 in the May. That's when we lost her . . . I kept the family together, on my own, going to school as well. And then I left school at 14 and went out to work on the farms.
>
> (G30)

and later in the interview described at length all the chronic illnesses and early deaths of her siblings. She herself – though by definition the survivor – suffered from chronic asthma. Nevertheless, when the conversation turned to general influences on health and illness, she had strongly held views:

> We were a healthy family. The country people are more healthy than the town people. They have more fresh air, there's not so much traffic, factories, things like that. And we lived off the land, more or less, there wasn't so much tinned stuff and things like that . . . Their whole way of life has a lot to do wi' it. You're up early in the morning, your work's not finished until maybe late at night, plenty o' fresh air.

Another example of many similar accounts was the woman who said:

> My father didnae work frae during the first war – he was hurt in the war, so my mother had to bring up eight of us – it wis just a case o' us getting – we got wur soup, we didnae get the best o' everything, we just got the cheapest o' everything, but it wis a' *good*. I suppose that would give us a' the chance o' better health.

At the same time, it would certainly be untrue to say that these women did not have a clear perception of the causes of their own specific, current chronic conditions lying in past circumstances. They seemed to be saying that their simple, healthy childhoods (leaving aside infectious disease, which was simply an ever-present but unavoidable danger, now removed by medical science) had provided them with a reserve of good health, better to withstand the attacks that later life circumstances might make. At the most difficult period of their lives, which most saw as their young married days, neglect of their own health had been inevitable. One woman was clear, for instance, about the cause of her long-term arthritis:

> Well, put it like this, when you've got young family you've got a lot of hard work. More so when you have five. It's nae easy work. And

we'd nae washing machines, nae hot water, nae sink – well, we had a
cold sink in the corner . . . there was a lot of hard work, there was stone
floors.

(G19)

Another had similar views about arthritis in her knees:

Gaun aboot wi' auld shoes on – gaun aboot getting my feet soakin' –
maybe, if I'd taken mair care o' mysel' earlier on. But wi' kids, no
money for yourself', you couldnae dae it.

(G23)

Later, however, this same woman talked at length of the simple, austere upbringing of her own children, and explained how 'healthy' their childhoods had
been by the same sort of reasoning that other women applied to their own
childhoods:

Well, my four was healthy. They was never pampered and wrapped up.
They niver wore scarfs and hats in the winter time. They were jist out
in a' weathers. And they jist ate a' thing that was going. And yet they
were healthy.

To neglect their own health in the way they now admitted they had done meant
that they were responsible, but on the other hand no one could have behaved
differently:

Three times in the city hospital with tuberculosis – I called it neglect.
Well, I had pleurisy before my twins were born, and I cracked my ribs
just before A. was born, and I had pleurisy, and I had naebody in, wi' six
o' them, you know. And I had pleurisy, and there was naebody to look
efter me, I just used to come an' get my poultice and heat it at the fire
and put it back on. It was really neglect – my own – well, no my own
fault, I had to look efter my bairns, you understand.

(G7)

Many other women similarly struggled to reconcile a strong sense of self-
responsibility with the conviction that all their health problems stemmed from
childbearing and the difficult days of early motherhood. To present the process as
one of self-sacrifice and 'good' motherhood was an obvious solution:

When they were young, if I was ill, I couldn't afford to be ill and that
was all there was to it. Because he was at sea and there was naebody.
There wasn't anyone to watch the kids. If I was ill I still had to get up and
work, you know – you couldn't be ill.

(G25)

[. . .]

Health as biography

[. . .] Behaviour was the simplest 'public' answer to 'what is the cause of illness', the known 'expected' answer, and the one which they believed was medically authorized (Cornwell 1984). To consider typical answers in this way, however, is largely to misrepresent the women's real thinking about cause. If, in a different manner of analysis, a single respondent's way of thinking is traced back and forwards throughout the hour or two of conversation, these answers are seen in context. In fact, nothing has one cause. Alternatives are tried out, rejected, associated with each other, traced from one period of life to another. Examples are given of different cases, and the different factors that might apply are reasoned out. An attempt is made to achieve that 'experiential coherence' (as distinct from abstract, theoretical coherence) which has been shown (e.g. Pinder 1992) to be sought by those trying to interpret their own chronic disease.

Obviously, this is less easy to illustrate briefly. However, two examples follow, confined to the single story of the woman's own current and most salient health problems, which illustrate some typical themes. In these stories, as Cornwell also found, causal theories move between internal and external factors: 'the illness was not portrayed as something that could be separated from the person or the circumstances of their personal biography' (1984: 161). The women seek to answer the 'Why me? Why now?' questions in a way which, in Herzlich and Pierret's (1984) words, 'transcends the search for causes and becomes a quest for meaning'.

G14 – aged 54, twelve children

The main complaint chronic bronchitis: began with 'change of life at the time'. But also began when husband, 'a war pensioner', could not work and she 'took on a really old house' with the idea of lodgers. 'And then I took ill. I had a' the work and a' thing, you see.' — *life stage / stress, social circumstances*

The bronchitis 'started off with flu, and developed from that.'

Doctors told her it was smoking, and 'I stopped for nine months!' (But claims was better when she started again.) — *(?) behaviour*

Second, later, account of beginning of bronchitis: had a bout of pneumonia and neglected it, because she will never 'give in' to illness. 'Cos that was me, wi' pneumonia and bronchitis, walking down to the City hospital' (very long account of resisting hospitalization, on this and other occasions). — *self-neglect*

'I said, I'm nae gaun intae nae bed, I've a' these bairns at hame, I'm gaun back.' 'It's got to beat me first afore I'll call the doctor.' — *life stage / 'not giving in'*

At about the same time she had a bad fall on ice in the street, 'Something gaed intae my leg'. Secondary trouble is still pains in the leg and arms. 'It wis after that I first got the cold, and it went to my chest.' — *effects of trauma*

At present has laryngitis, but 'I'm blaming the weather.' 'And   weather
    smoking disnae help.'   behaviour

The continued pain is perhaps 'just wear and tear on the   natural ageing
    spine'. Of course, 'You couldnae expect onything else, wi'
    all that bairns.' She had two children after 40, which was   childbearing
    'too auld, maybe'.

Also has 'a kinda knot at the back o' my neck', which may be
    affecting the spine, but 'I think it's just a cyst maybe'.

Also suffers from migraine. Considers whether it is perhaps   childbearing
    associated with her neck? But 'I've had migraine since the
    last one was born.'

Nevertheless describes self as healthy. 'The only recipe I say is   self-responsibility
    nae to lie down wi' the least little thing that's wrang wi' ye.   'not giving in'
    Sometimes, if ye ging awa' and do a little bit of washing or
    something, you forget a' aboot your pains.'

. . .

G19 – aged 43, five children

Major current problem is that she is waiting for a
    hysterectomy, 'I'm aye awfu' tired'. Ever since the fifth   childbearing
    child (at 30) 'I've felt really tired and done.'

Has also had bronchitis all her life. It 'comes back wi' the   weather behaviour
    weather'. 'And of course I smoke.' It started with 'teething   heredity
    bronchitis' and runs through the family: 'My father had it,
    and my sister and myself, had it, and my daughter has it aff
    me, and her baby here, seven weeks old and it already has a
    whistle, so it must be taking it aff the mother.'

Returns to gynaecological problems. 'It's mental strain – and   stress
    bringing up five kids is bound to leave something, I mean
    it's a' right for him [husband] – he gaed round the world
    when my kids was little, he cam home and put me pregnant
    and gaed awa' again!'

Further talk of family history of chest problems, which leads   heredity
    to story of own mother's death from cancer.

Gynaecological problems: the state she is in is largely 'my ain   self-neglect
    fault' for not consulting earlier. 'It's jist anither phase of   life stage
    life. There's different things in life occurs, and you go on to
    anither phase of life. Me, I've come through all I've come
    through, it's only me I'm hurting now' (by neglect of health).

Nevertheless 'healthy enough'. No reason to coddle self now.   stress
    In comparison with days when children were young, life is   social
    easy. At that time she was almost overwhelmed with   circumstances
    illness, but pulled herself through by her own efforts.

Returns to talk about mother. 'This is aye at the back o' my   some diseases
    mind. Naebody kens until you're actually opened.'   unpredictable

Seems to retreat to talk again of bronchitis, which is more   heredity
   familiar and understandable: 'I mean, we're all made of an
   impression on our ancestors, arn't we? So if you've a
   weakness it must come out some way.'

. . .

Chains of cause

Several themes run throughout these accounts. First, there is the constant emphasis on life events, especially those identified with their female roles: childbearing, the care of elderly parents and their deaths, the menopause, widowhood, the deaths of children. Almost every chronic condition had its 'real' origins in one of these events. In particular, childbearing had been the crucial event: 'a woman's never the same after she's had children' was a popular aphorism.

These were all links in the chain of cause. A second notable feature of the accounts was the strain to connect, to present a health history as a chain of cause and effect, with each new problem arising from previous ones. There was a common concept of one disease 'going into' another, and many causes were sought in past injuries. A cough would 'go into' bronchitis, meningitis was caused by 'a knock', accidents many years before were blamed for arthritis. Accidents, like surgery, were assaults upon the body, unnatural breakings or openings which would leave it susceptible. Occasionally, disease might be seen as striking randomly: cancer is the most common example, though it must be noted that the reluctance to discuss cancer at length seemed also to be an expression of a taboo. Often the disease was not directly named, or the voice was dropped to a whisper. For most diseases, however, cause was not random. The women resisted the idea that one part of their body might have 'gone wrong' at one time, and another at another, without there being any connection. One thing must lead to another: there must be a logical biography.

These chains of cause stretched back through generations. Thus heredity and familial patterns were another pervasive theme in the talk of their own disease. In part, this was simply a natural human tendency towards 'pattern making', and, since families in the past had been large and certain diseases very prevalent, there was a high likelihood that if patterns were sought they could be found. Family weaknesses often lay in stomachs, or chests, or some other part of the body: 'They've all been bothered with their legs.' Alternatively, families could have some inherent strengths, resilience to certain types of condition. These discussions of family history, often very long, were commonly quite sophisticated, with the women working out in great detail exact degrees of relationship, the evidence of changes in environment (many older members of families had emigrated), or the different likelihoods of infection, direct inheritance or 'susceptibility'. G37, for instance, explained:

> I think family traits have a habit o' – you know, cropping up. You might
> have a family that's prone to rheumatics. Rheumatics aren't infectious,
> but if it runs in a family, to me, you know, as it comes down the line,

there's always going to be somebody that's sorta inclined to take that. In this climate . . .

This was set in the context of a recital of the lives and deaths of her own parents, siblings and grandparents, and then of her husband's family. A digression considered the effects of voluntary lifestyles: her paternal grandfather died young, but he was a well-known drinker; on the other hand so did his father, 'and he was a very religious churchgoing man, he didn't smoke or drink'. The conclusion was:

> families can be long-living families or short-living families. I think it must be something to do with the genes.

This fondness for familial 'explanations', as for connecting up the events of their lives, could be understood as a liking for continuity, a desire to give meaning to their lives. Their family histories, together with their own experiences, constituted their identity. Their present health status, including all the emerging problems of middle-age, had to be accommodated into that identity.

Health as moral identity

In particular, they wished to present a moral identity. Moral opprobrium attached, not to *having* illnesses, but in 'lying down' to them. A woman who complained, who made a fuss, who allowed illhealth to interfere with her duties, was a 'poor thing', to be pitied or scorned. Almost without exception, they themselves were presented as models of stoicism:

> I never lie down to illness – I've gotten up in the morning wi' a migraine and gone to work. Nearly killed me, mind, but I've gone . . . I'd rather be out in the company, you know, an' you're busy. I mean, if you're in the house you've still to make a meal and light the fire – you just canna lie. Well, I canna, I canna lie if I know the fire wants cleaning, no matter how bad I am. I've never been off work, never. You get some that stops off with the least thing.
>
> (G22)

They were firm adherents to the Protestant ethic. Hard work was virtue, virtue was rewarded, and health must be the reward of industry. So almost all were quick to describe themselves as 'healthy', no matter how long the list of illness they then went on to describe. This applied to their family members as well, even though they may have had many chronic diseases and died at an early age:

> My mother was aye healthy – she wis up at 5 o'clock in the morning, she had a' her work done, she wis oot in the toon half-past 8, she had a' her shopping done. She was real healthy, like.
>
> (G7)

These attitudes may obviously be characteristic of the particular culture of NE Scotland. But perhaps it is also an example of one of the paradoxes of 'embodiment' noted by Turner (1984): that, while the whole Christian tradition of the West affirms that the body is but weak flesh, the location of sin, it is also 'an instructive site of moral purpose and intentions', with health as the sign of moral well-being.

Identity created through interaction

People do not, of course, create their biographies and their identities in a vacuum. It is obvious that the process not only takes place within a cultural context, but is also a continual interaction with others, especially parents, spouses, other family and neighbours. Although the data here were, ideally, collected in one-to-one private conversations between interviewer and subject, some evidence about this process did emerge. In crowded and gregarious households privacy was not always possible, and there are a few interviews where other family members – usually husbands or daughters – were present, at least for part of the time. It seems of interest to ask whether these presentations of self were – in a situation where they were being offered to a relative stranger – likely to be challenged, or likely to be reinforced.

Within the family, there were in fact frequent examples of support, and none of challenge. That this was how the woman *was* was a well-known fact. A few of the husbands who happened to hear part of the interview expressed some cynicism about 'all this women's talk', and provided a chorus of comment, sometimes with friendly bickering and sometimes with an undercurrent of spite, but never with any serious challenge to the woman's image as someone who would not 'give in' to illness. Moreover, several women (not in the presence of their husbands) suggested that these stoical attitudes were the direct result of being placed in women's roles, in a culture where men had expected their wives to serve them, and where men's household comfort and working capacity took priority. Men 'who has pampered their wives' were not spoken of with any particular favour: they did their wives no service. The women's daughters did not necessarily agree: times had changed. Nevertheless they, too, supported and amplified the 'strength through adversity' theme of their mothers' biographies, using as their evidence the often-heard stories of their childhoods.

These fortuitous occasions where family interactions were observed cannot necessarily be regarded as representative data. The joint creation of biographies within families is a topic deserving research in its own right. There did, however, seem to be glimpses here of the processes by which biographies evolve and are reinforced.

Identity and deprivation

This intensely moral view of health meant, of course, that – even while they were recounting all the health deprivations of the past – the women were as reluctant to describe their families as unhealthy as they were to label themselves. If actually challenged, they would reject ideas about class inequalities [. . .]:

> I dinna think their surroundings has onything to dee wi' it. I mean, you could have ony God's amount o' money and the best o' everything, and you could have the unhealthiest child in the world. An' you could hae nothing, and hae to work and bring them up yoursel', an' you'll find you've got the healthiest kids.
>
> (G40)

They were aware, as they offered their biographies, that they had little to boast of in terms of material success. They could, however, be proud of their large, close families and of the virtues – simplicity of lifestyle, hard work, triumph over adversity – which they saw as pre-eminent. Those in richer circumstances probably lacked these virtues, and could not be rewarded with better health.

Conclusion

In summary, it seems probable that if these women had been asked the brief direct questions of the Health and Lifestyle Survey, their answers would have been in accordance with the class patterns found. Illness was primarily one's own responsibility, not only at the superficial level of quickly-offered survey responses, but also at a deeper level of claiming responsibility for one's own identity. They did not dwell on class inequalities because, though they were very conscious of the perils of the environment in the past, by contrast life seemed to be largely without such dangers now. They were perfectly capable of holding in equilibrium ideas which might seem opposed: the ultimate cause, in the story of the deprived past, of their current illhealth, but at the same time their own responsibility for 'who they were'; the inevitability of illhealth, given their biographies, but at the same time guilt if they were forced to 'give in' to illness. With this emphasis on selfhood and self-responsibility, and their knowledge of greatly improved general social circumstances, a rejection of ideas about (contemporary) 'inequality' was understandable.

Many such qualitative studies have shown that people reconstruct bio-medical concepts, including those of aetiology, in the light of their own biographies. Perhaps sociologists and social epidemiologists may have to accept that their concepts, too, may have little reality at the level of individual perceptions.

References

Blaxter, M. (1990) *Health and Lifestyles*, London: Routledge.

Blaxter, M. and Paterson, E. (1982) *Mothers and Daughters*, London: Heinemann.

Cornwell, J. (1984) *Hard-earned Lives: Accounts of Health and Illness from East London*, London: Tavistock Publications.

Herzlich, C., and Pierret, J. (1984) *Illness and Self in Society*, Baltimore: Johns Hopkins University Press.

Pinder, R. (1992) 'Coherence and incoherence: doctors' and patients' perspectives on the diagnosis of Parkinson's Disease', *Sociology of Health and Illness* 14: 1.

Turner, B.S. (1984) *The Body and Society*, Oxford: Blackwell.

Chapter 3

Charlie Davison, George Davey Smith and Stephen Frankel

LAY EPIDEMIOLOGY AND THE PREVENTION PARADOX

The implications of coronary candidacy for health education

From *Sociology of Health and Illness*, 13 (1) 1991:1–19

Introduction

IT IS WELL KNOWN within contemporary British society that coronary heart disease is a major cause of pain, illness, disability and untimely death. Like all kinds of misfortune (undesirable events which occur to some people sometimes but not everybody always) heart disease is the subject of a variety of cultural operations and activities whose goal is to bring it under some measure of human control. A precursor to such control is the development of an explanation (or set of explanations) which can account for the occurrence of the misfortune itself. Over the past three decades a well defined explanatory paradigm has developed in medical and official circles in Britain concerning the misfortune known scientifically as coronary or ischaemic heart disease and to the non-medical public as heart trouble, heart attack, coronary, heart, dicky ticker etc. Before entering into a discussion of the daily cultural practice that we have labelled 'lay epidemiology', it is worth taking stock of the back-drop to the study reported here and particularly the 'official' line on heart disease in Britain.

During the course of the twentieth century, investigators have announced the discovery of many conditions and behaviours which have strong associations with the development of coronary heart disease (CHD) in individuals. Some have been identified as possible causal factors. The communication of these discoveries to the wider society and their implications for personal life and behaviour has become a major concern of many primary care professionals and a growing body of health educators and health promoters.

It has become common currency in modern Britain that many deaths attributed to heart disease are preventable. This general outlook has come to be broadly shared by people within and outside the various medical professions. The core of the notion is that, in many cases, damage to the circulatory system is caused by identifiable behaviours which could theoretically be modified or eliminated. Turning this theory into practice has been the task of a plethora of public and private bodies, large and small, academic and campaigning, whose activities have encompassed fund-raising, research, political and professional lobbying, and direct public education . . .

Against the back-drop of large-scale intervention, a complex debate has developed in public health and medical social science circles concerning the efficacy, politics and ethics of prevention strategies based on individuals and prevention strategies based on communities. There are two basic strands to this debate:

(a)   Should public health initiatives concerning chronic disorders be based on screening, whereby those identified as being 'at high risk' are discovered and appropriate personal interventions made? Or should public health initiatives be based on a general population intervention, whereby the entire population is treated as being 'at risk'?

(b)   Should prevention efforts be aimed at specific behaviours deemed to be under the voluntary control of individual citizens, or should prevention efforts be aimed at infrastructural upgrading and the improvement of general social conditions? . . .

This paper concerns the status of this professional/official ideology in the daily lives of people living in the southern half of Wales. The central focus is on the relationship between these ideas and the everyday cultural mechanisms which serve to explain illness and death attributed to heart conditions. The paper is based on a preliminary analysis of formal, semi-structured interviews with randomly sampled adult informants in two urban and one rural district of South Wales ($n = 180$) and from many hours of informal discussion and observation carried out in the same areas. Fieldwork has involved formal (taped semi-structured interview) and informal (observation, discussion) interaction with male and female adults from a wide range of socio-economic circumstances. Our general aim here is to explore one of the central themes of both scientific and lay theorising about illness and death associated with impairment of the heart and its functions – that of assessing the possibility and probability of an individual becoming a victim.

The individual and the social appear interwoven in this public discourse, much as they do in many professional debates concerning the aetiology and distribution of chronic disease. Unlike those debates, however, 'lay' theories may display a complex and thoughtful interest in the relationship between preventability and inevitability, an area sometimes glossed over by the confidence in control which pervades the ideology of modern Western medicine.

The professional, official and media messages concerning the preventability of heart disease to which the informants taking part in this project have been exposed are similar in nature to those directed at other British populations. Almost all the countries and regions of the United Kingdom have been the targets of mass communication exercises concerning the risks of everyday behaviour and the importance of individual action to gain better health. It is our observation, however, that the early launch and consequent high profile of Heartbeat Wales have led to a stronger local impact than other British campaigns. In a qualitative sense attitudes towards illness and its prevention amongst the informants taking part in this research can be seen as broadly representative of wider British society. Given that professional and state intervention in the area of heart disease has been stronger in Wales than the rest of the United Kingdom, however, and that other regions and countries are currently 'catching up', the South Wales data presented here are of particular interest as an indicator of future developments elsewhere . . .

Coronary candidacy and the study of health beliefs

In this paper we describe and attempt to analyse the use of one cultural mechanism which plays a central role in the explanatory systems employed in Britain to account for coronary heart disease. The idea which we address is that of the 'candidate for heart trouble', 'coronary candidate', or 'the kind of person who gets heart trouble'. Our aim, here, is to describe a general explanatory framework which we have observed in wide usage in everyday life, a framework which is based on a fusion of all aspects of the explanatory dilemma discussed above. We also seek to provide an illustration of the sophistication of the cultural mechanisms which are used to account for the misfortune of common chronic illness in a markedly scientific society.

Clearly, in a social world as highly differentiated and stratified as our own, the views and attitudes of individuals and cultural groups differ widely. The goal of our analysis, however, is to explore the overall structures within which differentiation occurs, rather than dogmatically to ascribe detailed and fixed ideas to all members of such a complex social formation.

In recent decades, there has been a growing level of interest in academic and clinical circles in the area of 'health beliefs' (see for example: Herzlich 1973, Blaxter 1979, Pill and Stott 1981, 1982, 1985). It has been suggested that there exist, in the public mind, a range of explanatory models (Kleinman 1980) which people employ to account for illness and poor health and which serve to identify appropriate paths of treatment. Further to this idea, it has been advanced that individuals and groups have at their disposal a 'repertoire' of health beliefs (Chrisman and Kleinman 1983, Chrisman 1989) on which they may draw under various circumstances. While a certain amount of work has been done on the actual contents of such beliefs (Helman 1978, Blaxter and Paterson 1982, Williams 1983, Cornwell 1984, Pollock 1988) and some investigations have been carried out into their social distribution (Pill and Stott 1985, Calnan 1987, Cox et al. 1987), the ways in which they influence or inform individual and group behaviour remain somewhat enigmatic (for a useful review see Dean 1984).

The idea of 'candidacy' is of particular interest to the study of health beliefs because it is one way in which a general knowledge about the causes and distribution of illness is placed in an operational field. Through its use, generalised information which is derived from an aggregation of many cases is returned to the realm of the individual. It is a mechanism that helps individuals to assess personal risks, obtain reassuring affirmation of predictability, identify the limits of that predictability (thus mapping un-predictability), devise appropriate strategies of personal behaviour and to go some way towards explaining events which, by their very nature, are deeply distressing. In the cultural edifice which our society has erected to make sense of coronary disease and death, 'candidacy' is a central pillar.

Candidacy and 'lay epidemiology'

In the course of our discussions with the informants taking part in our investigations, we have observed that the scientific medical fields of symptomatology, nosology, aetiology and epidemiology have identifiable counterparts in the thoughts and activities of people outside the formal medical community. As is the case with scientific areas of theory and practice, the lay schema is not a series of discrete units, but a complex and interactive system in which each branch can be both informed by and dependent on the others. Lay and scientific 'ologies' are not, of course, entirely congruent, but we discern a certain degree of overlap.

The notion of 'candidacy' belongs to the area of lay epidemiology and, as is the case with other areas of lay knowledge and belief, it shares much with its more strictly scientific counterpart. Individual cases (from personal observation or report) of people who are known to have suffered heart disease are purposefully linked to other circumstances surrounding the event. From this data, regularities are noted and these contribute to the generation of explanatory hypotheses which serve to challenge or support suspected aetiological processes.

Aetiological theories, in turn, dictate the type of information which is commonly communicated about each case. Thus, because hair colour is not linked to the onset of heart trouble in aetiological hypotheses, the hair colour of sufferers is not noted by observers nor is it communicated in conversation or mass media reportage. The widespread belief that obesity is strongly associated with many heart cases, on the other hand, leads to the noting and communication of the sufferer's stature or build. These ideas do not exist as individual snippets of information. They are given coherent form and substance by the use of an overall profile or image of the kind of person who tends to suffer from heart trouble. This person is a 'candidate'.

Clearly the development of these ideas is not an entirely individual affair. Rather it is a collective activity with many different types of input. The mass media and official bodies are the source of much processed scientific data; reports of illness and death are available from family, friends, work colleagues and neighbours; celebrities such as politicians and sports people suffer and die in the public gaze; individuals make their own observations of themselves and of those around them. None of this cultural activity takes place in a vacuum or is drawn tabula rasa by an individual. Such is the cultural condition of individuals in mass society that the opinions, attitudes and perspectives they hold tend to be personalised modifications of generalised systems passed on from agencies of the wider society.

In the context of a social formation so overtly conscious of its own technological advance, such modifications often contain the idea that received systems are inherently old fashioned or outmoded. In our experience, this is certainly true of explanatory mechanisms used in the field of health and illness. Here scientific/medical advance is seen as so rapid that there is a general expectation that new treatments, cures and prophilaxes will constantly appear. Those in tune with advances in the field of illness prevention through behaviour change are often labelled 'health conscious'; the obvious parallel being with the similarly fast-moving worlds of fashion and style in clothing and the arts.

The idea of candidacy in everyday life

As a mechanism which orders experience and observation, making sense of everyday events, the idea of candidacy appears in many different social and conversational contexts. We have identified four distinct uses of the candidacy idea:–

(i)   the retrospective explanation of other people's illness and death through heart disease;
(ii)   the prediction of other people's illness and death through heart disease;
(iii) the retrospective explanation of one's own illness through heart disease;
(iv)   the assessment of one's own risk from illness and death through heart disease.

As some of the excerpts from our interviews illustrate, the use of the idea of candidacy is often attended by laughter. We find that this aspect of the system is in keeping with a more general cultural tradition which employs humour to defuse danger and so allows the 'unthinkable' to enter everyday discourse.

Candidacy as restrospective explanation

In the first type of instance, a person who has suffered or died from 'heart' is being discussed:

INFORMANT: Mind you, he was always a bugger for his fry-ups and his cream-cakes, so he had to be well up for it, like.
INFORMANT: Of course, it was in the family, so it was to be expected really.
INFORMANT: Fit, skinny, young. The last person you'd expect to have a coronary!
CD: And you say that your uncle had a heart attack . . .
INFORMANT: Well, with him, frankly he was a walking heart attack waiting to happen! (laughter)

Where an individual's own suffering from heart trouble is being discussed or mentioned, the retrospective assessment of candidacy is less likely to be attended by laughter. The definition of the issue as humorous, though, is sometimes an option which the sufferer chooses. As the following excerpt indicates, the explanation of one's own heart trouble is essentially similar to the explanation of the misfortune in others:

CD: Do you think that there was luck involved, for example, in the onset of your, um, angina the first time you had it? Or of your heart thing the first time you had it?

INFORMANT: Not particularly no no I don't think so. I think that was a result of, of, uh . . . a definite sort of stress that was taking place in my life, as it does in so many others.

Candidacy as prediction

In the second type of instance, a person is referred to as being a likely candidate in connection with some event or story which is under discussion. When a local media news bulletin carried a report of a school bus crash precipitated by the driver's sudden heart attack, a teenager joked:

INFORMANT: God, half of our drivers look as if they might keel over at any moment! (laughter)

CD: Really?

INFORMANT: Yeah, big fat wheezy blokes huffing and puffing! (laughter)

Such comments may also refer to the special treatment (gentle, restrained or slow) deemed to be necessary when dealing with a candidate:

(*informant referring to a minor argument in a cinema queue*) I didn't like to say any more, 'cos she looked as if she might have a heart attack any minute! (laughter)

The predictive dimension of candidacy is also used in everyday conversation in a less humorous way, with such comments as 'he'll have a heart attack if he isn't careful', or 'she shouldn't be carrying that heavy box all that way, a big woman like that'.

Candidacy in personal risk assessment

The use of candidacy in the assessment of personal risk clearly involves the use of the construct for predictive purposes. There are, however, such marked differences in tone, context and 'flavour' between personal and general usage that we describe them separately here. We have observed that the personal assessment use of the candidacy idea is less common in everyday conversation than the other types. For those individuals who participate in this use, however, we would judge that it is of particular importance in assessing the appropriateness of behavioural change.

The language of this type is similar, however:

INFORMANT: Thinking about my parents and my job, I suppose I've gotta be a candidate for some kind of heart trouble.

CD: Do you think of yourself as being particularly at risk from these kinds of problems?

INFORMANT: I don't know why, exactly, but I've always thought of myself as a candidate for cancer, rather than heart.

. . .

Who is a candidate?

In the course of our investigations we have encountered a wide range of conditions and behaviours which our informants perceive as being causally linked to the onset of heart disorders. In many cases, the fact that an individual exhibits or partakes in just one of these factors is enough for them to be identified as a coronary candidate. This is particularly true in the case of retrospective candidacy, that is when acquaintances of a sufferer admit to 'not being surprised' that X had a heart attack, although they may not have actually predicted it.

In cases where an individual presents an extreme form of a risk condition or behaviour, a more complete form of candidacy emerges which includes a predictive as well as a retrospective dimension. This is also the case when a combination of different risks are identified in the conditions and behaviour of the individual in question. Thus, a person who is thought to be overweight (but not extremely so) may not be identified as a candidate in a predictive sense, but if they suffered a heart attack, their size may well be mentioned retrospectively as a possible cause. If that person also smoked and drank heavily, or held a particularly stressful job, or was subjected to worry through unemployment or debt, their candidacy would be enhanced and a predictive element appear. An *extremely* fat person, however, may well be identified predictively as a candidate, even if they were deemed to be entirely virtuous (and a strong moral dimension *is* present) in respect of behavioural risks and 'lucky' in respect of other risky conditions such as hereditary susceptibility.

It should be added here that many risky behaviours and conditions are closely linked to each other. A hereditary propensity to suffering from heart disorders, for example, may well go with an inherited tendency to be overweight. It is also widely assumed that poorer people eat 'badly' largely as a direct function of their poverty. Similarly people who are, by their nature, 'worriers' are likely to smoke more than others, thus doubly enhancing their candidacy. This type of linkage tends to give each individual candidacy an organic wholeness and a personal character. This accords well with the widespread notion that each individual is essentially unique and that each person's experiences and choices in life are different.

The full range of individual conditions and behaviours which we have recorded as being linked to coronary candidacy are listed in Table 3.1.

It is now clear, then, that the range of conditions and behaviours that are involved in the candidacy system is wide indeed. One of the striking aspects of this width is that almost any type of person could be a candidate. In occupational terms, there are risks attached to the lives of rich 'high-flying executives' and to those of impecunious manual labourers. A sedentary life is seen as risky, but so is a life of over-strenuous exercise. While we judge that, in general, women are seen as being at less risk than men, it is clear that the candidacy system can be and is applied across

Table 3.1 People who may be identified as coronary candidates

Fat people
People who don't take exercise and are unfit
Red-faced people
People with a grey pallor
Smokers
People with heart trouble in the family
Heavy drinkers
People who eat excessive amounts of rich, fatty foods
Worriers (by nature)
Bad-tempered, pessimistic or negative people
People who are under stress from – work
              family life
              financial difficulty
              unemployment/retirement
              bereavement
              gambling
People who suffer strain through – hard manual labour
              conditions of work/home
              excessive leisure exercise
              overindulgence
              (sex, dancing, drugs, lack of sleep, etc.)

gender boundaries. It could also be added that, after the age of about 40, candidacy is seen to increase with age.

Individuals, however, tend to place their own emphasis on various elements of the system, and it is unusual to encounter complete agreement between people as far as the finer details of candidacy and risk are concerned. The social distribution of these emphases (do 'executives', for example, tend to think that they or manual workers are at greater risk?) is at present under investigation as part of our continuing research project (for some limited but interesting data see O'Looney and Harding 1982).

Candidacy and the unpredictability of sudden death

A striking element of the notion of coronary candidacy is that it is recognised as being a fallible system. There are many coronary illnesses and deaths which occur to people who do not fit any particular candidacy profile, and this is widely noted. Indeed such comments as 'the last person you'd expect' or 'perfectly fit, and always led a healthy life' indicate that these events represent a violation of the candidacy system. It is also widely observed that not *all* candidates develop the illness.

Such violations, however, are readily incorporated into the explanatory model as a whole by the simple recognition that candidacy only indicates increased risk while death from heart attack remains famed for its caprice. A strong element of the public image of heart disease (and of the sudden fatal heart attack in particular) is that it is a random killer. In the course of our field investigation we have observed that, even though most of our informants have professed the opinion that heart disease is to some extent preventable or postponable, the idea that it could happen to anyone (at any time) is omnipresent.

Under these circumstances it could be said that the candidacy system has the second function of providing a simple classification of heart illness episodes. Some are explicable in terms of the conditions and behaviours described above whilst others are not. This second type belong in a residual bad luck category and are referred to through such phrases as 'one of those things', 'when your number's up', 'what's for you is for you', 'fate' or 'destiny'. People are said to have simply 'dropped dead' and the finality of this phrase somehow communicates both a random and sudden event. In the absence of an adequate aetiological hypothesis (the mechanism of misfortune is not understood), the answer to the more personal explanatory question (why this person and not that one?) is found in another rich field of British cultural life, that of chance.

The candidacy system, then, has two interwoven strands. On the one hand is a set of criteria which can be used in the post-hoc explanation of illness and death, the prediction of illness and death, and the assessment of risk. On the other hand, there exists the all-important knowledge that the system is fallible. It cannot account for all coronary disease and death, neither can it account for the apparently unwarranted longevity of some of those that the system itself labels as candidates. Thus the observation that 'it never seems to happen to the people you expect it to happen to' becomes integrated as a central part of the system itself.

Candidacy, population approaches and the prevention paradox

It can be seen from the description of the system given above that many of the factors that go into the assessment of candidacy are closely linked to those highlighted by contemporary health promotion campaigns. But to see quite how compatible the systems are, it is necessary to examine the theory and rationale underpinning strategies which treat the entire population as being at risk.

The essence of the population approach to heart disease prevention is the recognition that screening individuals to identify those at high risk is a strategy which can deliver only limited success. This is because most fatal heart attacks happen to people outside the high risk group. Even if screening were well attended, identified high risk subjects accurately and led to successful intervention in all of the high risk cases it discovered, the total number of heart deaths prevented would be relatively small.

Where the bulk of deaths from CHD occur in the middle range of the population distribution of any given risk factor, a strategy must be followed which brings about a general diminution of a given risk in the population as a whole. Such a strategy, however, leads to a situation in which many individuals change their lives to no personal end – they would not have had a heart attack anyway. Rose terms this the 'Prevention Paradox', that is that 'a preventive measure which brings much benefit to the population offers little to each participating individual' (Rose 1985).

The prevention paradox poses some problems for those involved in the development of population approaches to heart disease prevention, in that if people are told that behavioural change is statistically unlikely to benefit them as individuals, they are unlikely to take part. Simultaneously, it is recognised that the most efficient method of mass behavioural change is to change the norms or rules of behaviour – in short to change culture itself. As Rose points out: 'If non-smoking eventually becomes "normal", then it will be much less necessary to keep on persuading individuals. Once a social norm of behaviour has become accepted and (in the case of diet) once the supply industries have adapted themselves to the new pattern, then the maintenance of that situation no longer requires effort from individuals. The health education phase aimed at changing individuals is, we hope, a temporary necessity, pending changes in the norms of what is socially acceptable' (Rose 1985: 37).

Rather than communicate the paradoxical nature of population strategies to the general public, the response of health educators and health promoters in Wales and elsewhere has been to disseminate simple messages suggesting that 'saturated fat is bad for you – eat less', 'obesity is dangerous – stay slim', 'exercise is good for you – do more', etc. The strong implication that flows from the contemporary 'health lifestyles' movement is that, for example, all saturated fat is always bad for everyone. The fact that this type of message is at best a distortion of the epidemiological evidence (see for example Oliver 1987) appears not to have diminished the zeal of its delivery.

The strategists of modern population approaches, however, have overlooked the existence and operation of lay epidemiology. The fact that ordinary people notice illness and death, talk about these events and partake in individual and group explanations has important implications for the cultural engineering activities of the health promoters. Whether or not coronary mortality drops, heart attacks will continue to kill people who were apparently not at risk and people who are at risk will continue to avoid heart attacks.

The basic result of the cultural engineering approach to coronary prevention is that publicly recognised risk thresholds are lowered. People who, before the onset of whole population health education, never thought of themselves as being at risk (from their diet, for example) now do. In the course of our discussions with informants and our observations of social responses to health education, we have identified two important outcomes of the public lowering of risk thresholds. Firstly, the number of individuals who survive risky behaviours becomes greater. Secondly, while the number of coronary cases who were not apparently at risk diminishes, there is a heightening of their public profile.

As we have seen, lay epidemiology detects these anomalous deaths and unwarranted survivals and cultural systems of explanation exist to account for them. Those who have lived beyond publicly recognised risk thresholds and survived into a healthy old age are seen as being 'lucky' because their individual 'constitution' allowed them to enjoy themselves and remain alive. Those who have led safe lives yet not 'died of old age', have their passing put down to 'bad luck', 'just one of those things', or the mysterious activities of the 'grim reaper'. It is ironic that such evidently fatalistic cultural concepts should be given more rather than less explanatory power by the activities of modern health education, whose stated goals lie in the opposite direction.

Aside from irony, however, there are also important political implications to be found in the interaction between lay epidemiology and the prevention paradox. It is clear that modern British health education has never come to terms with the complex relationship between the individual and the collective in the field of health and illness. Rather it has opted for a form of worthy dishonesty based on two simple premises. First, that individual citizens cannot or will not take part in behavioral change unless they are encouraged to anticipate an individual benefit. Second, that the broadcasting of propaganda based on half-truth, simplification and distortion is a legitimate use of public funds, so long as the goal of the enterprise is the good of the community.

The responses of the lay public in Britain to the current health education campaigns concerning individual behaviour and the risks of CHD reveal a sharp conflict between self-interest and shared values. While the operation of lay epidemiology ensures that it is impossible to fool all of the people all of the time, the central political issue remains unresolved. It will only be with the socialisation of health, when it is seen as a collective and not an individual phenomenon, that the problems of the prevention paradox will be overcome.

References

Blaxter, M. (1979) Concepts of Causality: lay and medical models, In D.J. Oborne, M.M. Gruneberg and J.R. Eiser (eds) *Research in Psychology and Medicine (2)*, London: Academic Press.

Blaxter, M. (1983) The Causes of Disease: Women Talking, *Social Science and Medicine*, 17, 59–69.

Blaxter, M. and Paterson, E. (1982) *Mother and Daughters: a three generational study of health attitudes and behaviour*. London: Heinemann Educational Books.

Calnan, M. (1987) *Health and Illness: the lay perspective*. London: Tavistock.

Christman, N. (1989) Dental Difficulties – Americans explanations of peridontal disease. *Anthropology Today* 5, 14–16.

Chrisman, N. and Kleinman, A. (1983) Popular health care, social networks and cultural meanings, in D. Mechanic (ed.) *Handbook of Health Care and the Health Professions*. New York: The Free Press.

Cornwell, J. (1984) *Hard-earned Lives – Accounts of Health and Illness from East London*, London: Tavistock.

Cox B.D. *et al.* (1987) *The Health and Lifestyle Survey – Preliminary results*. London: Health Promotion Research Trust.

Dean K. (1984) Influence of health beliefs on lifestyles: What do we know? *European Monographs in Health Education Research* 6, 127–50, Edinburgh: Scottish Health Education Group.

Helman C. (1978) 'Feed a cold, starve a fever': Folk models of infection in an English suburban community. *Culture Medicine and Psychiatry*, 2, 107–137.

Herzlich C. (1973) *Health and Illness: a social psychological analysis*, London: Academic Press.

Kleinman A. (1980) *Patients and Healers in the Context of Culture*. Berkeley: Univ. of California Press.

Oliver M. (1987) Diet and coronary heart disease. *Health Trends*, 19, 8–11 May.

O'Looney B. and Harding M. (1982) Coronary Heart Disease – the view of a group at risk. *Journal of the Institute of Health Education*, 20, 13–21.

Pill R. and Stott N.C.H. (1981) Relationship between health locus of control and belief in the relevance of lifestyle to health. *Patient Counselling and Health Education*, 3, 95–99.

Pill R. and Stott N.C.H. (1982) Concepts of illness causation and responsibility: some preliminary data from a sample of working class mothers. *Social Science and Medicine*, 16, 43–52.

Pill R. and Stott N.C.H. (1985) Choice or chance: further evidence on ideas of illness and responsibility for health. *Social Science and Medicine*, 20, 981–991.

Pollock K. (1988) On the nature of social stress: Production of a modern mythology. *Social Science and Medicine*, 26, 381–392.

Rose G. (1985) Sick individuals and sick populations, *International Journal of Epidemiology*, 14, 32–38.

Williams R. (1983) Concepts of health: an analysis of lay logic, *Sociology*, 17, 185–205.

Chapter 4

Michael Calnan

"LIFESTYLE" AND ITS SOCIAL MEANING

From G. Albrecht (ed.) *Advances in Medical Sociology, Volume 4*, Greenwich, Conn.: JAI Press (1994)

IT IS ONLY IN RECENT YEARS sociologists have tended to focus in any great depth on health-related behavior. Prior to that this area was the territory of social psychologists, where the emphasis was on explaining "individual" behavior and behavior change. The aim of this paper is to highlight these emerging sociological perspectives but specifically focusing on patterns of health-related behavior, the factors that shape it, the context in which behavior changes and the barriers to behavior change. The paper begins with examining the significance of health beliefs because up until recently this was the traditional approach for explaining patterns of health-related behavior. It looks at the theoretical assumptions that underpin some of the social–psychological frameworks and assesses the empirical support for these frameworks. It also identifies other dimensions of health beliefs that may be significant but are, as yet, untested. The aim in the second part of the paper is to examine alternative explanations. The discussion begins with some consideration of other social–psychological models but the bulk of the second part of the paper focuses on how important it is to see health-related behavior and the meaning placed on it within its socioeconomic context.

The significance of health beliefs

There are a number of models or frameworks that have suggested that health beliefs may be useful for explaining health-related behavior. Perhaps, the most popular of these is the health-belief model. According to a formulation of the health-belief model (Janz and Becker 1984), preventive health behavior will be predicted by three sets of beliefs: perceived susceptibility (subject's perception of the risk of contracting the disorder), perceived severity (perceived seriousness of the illness/ leaving it untreated—including both medical and social consequences), and perceived benefits/barriers (perceived benefits and costs of taking the recommended health actions). The idea is that these beliefs work in concert to produce a decision to carry out the behavior or not.

An alternative construct or framework that had similar origins as the health-belief model in learning theory is the health locus of control. The general principles behind the health locus of control is that people who feel they control their own health are also more likely to engage in healthy behavior, while those who feel powerless to control their own health will be less likely to act in accordance with the recommendations of official health agencies. Since its original inception the general construct of the health locus of control has been modified (Wallston et al. 1978) and the favored approach is now the multidimensional health locus of control. This construct consists of three different dimensions of belief about the source of control of health: the internal, powerful other, and chance. People who score high on the internal scale are more likely to believe that health is the result of their own behavior, while high scores on the other two suggest either that health depends on the power of doctors or on chance, fate, or luck.

While both these approaches have been popular there are some fundamental problems with them. These problems occur at both the conceptual and empirical levels. At the empirical level studies have shown that both models have limited explanatory power. For example, a recent study (Calnan 1989), using data drawn from two large-scale community surveys ($N = 4,224$), examined the relationship between the multidimensional health locus of control (MHLC) and exercise, cigarette smoking, and alcohol use. The results showed that none of these relationships was more than modest in strength even within different social and economic contexts.

Similarly, in studies examining the predictive power of the health-belief model the evidence suggests only a modest relationship between the belief dimensions and behavior (Langlie 1979). Calnan and Rutter (1986) in their prospective study examined the predictive power of the health-belief model for explaining changes in the practice of breast self-examination. Three groups of women were investigated— 278 who accepted an invitation to attend self-examination classes and were taught the techniques in detail, 262 who declined the invitation, and 594 controls to whom no classes were offered. Beliefs and self-reported behavior were measured shortly before the classes took place and again a year later. The results suggested that beliefs do predict behavior, for both perceived susceptibility and perceived benefits/ barriers made significant contributions to the belief–behavior equations, and the relationships were generally highly reliable statistically. To that extent, the model was supported, however, the evidence also suggests that the relationship between the behavior and the dimensions of belief which the model stresses was not a strong or a simple one. There were two pieces of evidence in particular. First, only a small proportion of the variance was explained in the analyses, which appears to be a common finding in studies using the health-belief model. The figure was never higher than 25 percent and it was generally much lower. It was also noticeable that the greatest amount of variance was explained in the control group, where the smallest amount of behavior change was found. In fact, changes in beliefs were generally poor predictors of changes in behavior.

The second piece of evidence was that a supplementary analysis of the data showed that prior behavior was a stronger predictor of subsequent behavior than were beliefs. When prior behavior was introduced into the analysis, the proportion of variance explained was increased markedly—as much as 48 percent in one case.

In summary, this empirical evidence suggests that the health-belief dimensions identified in the health-belief model and the health locus of control have limited explanatory value. In addition to the weaknesses at the empirical level there are also problems at the conceptual level.

Some of these weaknesses in relation to the health-belief model have been discussed elsewhere (Calnan 1987). One, however, that illustrates these conceptual weaknesses is an examination of the concept of perceived vulnerability. The concept of perceived vulnerability to illness in general or to a specific disease is central to the health-belief model (Janz and Becker 1984). The concept appears to be derived from epidemiological models, which, using probability theory as their basis, identify the range of factors that might influence a population's or individual's vulnerability to disease in general or to a specific disease. This concept of perceived vulnerability has been exported to the area of health behavior where it is argued that certain levels of vulnerability are associated with a greater likelihood of compliance with officially recommended health actions. This approach has been accepted and adopted by those who are involved in designing health education campaigns where one of the major objectives is to educate the individual into awareness of how "at risk" he or she is to certain disease. . . .

Are health beliefs important for explaining patterns of health-related behavior? This is a difficult question to answer given the lack of strong empirical evidence. Certainly, there are other dimensions of health beliefs which have been explored and might be incorporated into the model. In addition to specific beliefs, more general beliefs might be introduced, such as the value placed on health (where health is often only one of many competing values), the way health is defined, beliefs about the extent to which the individual feels responsible for his or her own health and in control of it, and beliefs about the value of disease prevention and health promotion (Calnan 1987). For example, as Crawford (1984) showed in his study of concepts of health amongst middle-class Americans, there are two apparently contradictory definitions of health that are prevalent. On the one hand, to be healthy is to demonstrate that there is a concern for the virtues of self-control, self-discipline, self-denial, and will-power. On the other hand, health means being happy, enjoying oneself, and being free to indulge as one wishes. And, it appears in Western society there is ambivalence about the use of drugs.

Some logical connection between concepts of health and beliefs about health maintenance is evident in that a dimension of health, which is very prevalent in lay concepts of health, is health as being fit, active, and strong. This is at least logically connected with lay ideas about health maintenance. Small-scale sociological studies (Calnan 1987) and large-scale surveys (Blaxter 1990) have shown that diet and exercise are the most popular activities for maintaining health. For example, evidence from the National Health and Lifestyle Survey (Blaxter 1990) showed that exercise, either in the form of active sports or keep fit, was the type of behavior which the majority of the sample thought was the key to maintaining or improving health. Among the elderly, activities such as gardening were important in maintaining health where among the young, active sports or keep fit were important. The next most important category was diet and this was favored more by females than males. Regular exercise is clearly logically linked with health as fitness and health as activity. The link between food and diet might also be seen as important for maintaining levels of energy and providing the resources necessary to keep active and fit to perform their daily tasks. . . .

While there appears to be some evidence of a logical connection between concepts of health and beliefs about health maintenance, how far do these concerns about health influence patterns of health-related behaviors? This particular question was the focus of a recent study (Calnan and Williams 1991) which, using ethnographic methods, attempted to identify how salient health was in people's daily lives. A novel methodology, at least in this area of research, was adopted in that the respondents were asked to describe, in detail, a day in their life (spontaneous discourse) and this was followed by more specific questions (probed discourse) about health and "lifestyle."

The evidence from the study showed that, irrespective of socioeconomic circumstances, matters of health rarely surfaced in people's descriptions of their daily lives. Neither did a concern with health in the context of behavior. Moreover, the emphasis placed within the first part of the interview upon spontaneous discourse left open the possibility that alternative forms of health-related behavior may emerge. However, this did not prove to be the case, and it was only at the level of probed discourse that discussions of health matters seem to emerge.

One interpretation of this evidence, and the most likely, is that health is not a priority for most people in the course of their daily lives and only surfaces when "health problems emerge or when trouble looms large." Thus, general discussions of health-related matters only seemed to surface spontaneously within respondents' accounts when they themselves, or their families, suffered actual health problems. This is well illustrated in the following accounts.

> As I think I said . . . I'm diabetic, so I have to do my injections in the morning and in the evening . . . Make a cup of tea, had some cod liver oil for me aches and pains . . . A teaspoonful a day . . . It seems to have stopped me joints aching and burning.

This highlights the taken-for-granted nature of health in routine daily life and the manner in which, paradoxically, it is only spoken about in its absence. For example, as one man remarked later on in the interview when asked to define health

> It's very difficult to say what you define as "fit" and "well." If what you have you take, I mean it is easy to take it for granted. I mean, if you take a man who, for argument's sake, has suffered with rheumatism, then you appreciate that you are presumably better off and fitter. It is very difficult to describe, something that I suppose you take for granted.

Moreover, as other studies have shown (Cornwell 1984), respondents may have different bodies of knowledge which they use in different contexts. This might be explained by the framework suggested by Young (1981) who argues that health and illness should be seen in the context of process and practice rather than in abstract terms. In his analysis of the nature of medical knowledge, Young makes a distinction between respondents' representational knowledge ("knowledge of something") and their practical knowledge ("knowledge produced in response to something"). Thus, when respondents are asked "What is health?" they produce a range of concepts (Calnan 1987) which seem to vary by social position. This might be seen as abstract or representational knowledge that was clearly present in the prompted questions on health and behavior. However, in everyday life such concepts are rarely adopted and more functional concepts such as the absence of incapacitating signs and symptoms are utilized. The evidence from this study (Calnan and Williams 1991) showed that the only exception to this was in relation to exercise, where clearly, among middle-class men and women, there was an emphasis on "well-being" and "relaxation," and physical exercise was used as a resource to achieve that end.

A further, related, explanation for the absence of discussion of matters of health in people's descriptions of their lives is that the social organization of people's everyday lives is based on decisions which have been taken in the past and have now become routinized and taken for granted. That is to say, it is only when these taken-for-granted features of daily life are called into question that they become readily apparent. In this respect, that which remains unspoken becomes just as important and revealing, perhaps more so both analytically and practically, as that which is cognitively organized (Locker 1981) in some shape or form. Certainly, as the responses to the prompted questions showed, the majority of people, irrespective of socioeconomic circumstances, did believe there was an association between these behaviors and health. However, given that respondents were clearly aware of the fact that the study was concerned with health, it might have been expected that more health-related knowledge would surface within the spontaneous talk. Certainly, in recent years "health" as an issue has received extensive media and advertising coverage and there are increasing "opportunities" for people to talk about health and, as Crawford (1984) points out, health is linked with wider social meaning.

> The body is not only a cultural object in illness or affliction. Bodily experience is also structured through the symbolic category of health. Health, like illness, is a concept grounded in the experiences and concerns of everyday life. While there is not the same urgency to explain health as there is to account for serious illness, thoughts about health easily evoke reflections about the quality of physical, emotional and social existence.

In summary, the evidence that has emerged from this analysis of health beliefs and their possible association with health-related behavior was that the importance of health beliefs may be over emphasized. Thus, it is necessary to explore other possible explanations for patterns of health-related behavior in the absence of health problems.

Explaining health-related behavior

Evidence from empirical research has shown that the strength of the statistical interrelationships between types of health-related behaviors are at best modest. For example, in one study (Calnan 1989) using a random sample from a community population, it was found that the correlation between alcohol use and smokers (0.19) and alcohol use and exercisers (0.15) was positive but only modest in strength. A similar pattern emerged in a large National Health and Lifestyle Survey (Blaxter 1990), that examined the interrelationship between smoking, alcohol use, diet, and exercise. This study examined the interrelationships between behaviors in different age and gender groups. The highest correlations were between smoking and diet, with those who smoke being more likely to have a poor diet, and those who do not smoke a better one. Smoking and alcohol were also associated, but less strongly, and alcohol consumption was associated with a high level of exercise. For men, drinking was correlated with a poor diet but diet was not correlated with exercise. However, for women, a good diet was correlated both with a high level of exercise and a low level of drinking. But, once again, the overall strength of the correlations was never more than modest ($< .25$). The implication of this is that health-related behavior cannot be conceptualized as a unidimensional phenomenon.

Evidence from a wide variety of sources (Blaxter 1990; Townsend et al. 1988) has also shown that patterns of health-related behavior vary markedly by socio-demographic characteristics such as social class, age, gender, and educational background. Not only that, but clusters of behaviors tend to be found among certain social groups. For example, Blaxter (1990) shows that those who were smokers, drinkers, had a poor diet, and carried out a low level of exercise, were more likely to be men, to be unskilled manual workers, to be unemployed among the young, and living alone among the elderly. Twice the average rate of this pattern of behavior was found in the Northern and Yorks/Humber regions of England. However, as Blaxter (1990) clearly shows, this type of group was in the minority and the majority did not have totally healthy or unhealthy lifestyles.

One interpretation of these pieces of evidence is that while individual beliefs about health-related behaviors or beliefs about the consequences of the behavior may influence the decision to adopt the behavior in question, social and economic circumstances may provide a setting which can act to enable or constrain the practice of health-related behavior. . . .

Social position and health-related behavior

Evidence, as has been previously presented, also shows that patterns of health-related behavior vary markedly by social position and it is therefore necessary to concentrate on the structural factors which modify beliefs and circumstantial factors.

Social and economic factors may act in a variety of ways. For example, studies such as that of Cornwell (1984) show how ideas about matters of health are grounded in everyday life, in turn, structured by social and economic circumstances. Cornwell in her ethnographic study in East London found that the set of moral and philosophical assumptions which underlay beliefs about work almost replicated those which underlay beliefs about health and illness. However, as was illustrated in the previous section the relationship between health beliefs and health-related behavior is a problematic one. Thus, it might be more useful to look at the approach that places greater emphasis on the direct impact of the material circumstances in which people live and work rather than on mental structures.

This approach is well illustrated in the work of Graham (1989) who showed how the interrelationship between socioeconomic circumstances and gender influenced the individual's attitude to smoking. Graham (1989) shows that at both household and individual levels, the evidence points to substantial spending on tobacco by low-income households. For example, low-income households with two adults and two children devote an average of 5 percent of the weekly household income to tobacco, compared with 2 percent in all households with two adults and two children. In addition, they spend absolutely more on tobacco than other house-holds. Also, spending among low-income households with children is higher than among those without children. The highest expenditure on tobacco, calculated on a per capita basis, is among one-adult households with children; 90 percent of these are headed by women. Studies have also shown (Baldwin 1985) that there are higher levels of spending on tobacco among households with a disabled child at all income levels. Thus as Graham points out:

> The research indicates that spending on tobacco is strongly related to particular forms of inequality, and specifically with caring for children in poverty.

Graham (1989) through her qualitative investigation, also provides an explan-ation for this pattern. In her study of 57 women she showed how in some families smoking was associated with breaks from care, when they rested and refuelled. She showed that cigarettes were also associated with breaks in their pattern of care when the demands of the children were too much to cope with. As one woman stated (Graham 1989):

> Sometimes I put him outside the house, shut the door, and put the radio on full blast, and I've sat down and had a cigarette, calmed down and fetched him in again.

In the context where women had to cut back on any luxury goods for them-selves such as shoes, haircuts, etc., cigarettes could be a woman's only purchase for herself. Thus, smoking reflects the social isolation and stress of caring for children in poverty. As Graham (1989) concludes:

> Where smoking is part of an individual's response to disadvantage, it is likely to function as part of a complex array of coping strategies that maintain the fragile equilibrium of everyday life. In these circumstances

increasing the pressures on women to become non-smokers may have wider implications for individual and family well-being. These may be missed by people concerned only with smoking cessation.

In these situations, the social benefits of habits such as smoking outweigh the known costs and even if some of these women would like to give up smoking, changing their health habits is difficult given the barrier of lack of resources such as time, energy, and finance.

Another study (Gabe and Thorogood 1986) also focused on smoking but also examined tranquilliser use among black and white working-class women. Their study also focused on the use of resources but the concept of resources was used to bridge the theoretical gap between social structure and everyday life. They argue that in contrast to Graham, resources should not be seen as external, inert materials possessed by individuals, but as a part of a process or set of relations. Resources can enable and constrain and are differentially distributed. Thus, they conceptualize "drugs" as resources, along with other material and sociocultural resources, that are both differentially available and variously experienced. They showed how patterns of drug use related to women's varying access to a range of other resources such as paid work, social support, leisure, cigarettes, alcohol, and religion.

Similarly, in a study by Calnan and Williams (1991) smoking appeared to be used by working-class women as a resource for relaxation and for handling the stresses and strains of everyday life. In contrast, all of the men who smoked stressed the habitual and sociable nature of smoking. For example, this was what one working-class man said:

> Well, I suppose it's just a habit I've got into and you just, playing cards, you just simply light up, don't you and that's it. Somebody offers you one and you just sort of take it, you know.

. . .

Attitudes or social circumstances?

Explanations for variations in patterns of health-related behavior, as was shown in the previous sections, either tend to emphasize the importance of individual attitudes toward behavior and its consequences or the importance of the social contexts and circumstances in which the behaviors are carried out. The evidence suggested that both explanations were significant and probably related. However, Blaxter (1990) in her analysis of data from the U.K. National Health and Lifestyle Survey, attempts to estimate the relative effects of circumstances and attitudes on behavior. In her study she found that health beliefs, such as a general, positive orientation toward responsibility for health, or internal locus of control, or measured in terms of belief about the importance of specific behavioral factors for health were associated with behavior. People with positive attitudes or beliefs that behavior is important were most likely to adopt "healthy" lifestyles. The aim of this analysis was to find out to what extent the connection between attitudes and behavior is due to intervening characteristics such as income, education, family, social class, or region of residence.

Some of the evidence which emerged from the analysis suggested that attitudes have rather little effect on behavior if social circumstances were controlled. For example, in her causal analysis examining differences between "healthy" and "unhealthy" behavior she examined the relative importance of attitudes such as the internal locus of control against social class and income. The causal analysis shows that, within social class and income groups, locus of control has a negligible effect on behavior. The total effect of social class is partly through income and partly through education.

In conclusion, this chapter has shown how there has been a shift in emphasis away from explaining health-related behavior in terms of medical rationality, that is, the assumption that health beliefs will and should explain health-related behavior toward attempting to understand the lay person's actions in terms of their own logic, knowledge and belief, and the context of their daily life. As a result, recent research has concentrated on the meaning placed on the behavior itself and how the social circumstances in which people live and work shape their "style" of life. This research is beginning to unravel the link between social structural factors such as social class, age, gender, and education; beliefs about behavior and its meaning and patterns of health-related behavior. Research up until now has tended to focus on health-related behavior in the context of domestic life. Future research might investigate the relationship between the work environment, beliefs about control and health-related behavior, and might begin by focusing on the process or the way the structure of the work environment influences beliefs about control. Perceived lack of control over the work environment might in turn shape beliefs about control over aspects of life such as health and which may have implications for health-related behavior.

Alternatively, rather than focus on the contexts and circumstances that limit "health choices" it might be beneficial to examine the circumstances that generate patterns of health-related behavior. For example, it has been argued (Calnan et al. 1993) that in the United Kingdom during the 1980s there were broad social changes in the relations of consumption. An increase in disposable incomes among middle-class and working-class households has created the conditions that have led to a widespread desire for personal control in the sphere of consumption. This, it is claimed, has led to increasing consumer expectations about health care which involve not only demands for higher standards of health care but a demand for greater personal control over health and its management that clearly has implications for health-related behavior. As yet, there is little evidence to substantiate this theoretical argument although it clearly points to a possible relationship between socioeconomic circumstances and health-related behavior.

The evidence from this paper has also suggested that for those intent on changing behavior, a strategy of attempting to change individual behavior through tapping salient beliefs may not be sufficiently effective given that many health-related behaviors are closely tied to social contexts and social circumstances. Thus, it is necessary to pursue policies which are aimed at social change as well as individual change. Also, as the ethnographic evidence suggests, these social policies may be more effective if they are tailored to the needs and perceptions of the community itself rather than top-down, paternalistic policies that might attempt to impose inappropriate policies on to the "target" population (Calnan 1991).

References

Baldwin, S. 1985. *The Costs of Caring: Families with Disabled Children*. London: Routledge.

Blaxter, M. 1990. *Health and Lifestyles*. London: Routledge.

Calnan, M. 1987. *Health and Illness: The Lay Perspective*. London: Tavistock.

——, 1989. "Control over Health and Patterns of Health-related Behaviour." *Social Science and Medicine* 26(4): 435–55.

——, 1991. *Preventing Coronary Heart Disease: Prospects, Policies and Politics*. London: Routledge.

Calnan, M. and D. Rutter, 1986. "Do Health Beliefs Predict Health behaviour?" *Social Science and Medicine* 22: 673–8.

Calnan, M. and S. Williams. 1991. "Style of Life and the Salience of Health." *Sociology of Health and Illness* 4: 506–29.

Calnan, M.S. Cant, and J. Gabe, 1993. *Going Private*. Milton Keynes: Open University Press.

Cornwell, J. 1984. *Hard Earned Lives*. London: Tavistock.

Crawford, R. 1984. "A Cultural Account of Health–Control, Release and the Social Body." In *Issues in the Political Economy of Health*, edited by J. McKinley. London: Tavistock.

Gabe, J. and N. Thorogood. 1986. "Prescribed Drug Use and the Management of Everyday Life: The Experience of Black and White Working-class Women." *Sociological Review* 738–72.

Graham, H. 1989. "Women and Smoking in the UK: The Implications for Health Promotion." *Health Promotion* 3(4): 371–81.

Janz, N. and M. Becker. 1984. "The Health Belief Model: A Decade Later." *Health Education Quarterly* 11: 1–47.

Langlie, J.K. 1979. "Interrelationships Among Preventive Health Behaviors: A Test of Competing Hypotheses." *Public Health Reports* 94: 216–20.

Locker, D. 1981. *Symptoms and Illness: The Cognitive Organisation of Disorder*. London: Tavistock.

Townsend, P., N. Davison, and M. Whitehead. 1988. *Inequalities in Health*. London: Penguin.

Wallston, K., B. Wallston, and R. De Veilra. 1978. "Development of the Multidimensional Health Locus of Control Scales." *Health Education Monograph* 6: 160–73.

Young, A. 1981. "When Rational Men Fall Sick." *Culture, Medicine and Psychiatry* 5: 317–35.

Chapter 5

Phil Brown

POPULAR EPIDEMIOLOGY, TOXIC WASTE AND SOCIAL MOVEMENTS

From J. Gabe (ed.) *Medicine, Health and Risk: Sociological Approaches,* Oxford: Blackwell (1995)

Introduction

EPIDEMIOLOGY HAS CHANGED dramatically from the original shoe-leather epidemiology of John Snow, a committed and passionate discoverer of the causes of human suffering and death. In recent decades epidemiology has been shaped on a laboratory science model, often more concerned with protecting the increasingly rigid standards of scientific procedures than with safeguarding public health. At present, there is a countervailing approach – that of popular epidemiology – which returns to the roots laid down by Snow. By examining popular epidemiology, I intend to illustrate the changing nature of discovery involving environmental hazards and diseases.

In particular, I want to show that the current efforts of lay people and certain scientists represent a significant contribution to both human health and scientific endeavour. These people are discovering disease clusters, agents which cause those diseases, and vectors by which the agents reach humans. They are also discovering a variety of social structural features: corporate dumping and cover-up, governmental complicity or at least failure to act appropriately, and local boosterism which pits co-residents against the lay investigators. And, they are engaging in self-discovery: finding the strength to carry out incredibly difficult and lengthy researches, learning to work collectively and cooperatively, and for some, redefining themselves as social activists with a larger political awareness.

Origins of epidemiological discovery

Shoe-leather epidemiology

Epidemiology begins for most of us with John Snow's 1854 discovery of the relationship between water contamination and a cholera epidemic in Soho, London. Snow listened to other people's anecdotal evidence about connections between water and cholera, and then made his own observations of such connections. He determined a localised area where the epidemic was most severe, and then surmised that the water pump at Broad Street was the cause (Goldstein and Goldstein 1986).

Snow conducted a health survey which showed him that mortality among people living further from the well occurred only when they specifically used that well. Mortality away from the well was at the pre-epidemic rate. To account for cholera among two groups of people who were believed to have not drunk contaminated water, Snow tracked down the indirect sources of water intake. To account for lack of cholera, he found that workhouse residents had their own water supply, and that brewery workers were drinking beer instead of water. Snow determined the source of the water as being one of two companies, identifiable by pipes and further confirmed by chloride concentration. The tabulation of cholera rate by water company provided proof of the source. Snow's famous removal of the handle from the Broad Street pump actually occurred after the epidemic had peaked, though that by no means diminishes the significance of his action (Goldstein and Goldstein 1986).

Note how advanced Snow was in his recommendations: 'The communicability of cholera ought not to be disguised from the people, under the idea that the knowledge of it would cause a panic, or occasion the sick to be deserted.' Such withholding of information is today one of the major problems in present-day relations between contaminated communities and government (Goldstein and Goldstein 1986). . . .

Popular epidemiology

Traditional epidemiology studies the distribution of a disease, and the factors that influence this distribution, in order to explain the etiology, and to provide preventive, public health, and clinical practices. Popular epidemiology is a broader process whereby lay persons gather data, and also collaborate with experts. To some degree, popular epidemiology parallels scientific epidemiology, such as when lay people conduct community health surveys. Yet it is more than public participation in traditional epidemiology, since it usually emphasises social structural factors as part of the causal disease chain. Further, it involves social movements, utilises political and judicial approaches to remedies, and challenges basic assumptions of traditional epidemiology, risk assessment, and public health regulation.

Popular epidemiology efforts do not *require* epidemiological health studies, even though these may occur. Indeed, activists generally want the hazards avoided and remediated. If the government and/or corporations involved would admit the problem and take appropriate action, activists would have no need for or interest in health studies. But the activists experience much resistance to their claims, and require the kind of public, political and scientific support that often presses for more concrete evidence of causation.

Popular epidemiology is similar to other lay advocacy for health care, in that lay perspectives counter professional ones and a social movement guides this alternative perspective. Some lay health advocacy acts to obtain more resources for the prevention and treatment of already recognised diseases (e.g. sickle cell anemia, AIDS), while others seek to win government and medical recognition of unrecognised or under-recognised diseases (e.g. black lung, post-traumatic stress disorder). Still others seek to affirm the knowledge of yet-unknown etiological factors in already recognised diseases (e.g. diethylstilbestrol [DES] and vaginal cancer, asbestos and mesothelioma). Popular epidemiology is most similar to the latter approach, since original research is necessary to document both the prevalence of the disease and the putative causation.

This leads us to consider popular epidemiology as having two elements. The first is a general description of the phenomenon of lay discovery of disease. This is often environmental or occupational, though it need not be. The second is the more specific participation of activists in epidemiological studies. It is important to note, however, that lay people who embark on a process of social discovery of toxic contamination do not typically have any idea of the extent of their future involvement. Hence, the more 'routine' popular epidemiology (general discovery) cannot be so easily distinguished from the more 'formal' type (involvement in health studies).

From studying contaminated communities where well-organised citizens' groups have discovered toxic contamination, we observe a typical set of stages. My chief model is the Woburn, Massachusetts case, where citizens discovered a leukemia cluster, pushed for government action, collaborated with scientists to conduct a health study on leukemia, reproductive disorders, and birth defects, and also filed suit against the companies they believed to be responsible. These stages may vary in different locations, and may overlap each other:

1   *Lay observations of health effects and pollutants.* Many people who live at risk of toxic hazards have access to data otherwise inaccessible to scientists. Their experiential knowledge usually precedes official and scientific awareness.
2   *Hypothesising connections.* Activists often make assumptions about what contaminants have caused health and ecological outcomes.
3   *Creating a common perspective.* Activists begin to piece together the extent of the problem, and to organise it coherently. 'Lay mapping' of disease clusters is a typical feature of this stage. Citizens also make discoveries of actual pollution sources.
4   *Looking for answers from government and science.* Activists expect government health agencies and their scientific colleagues to investigate the problem. Citizens are often given little or no support from officials and scientists. In-depth epidemiological studies are rarely done. Rather, officials may merely make statements about the relationship of rates in the toxic community to state or national rates.
5   *Organising a community group.* Citizens formalise their social action by setting up an organisation to provide social support and information for toxic victims,

deal with local, state, and federal agencies to attract media attention, and often enough to make connections with other toxic waste groups.

6   *Official studies are conducted by experts.* Additional pressure leads to more detailed studies, but these tend to continue the denial of toxic waste-induced disease.

7   *Activists bring in their own experts.* Here is where the more 'formal' popular epidemiology efforts begin. With official support for their claims of toxic contamination, citizens find sympathetic scientists who are willing to help them in health studies. There are differing degrees of lay involvement in these studies.

8   *Litigation and confrontation.* Often, citizens file suit against corporations they believe are responsible for the contamination. They may also take other political action, such as picketing, boycotting, and lobbying.

9   *Pressing for official corroboration.* When lay-supported or lay-involved health studies are completed, citizens attempt to use that data to confirm their claim. They typically meet even more resistance, often from a growing number of national actors such as professional organisations, federal agencies, and disease philanthropies.

10   *Continued vigilance.* Whether or not activists have been successful in making their case, they find the need to be continually involved in cleanups, additional official surveillance, media attention, and overall coordination of efforts.

Throughout these stages, lay and professional disputes occur. I now turn to the main elements of those disputes: lay participation, standards of proof, constraints on professional practice, disputes over the nature of risks and hazards, quality of official studies, and professional autonomy.

Struggles over scientific discovery

Popular participation and the critique of value-neutrality

Popular epidemiology practitioners disagree that epidemiology is a value-neutral scientific enterprise. Traditional epidemiologists criticise health studies where citizens play a role, as in the case of Woburn where activists worked with bio-statisticians to conduct a large health survey. That study determined that exposure to contaminated well water was associated with increased childhood leukemia and a variety of birth defects and reproductive problems (Lagakos *et al.* 1984). The critics who argued that the study was biased upheld the notion of a value-free science in which knowledge, theories, techniques, and applications are devoid of self-interest or bias. Sociological and other social scientific studies of science dispute such claims, arguing that scientific knowledge is not absolute, but rather the subject of debate among scientists. As well, scientific knowledge is shaped by media influence, economic interest, political pressure, and social movement activism (Dickson 1984). On a more practical level, science is limited by financial and personnel resources; lay involvement often supplies the labour power needed to document health hazards. Science is also limited in how it identifies problems worthy of study. It does not typically take its direction from the lay public, but from established professional and organisational routines.

Toxic activists see themselves as working to correct problems not dealt with by the established scientific community. The centrality of popular involvement is evident in the history of the women's health and occupational health movements which have been major forces in pointing to often unidentified problems and working to abolish their causes. Among the hazards and diseases thus uncovered are DES, Agent Orange, asbestos, pesticides, unnecessary hysterectomies, sterilisation abuse, and black lung.

Some epidemiologists who support lay efforts to uncover environmental health effects put forth a distinctively value-laden epidemiology. Wing (1994) best exemplifies this alternative conceptualisation of epidemiology:

1   It would ask not what is good or bad for health overall, but for what sectors of the population.
2   It would look for connections between many diseases and exposures, rather than looking at merely single exposure–disease pairs.
3   It would examine unintended consequences of interventions.
4   It would utilise people's personal illness narratives.
5   It would include in research reporting the explicit discussion of assumptions, values, and the social construction of scientific knowledge.
6   It would recognise that the problem of controlling confounding factors comes from a reductionist approach that looks only for individual relations rather than a larger set of social relations. Hence, what are nuisance factors in traditional epidemiology become essential context in a new ecological epidemiology.
7   It would involve humility about scientific research, combined with a commitment to supporting broad efforts to reform society and health. . . .

Lay–professional differences concerning risks and hazards

Scientists have been professionally socialised to believe that science and technology are best left to scientists and engineers. Growing public fears of toxic wastes – quite often realistic – have encountered much epidemiological disagreement. Communities which believe themselves to be contaminated or at risk have found that the epidemiological response is often defensive and hostile, based on a view that alternative hypotheses are threats to scientific inquiry. In particular, scientists often cite what they view as erroneous public beliefs concerning increases in cancer rates, the extent of environmental causes of cancer, and the existence of cancer clusters. Scientists often charge lay people with being 'anti-scientific', when in fact citizens may simply work at science in a nontraditional manner, or else are critical of official practices. Indeed, surveys of toxic activists show that they express support for scientists as important sources of knowledge (Freudenberg 1984).

Professionalist practices of excluding the public are particularly ironic in the case of epidemiology, since the original 'shoe-leather' epidemiological work that founded the field is quite similar to popular epidemiology. Yet modern epidemiology has come far from its origins, turning into a laboratory science with no room for lay input. Along the way, the passionate discovery has been transformed into a routinised science establishment.

This clash of rationalities discussed above is particularly evident in risk assessment. Langdon Winner (1986) views the rise of risk assessment in the 1970s as a backfire against environmentalism, with 'health hazards' redefined as 'health risks'. Thus, he notes, 'What otherwise might be seen as a fairly obvious link between cause and effect, for example, air pollution and cancer, now becomes something fraught with uncertainty.'

The early approaches to risk, which continue to dominate, came from engineers and cognitive psychologists. These risk assessment experts employed questionnaires, in tandem with actual hazard rates, to argue that respondents overestimate 'flashy' causes of death and those which receive more media coverage. At the same time respondents underestimate less 'flashy' ones. Scholars explained this by noting that people rely on anecdotal evidence, have an emotional involvement in the issue, have deep distrust of social authorities, are overconfident in their personal ability to actively avoid hazards, have difficulty imagining low probability/high consequence events happening to them, and have trouble taking in new information, and often stick with past judgements. Lay people are more likely to assess high risk when the activity is seen as involuntary, catastrophic, not personally controllable, inequitable in distribution of risks and benefits, unfamiliar, and highly complex. The risk assessors calculated these dimensions of risk as falling into three factors: their familiarity with the hazard, the conceptual 'dread' associated with it, and number of people exposed to the hazard (Fischoff et al. 1982). . . .

It is important, especially when studying race and class differences, to add another concern – the population studied. Risk assessment, as well as epidemiological research, typically treats race and class burdens as variables to be controlled, rather than as special features of populations. Yet populations are not random; they are stratified according to social structural features such as race and class. The context of this stratification means that the hazard exposures are not random, and hence we cannot accurately find universal dose–response relationships (Wing 1994). Because of the stratification of society, hazards are inequitably grouped together and people experience them as collective assaults rather than as individual probabilities.

These contextual issues can be seen in Martha Balshem's (1993) study of how a Philadelphia cancer prevention project clashed with the white, working-class neighbourhood's belief system. The project identified excess cancer in this area, a fact widely known by the residents and the media. The medicalised approach of the health educators focused on individual habits, especially smoking, drinking, and diet. Tannerstown residents countered this worldview with their belief that the local chemical plant and other sources of contamination were responsible.

The professionals approached the working class as a monolithic mass of people with many unhealthy behaviors and nonscientific attitudes. What professionals call working class 'fatalism' appears more sensible as a response to economic insecurity in the face of Philadelphia's declining industrial workforce. The health educators medicalised working-class fatalism as a 'disease' that prevents people from complying with cancer prevention experts' prescriptions. To change lifestyles appeared merely to be what Balshem (1993: 57) notes is 'to adapt to life in the "cancer zone".'

Balshem recounts one woman's tale of agony over her husband's death from pancreatic cancer. Jennifer fights for the right to see John's medical record. When she finds a line about his smoking and drinking, she asks the doctor, 'What's this on here?' He responds 'That's not important.' Jennifer retorts, 'It's important to me. You're going to take this report saying he's an alcoholic and he smokes and this is what causes cancer. Then you wonder why we get upset because the statistics are wrong.' Jennifer struggles to get his medical record rewritten, and she demands an autopsy to show that he didn't die of lung cancer, but of metastatic pancreatic cancer, and hence is not blamed for smoking-induced cancer. Jennifer, like toxic waste activists, wants justice and fairness, and will use science if it can be of help. But they do not desire a science 'above' ethics and morality. That is a contradiction in terms for them.

Scientific contributions of popular epidemiology

Lay epidemiological approaches have changed the nature of scientific inquiry in various ways.

1   Lay involvement identifies the many cases of 'bad science,' e.g. poor studies, secret investigations, failure to inform local health officials, fraud and coverup.
2   Lay involvement points out that 'normal science' (Kuhn 1963) has drawbacks, e.g. automatically opposing lay participation in health surveys, demanding standards of proof that may be unobtainable or inappropriate, being slow to accept new concepts of toxic causality.
3   The combination of the above two points leads to a general public distrust of official science, thus pushing lay people to seek alternate routes of information and analysis.
4   Popular epidemiology yields valuable data that often would be unavailable to scientists. If scientists and government fail to solicit such data, and especially if they consciously oppose and devalue it, then such data may be lost. This goes against the grain of traditional scientific method.
5   Popular epidemiology has pioneered innovative approaches. For example, the Environmental Health Network is testing a new way to ascertain quickly the relationship between disease clusters and toxic wastes by using the Environmental Protection Agency's (EPA's) Toxic Release Inventory, a computerised database accessible to all citizens in public libraries.

These five elements have been common to many contaminated communities, but in Woburn the lay contribution to scientific endeavour has been dramatic. The Woburn case was the major impetus for the establishment of the state cancer registry. Of particular value is the discovery of a trichloroethylene (TCE) syndrome involving three major body systems – immune, cardiovascular, and neurological – which is increasingly showing up in other TCE sites.

Activism has also contributed to increasing research on Woburn: the Department of Public Health (DPH) and Centers for Disease Control (CDC) are conducting a major five year reproductive outcome study of the city, utilising both prospective and retrospective data, and citizens have a large role in this process. The DPH is conducting a case-control study of leukemia. Toxic waste activism in Woburn has also led to several Massachusetts Institute of Technology (MIT) studies. One group of projects, totalling $3.33 million in federal support, will produce a complete hydrogeological study; a history of the tanning industry, a major polluter; and an innovative genetic toxicology study based on human cell mutation assays, which will endeavour to produce a 'unique chemical fingerprint' of a large number of known and suspected toxic substances (Massachusetts Institute of Technology 1990). A second MIT effort is a three year study funded by the Agency for Toxic Substances and Disease Registry and the National Institute for Occupational Safety and Health. It will examine the scientific, ethical, and legal issues in monitoring residents and clean-up workers in three Superfund sites, one of which is Woburn. It is significant that both public officials and university scientists attribute the strength and innovativeness of this variety of research to the strong community involvement.

How do we know if lay investigations provide correct knowledge?

Toxic activists are not anti-scientific. In many cases, popular epidemiology findings are the result of scientific studies involving trained professionals, even if they begin as 'lay mapping' of disease clusters without attention to base rates or controls. This lay mapping phenomenon is almost an instinctual reaction. Patricia Nonnon did it when she noticed high rates of leukemia in the Pelham Bay section of the Bronx in New York City (Lorch 1989). In Staten Island, another New York City borough, a landfill worker tracked down the health status of his workmates when he discerned an elevation in cancer and other diseases. A Coeur d'Alene, Idaho woman tracked down several entire high school graduating classes when she noticed a huge cancer increase. Leon and Juanita Andrewjeski kept what they termed a 'death map' of cancer deaths and illness and of early heart attacks among farmers downwind of the Hanford, Washington nuclear reservation (Kaplan 1991). In Leominster, Massachusetts, a doctor told a woman, 'You do so well with your [autistic] children, you should talk with other parents on your block who have autistic children.' This led to lay mapping of 35 cases in a small area (Lang 1994).

At the scientific level lay-involved surveys are sometimes well-crafted researches with defendable data. Lay people may initiate action, and even direct the formulation of hypotheses, but they work *with* scientists, not in place of them. Thus, the end results can be judged by the same criteria as any study. But since all scientific judgements involve social factors, there are no simple algorithms for ascertaining truth. Scientific inquiry is always full of controversy; what is different here is that lay people are entering that controversy.

To err on the side of caution

Toxic activists believe that epidemiology needs to return to its roots. One central part of that is the elevation of public health over abstract canons of science. Doing that means, among other things, to err on the side of caution. A society more concerned with overall well-being will conduct research differently, and act on it differently. When the Swedish government found a connection between power lines and childhood leukemia, the government immediately made plans to alter power lines. The alternative in the US would be, at best, to appoint a National Cancer Institute or Department of Energy panel to study this question for several years, with a host of lobbying efforts to make sure the utility companies received adequate representation. That would be similar to the situation in 1992 when the tobacco industry got the EPA to throw certain scientists off a second-hand smoke panel because they were considered too vocal in their beliefs that tobacco caused lung cancer.

The elevation of public health concerns also means a more powerful role for social activists in setting the health agenda. We remember the importance of veterans' organisations in confronting Agent Orange. Women's health activists were central in showing links between DES and vaginal cancer. Recently, activists won a large federal research effort to study excess breast cancer in Long Island, New York, and forced President Clinton to publicly support more funding.

Sociologically, we may situate research silences and scientific/governmental resistance in a large context of professional resistance to controversial discoveries concerning such problems as drug side effects, unnecessary surgery, and environmentally induced diseases. Normal science and its supporters do not like to challenge political, economic, and intellectual sources of power. Nor do they want to change the theories and methods to which they are accustomed. They do not want alterations in their professional and institutional arrangements which might threaten funding, power, influence, and tradition. They most certainly do not like lay input, and lay input is pervasive in the discussions of environmentally caused disease.

Toxic waste activism and environmental justice

My definition of popular epidemiology early in this chapter included the centrality of political action and social movements. Many local toxic action groups do not initially view themselves as part of a national or international movement. Rather, they are only dealing with what they perceive as local problems. But the initial groups, such as the Love Canal activists, set in motion a new movement. As well, the subsequent prevalence of these groups contributes to an already existing movement which has some more consciously political centres of activity. While most of these groups would not style themselves as popular epidemiology practitioners, this is what they are doing in their lay efforts to uncover disease and act on that discovery. The toxic waste movement represents a solidification into broader social action of popular epidemiology's critique of traditional science . . .

A new type of social movement

The toxic waste movement has been a dramatic force in US society in the last two decades. Unlike other social movements, this one is not characterised by national organisations. The toxic waste movement is highly decentralised, composed of thousands of small community-level groups. Its few national organisations, such the Citizens' Clearinghouse Against Hazardous Waste and the Environmental Health

Network, are sources of inspiration and resources, rather than officials and organisa-tions exerting influence over local groups. There are also some statewide toxic activist coalitions that play similar roles.

Some local organisers have become highly politicised, such as Lois Gibbs, whose experiences at Love Canal inspired her to form a national group. Patty Frase, without prior political experience, started as a local organiser in her home town of Jacksonville, Arkansas, site of the Vertac Chemical Corporation which produced herbicides and pesticides. She moved on to organise a statewide toxic waste coalition (Capek 1993). Some local activists have become somewhat professionalised – two staff members of Woburn's For a Cleaner Environment (FACE) group later worked for a national non-profit organisation that provides consultation to local groups engaged in lay epidemiology. Even when local activists lose their political naivety, they still may cease their activism when they attain their goals. Yet while many groups have a short life, their large number guarantees increasing strength to the overall movement.

There are several reasons for the lack of national participation. Without a history of radical political action, local activists do not automatically see the benefits of a national organisation. Local activists have often suffered family injury or death directly, and they spend enormous time on arranging health care and organising their lives around a debilitating or fatal disease. Local groups are bogged down in lengthy and difficult efforts at discovery, remediation, litigation, and organising. For example, Woburn's Ann Anderson began her 'shoe-leather epidemiology' in 1973. As of 1994, the two Woburn Superfund sites are still not cleaned up, and the litigation appeal only ended in late 1990. In the Velsicol case in Hardeman County, Tennessee, a state regulatory agency brought the problem to light in 1964; in 1966 the United States Geological Survey got involved; in 1972 Velsicol was ordered to close the dump; in 1977 residents began to organise, and in 1988 the final appeal of the case was heard (Brown and Mikkelsen 1990: 71–2). Such lengthy processes diminish groups' potential for broader activism.

Some critics argue that the toxic waste movement is too motivated by narrow self-interest – protection of one's own 'backyard' rather than the larger common good. It is true that toxic waste activists are not usually motivated by global environmental concerns, although a good number quickly come to understand their local problems in that larger context. As Lois Gibbs (1991) points out, 'NIMBY has now become NIABY, Not in Anyone's Backyard.' In other words, these groups seek the protection of all people against toxic waste hazards through minimal environmental discharge, on-site mobile disposal, and the banning of entire dangerous categories of chemicals and metals. As the 'NIABY' approach becomes more dominant, local activists grasp their role as one of many groups which have altered the national political life (Freudenberg and Steinsapir 1992). In Lois Gibbs' (1991) words, 'We're working locally and affecting national policy.' Local toxic waste activist groups have been mistrustful of the global emphasis of mainstream environmentalism, since those national organisations have taken up global issues at the expense of local matters of human health . . .

Successes of the toxic waste movement

Toxic waste organising has had considerable success. Toxic activist organisations have provided desperately needed support and encouragement to their own members and to activists in other locations. Groups have catalysed clean ups of hazardous waste sites, blocked hazardous facilities, halted pesticide spraying, and forced companies to upgrade pollution management technology. Through these successes, the movement has forced corporations to consider the environmental effects of their production and disposal practices, resulting in source reduction. At the government level, groups have won legislation, as well as the right-to-known about local hazards and the right-to-participate in decision making. For the overall public, the toxic waste movement has increased public support for environmental protection (Freudenberg and Steinsapir 1992).

Activists observe science in practice as being a servant of corporate and governmental interests, and thus seek a lay, democratic science which we see in popular epidemiology. As with other social movements in health, the toxic waste movement alters accepted scientific definitions of the problem, and leads to significant advances in scientific knowledge. In doing so, it challenges normal routines of corporate power, political authority and professionalism.

The toxic waste movement, especially under the influence of the environmental justice perspective, helps steer the environmental movement clear of an emphasis on personal solutions and recycling; it emphasises the well-being of humans as a crucial issue, as opposed to wildlife and wilderness; it forces awareness of the Third World ramifications of toxic waste dumping; it introduces a different class and racial awareness based on the groups most affected; it places gender in a central role, due to the predominance of women activists and their particular approaches to social problems; it offers political participation to many who would otherwise not be recruited, especially minorities and working-class people (Dunlap and Mertig 1992, Brown and Masterson-Allen 1994).

Conclusion: causes and implications of popular epidemiology

Dramatically increasing scientific, as well as lay, attention to environmental degradation, may make it easier for many to accept causal linkages previously considered too novel. Similarly, many more disease clusters are being identified as a result of this expanding attention and its related social movements. Growing numbers of similar cases containing small sample sizes and/or low base-rate phenomena may allow for more generalisability. These increasing cases also produce more anomalies, allowing for a paradigm shift.

Causal explanations from outside of science also play a role. Legal definitions of causality, developed in an expanding toxic tort repertoire, are initially determined by judicial interpretation of scientific testimony. Once constructed, they can take on a life of their own, setting standards by which scientific investigations will be applied to social life, for example, court-ordered guidelines on claims for disease caused by asbestos, nuclear testing, DES, and radiation experimentation.

Popular epidemiology stems from the legacy of health activism, growing public recognition of problems in science and technology, and the democratic upsurge regarding science policy. Communities face difficulties in environmental risk assessment due to differing conceptions of risk, lack of scientific resources, poor access to official information, and government policies which oppose or hinder public participation. In popular epidemiology, as in other health-related movements, activism by those affected is necessary to make progress in health care and health policy. In this process there is a powerful reciprocal relationship between the social movement and new views of science. The striking awareness of new scientific knowledge, coupled with government and professional resistance to that knowledge, leads people to form social movement organisations to pursue their claims-making. In turn, the further development of social movement organisations leads to further challenges to scientific canons. The socially constructed approach of popular epidemiology is thus a result of both a social movement and a new scientific paradigm, with both continually reinforcing the other.

References

Balshem, M. (1993) *Cancer in the Community: Class and Medical Authority*. Washington D.C.: Smithsonian Institution Press.

Brown, P. and Masterson-Allen, S. (1994) Citizen action on toxic waste contamination: a new type of social movement, *Society and Natural Resources*, 7, 269–86.

Brown, P. and Mikkelsen, E.J. (1990) *No Safe Place: Toxic Waste, Leukemia, and Community Action*. Berkeley: University of California Press.

Capek, S.M. (1993) The environmental justice frame: a conceptual discussion and an application, *Social Problems*, 40, 5–24.

Dickson, D. (1984) *The New Politics of Science*. New York: Pantheon.

Dunlap, R.E., and Mertig, A. (1992) The evolution of the U.S. environmental movement from 1970 to 1990: An overview. In Dunlap, R.E. and Mertig, A. (eds) *American Environmentalism: The U.S. Environmental Movement*, 1970–1990. Philadelphia: Taylor and Francis.

Fischoff, B., Slovic, P., and Lichtenstein, S. (1982) Lay foibles and expert fables in judgments about risk, *The American Statistician*, 36, 240–55.

Freudenberg, N. (1984) Citizen action for environmental health: report on a survey of community organizations, *American Journal of Public Health*, 74, 444–8.

Freudenberg, N. and Steinsapir, C. (1992) Not in our backyards: the grassroots environmental movement. In Dunlap, R.E. and Mertig, A. (eds) *American Environmentalism: The U.S. Environmental Movement, 1970–1990*. Philadelphia: Taylor and Francis.

Gibbs, L. (1991). Keynote address. 1991 conference of Massachusetts Campaign to Clean up Hazardous Waste. Boston, Massachusetts, 13 April.

Goldstein, I. and Goldstein, M. (1986) The Broad Street pump. In Goldsmith, J.R. (ed.) *Environmental Epidemilogy*. Boca Raton, Florida: CRC Press.

Kaplan, L. (1991). 'No more than an ordinary X-ray': a study of the Hanford Nuclear Reservation and the emergence of the health effects of radiation as a public problem. Ph.D. Dissertation. Heller School, Brandeis University, Waltham, MA.

Kuhn, T. (1963) *The Structure of Scientific Revolutions*. Chicago: University of Chicago Press.

Lagakos, S.W., Wessen, B.J., and Zelen, M. (1984). An analysis of contaminated well water and health effects in Woburn, Massachusetts, *Journal of the American Statistical Association*, 81, 583–96.

Lang, M. (1994) 'Welcome to the Plastic City': Community responses to the Leominster, Massachusetts autism cluster. Presentation at American Sociological Association, Los Angeles. 8 August.

Lorch, D. (1989) Residents force start of cleanup at Bronx dump, *New York Times*, 14 Nov.

Massachusetts Institute of Technology (1990) Center for environmental health sciences at MIT. Cambridge: Massachusetts Institute of Technology.

Wing, S. (1994) Limits of epidemiology, *Medicine and Global Survival*, 1, 74–86.

Winner, L. (1986) *The Whale and the Reactor: A Search for Limits in an Age of High Technology*. Chicago: University of Chicago Press.

Chapter 6

Evelyn Parsons and Paul Atkinson

LAY CONSTRUCTIONS OF
GENETIC RISK

From *Sociology of Health and Illness,* 14 (2) 1992: 437–55

Introduction

'**R**ISK' ENTERS INTO MANY CONTEXTS of medical discourse and decision-making. It is especially pertinent to genetically transmitted disorders, where the calculation of risk of transmission from one generation to the next is both the outcome and the preliminary to a great deal of intervention on the part of medical geneticists. It is also the basis for important issues of understanding and action on the part of lay social actors who may be the agents of genetic transmission. This paper will address the construction of 'risk' in relation to one particular genetic disorder, Duchenne Muscular Dystrophy (Duchenne).

Carrier risk and reproductive risks in Duchenne raise a number of issues relevant to the medical sociologist, from the professional work that goes into their production, to the lay understandings of the values and their relevance for reproductive behaviour. In this paper attention will be focused on lay definitions and understandings of 'risk' values that are provided by genetic counsellors and medical practitioners.

The research reported here is based on a purposive sample of two-generational pairs of women in families with Duchenne. Respondents were identified initially from their personal files held in the Institute of Medical Genetics on the basis of their relationship to a boy with Duchenne. The sample consisted of a group of mothers whose sons had manifested Duchenne and their daughters who were old enough to face the issue of their own reproductive behaviour in the light of their reported risks. Interviews were conducted with 22 mothers and 32 daughters and in all cases significant social details have been changed and pseudonyms used. Full details of the sample and the conduct of the research are reported elsewhere (Parsons, 1990). The interviews were unstructured, lasting between two and four hours, and were conducted in the women's own homes. They covered many aspects of their experiences of having a son or a brother with Duchenne. The information gathered included the women's understandings of what it meant to be 'at risk', their reproductive behaviour or intentions, their attitudes to abortion, the explanations they gave for a genetic disease in their family and their understanding their past or present risk status.

The focus of this paper is the women's own constructions of genetic risk rather than the detailed processes whereby risk figures are produced and negotiated between the laboratory scientists and medical geneticists. The issue of the social construction of medical risk values will be discussed in another paper. Its absence from this discussion, however, does not mean that the 'risk' figures in question are to be regarded as values independent of judgement, inference and practical reasoning.

Duchenne Muscular Dystrophy

Duchenne is a genetically transmitted disorder that only physically manifests itself in males but is transmitted by females. It is a muscle wasting disease which begins to show itself in early childhood. There is a progressive deterioration; death in late adolescence is the predictable outcome.

Women who have a male member of their family affected by Duchenne are either obligate carriers or are classified as being 'at risk' of carrying the defective gene. It is the task of medical geneticists to generate estimates of a woman's carrier risk, based on a combination of family history, results from creatine kinase testing and DNA studies. It is only women who are obligate carriers who can know their carrier status with any certainty. For other women the figures that they are given by geneticists and counsellors are estimations based on the family information available and scientific knowledge operating in a particular genetics laboratory at a specific point in time. Carrier risk figures are often modified as a result of changes in a family situation (for example the birth of an affected boy or the detection of a deletion in a male fetus), or advances in molecular biology (for example the availability of new probes to detect deletions, see Rhona et al., 1991).

Carrier risks are expressed as a percentage, ranging from 0.1 per cent to 99.9 per cent. It is on the basis of a woman's carrier risk that her risks in reproduction are calculated. For example an obligate carrier with a 100% liability in terms of carrier status has the following reproductive risks:

- 1 in 4, or 25 per cent chance in any pregnancy of having an affected boy
- 1 in 4, or 25 per cent chance in any pregnancy of having a carrier girl
- 1 in 2, or 50 per cent chance in any male pregnancy of having an affected boy
- 1 in 2, or 50 per cent chance in any female pregnancy of having a carrier girl.

The calculations of reproductive risk for the rest of the women are more complex.

For example a woman with a carrier risk of 44 per cent translates into the following risks in reproduction:

- 1 in 9, or an 11 per cent chance in any pregnancy of having an affected boy
- 1 in 9, or an 11 per cent chance in any pregnancy of having a carrier girl
- 2 in 9, or a 22 per cent chance in any male pregnancy of having an affected boy
- 2 in 9, or a 22 per cent chance in any female pregnancy of having a girl carrier.

For any woman in the family there are two sets of risk figures: her carrier risk which expresses her chances of carrying the defective gene and her reproductive risks which indicate her chances of having an affected male or carrier female in a particular pregnancy.

Definitions of carrier risk rates

Women's accounts of risk

All the women in the study had, at some time in their lives, been given a figure which represented their carrier risk. It was possible, from their personal files, to ascertain their current risk figure and how and when that information had been given to them. During the course of the interview 48 women were asked what their risk figure was. The purpose was not to evaluate their recall capacity or the effectiveness of genetic counselling. It was rather to hear how they talked about their risk in the course of an informal conversation, and to see how they had incorporated a carrier risk rate into their everyday reality. In particular, it was intended to explore whether they retained it in mathematical form, or had translated it into a descriptive category.

There was no evidence during the study to indicate that any respondents were affected by a general lack of numeracy. Mrs Poole and her daughter Victoria were interviewed together. Mrs Poole had been given a carrier risk of 92 per cent and her daughter Victoria one of 27 per cent. The discussion on risk and probability went like this:

> MRS POOLE: They do say that your risks have gone down a bit, what are you now – 1 in 7 or 1 in 8?
> VICTORIA: No – 75 – (Silence.)

Later in the interview EP tried again:

> EPP: Do you know what your carrier risk is, Victoria?
> VICTORIA: Well I think it's about 70 something, it's over 70, it's not 50:50, it's over 70.
> MRS POOLE: No she's definitely got it –
> EPP: What's that, she is a carrier?
> MRS POOLE: Oh she is a carrier.

VICTORIA: Oh I am a carrier – yes – if it's a boy it's 70 per cent chance that he would be.

Victoria was convinced that she was a carrier and that there was a 70 per cent chance, in any male pregnancy, that the foetus would be affected. Both mother and daughter had translated Victoria's carrier risk into a routine recipe of certainty: 'Oh she's definitely got it': 'Oh I am a carrier'.

Jean Moffoot, a daughter, had been given a carrier risk of 80 per cent. This meant there was a 20 per cent chance she was not a carrier and a 60 per cent chance that any male pregnancy would be unaffected. She had been told by her mother that all boys would be affected and had taken that definition without question. She made no attempt to explore carrier risk or its significance:

EPP: What are your carrier risks?

JEAN: I – um was it 50:50 or something?

She continued:

JEAN: Now when my mother had the test at the same time as me she was 75 per cent, so there, and I was 50 per cent.

EPP: Do you know what that means?

JEAN: It was just half and half – all I know, I am totally blind really . . .

She had confused her carrier risk with the reproductive risks of an obligate carrier. Her husband joined in and said that the 50 per cent chance was of the baby being affected, but Jean insisted:

JEAN: Oh no, I didn't take it that way, oh definitely – you had the risk – and I was just under that, you couldn't all my mother told me was that if it was a boy then it would be like Clive and I couldn't live with it like Clive.

She had passed this message on to her husband before they got married:

JEAN: You knew I just said to him – 'If we have children we can only have girls.' . . . I think that all he thought was that he couldn't have a son.

There had been a translation of risk and uncertainty into a binary statement: 'We can only have girls.' This use of a definitive statement, or a 'one liner' was also evident in the Cope family. When Gillian (a daughter) was asked what her carrier risks were she said:

GILLIAN: I was given a percentage, but I can't remember it, that was when I was eighteen . . . I think it was quite a risk . . .

Later in the interview she talked about risk again:

> GILLIAN: Well it was more or less that I couldn't really have a boy.

Her sister Penny was unable to give her risk figure either, but she admitted:

> PENNY: I can always remember when I was small I can always –
> although you (referring to her mother) hadn't said to me, I
> always used to have that in my mind that if I had a boy he was
> going to be the same as Roy, I always thought that, you know
> without being told, that was always in my mind.

None of the three women had retained her carrier risk as a mathematical figure. They had translated them into descriptive categories that had become routine recipes for their reproductive behaviour: 'I can't really have a boy.' . . .

Women's understandings of clinical explanations

Several of the women talked about how the clinicians had tried to simplify their carrier risks by the use of ratios. Kitty Bain (a daughter) had a medically defined carrier risk of 33 per cent and this is how it had been explained to her:

> KITTY: They gave me odds, I can't remember the actual odds, I was
> classed, I think, as high risk . . . he did tell me about the blood
> test and what they looked for, the abnormalities and then how
> they calculated my risk . . . they said I've got to have eight
> children to have one affected, I thought – 'Do I have to have
> eight children to prove them wrong?

Again Kitty did not use a percentage figure in talking about her risk but a ratio and a descriptive category.
Mrs White said her daughter Pamela had been confused by the explanation she had received:

> MRS WHITE: They said it's 100 to 1, so Pamela said, 'If I had a hundred
> babies would it only happen to one of them?'
> Never understood them (referring to carrier risks) and still
> don't understand them.

Her other daughter (Joan) had obviously been equally confused:

> JOAN: They used to say things like 'Oh 1 in a 1,000' and you think –
> 'Oh well have I got to have a thousand babies before I have one
> that's like that?' you know.

The same method of explanation had been used when Janet Hargreaves had been told:

JANET: At one time this doctor was telling me the chances I had, that
              was no good to me, I remember saying to them – 'What good is
              that to me, I would never want a load of children anyway, my
              mother had six.'

Abigail Hayward had been given a risk of 22 per cent and this is how she talked
about it:

ABIGAIL: Um – I think about half a per cent – 50 per cent or
              something . . .

Asked her if she understood those figures, she continued,

ABIGAIL: (pause and laughter) – well not really, all I know – he (the
              doctor) said to me did I understand it and I said 'Well no.' So
              he said to me – 'Well if you got pregnant five times that means
              four out of the five could be boys.' That's how he explained it
              to me in other words. But it can affect you in different ways
              can't it?

Abigail recognised the potential of a 50/50 risk in reproduction but had not retained
accurately her carrier risk rate. . . .

Risk, relevance and recipe knowledge

There are several issues relevant to lay understandings of risk highlighted in the
women's accounts. First, there were 28 of the 48 women who talked about their
risk using some form of mathematical or probability ratio. There were 13 who
quoted it with a degree of accuracy (i.e. within plus or minus 2 per cent). The
majority of these were the younger women who were still family building, which
could well be a feature of the increasing availability of genetic counselling. It also
illustrates Schutz's concept of zones of relevance in the structuring of personal
stocks of knowledge (Schutz, 1946). Women who were involved, or potentially
involved, in reproductive decision making retained risk information in a zone of
high relevance because it was defined by them as something of immediate personal
concern. The relevancy of risk is also noted by Lippman-Hand and Fraser
(1979: 55):

> it would seem that recall of rate information depends on the relevance of
> this information to the family at the time they are asked to remember it.

Second, there were 15 women who quoted a figure for their carrier risk which
did not correspond to the one in their medical records. It was clear that nearly
half had confused carrier and reproductive risk figures. This difference is not
only mathematically significant (a reproductive risk in any pregnancy is 25 per cent
of a carrier risk) but points to a potential difference between medical and
lay perspectives. In the laboratory the scientists calculate carrier risk figures and

their ultimate concern is to establish definitive indicators of carrier status. This focus is translated to the clinicians who retain a 'carrier' perspective in the genetic counselling discourse. In total contrast the primary focus for many women is not their carrier risk but their risks in reproduction.

Third, there were 36 of the women who talked about their carrier risk using a descriptive ranking: that is they referred to them as either 'high' or 'low', 'bad' or 'not so bad'. It was possible to take this informal ordinal scale and see where they placed significant thresholds. There were two main watersheds: women ranked risks below 5 per cent as 'low' and those above 20 per cent as 'high'. Risks between 5 per cent and 20 per cent were defined by three women as 'low' and by two as 'high'. Details of the way the women ranked their own risk on an ordinal scale is shown in Table 6.1.

Fourth, in conversation a number of women talked about their risk using routine recipes, or 'one liners', such as 'I can only have girls', or 'I can never have boys'. Mathematical percentages and ratios were translated into meaningful everyday statements for reproductive action. This was particularly noticeable at the polarities where risk was resolved into either certain carrier or certain non-carrier status. . . .

The evidence from this study in Duchenne would indicate that the resolution was towards greater *certainty* rather than greater uncertainty. Women, in their assessment of risk, adopted descriptive statements that were recipes appropriate for genetic decision making. They assessed their risk in terms of 'being a carrier' or 'not being a carrier', as 'being able to have boys' or 'not being able to have boys'. This resolution of risk meant that the women were not constantly living with uncertainty in genetic decision making. Lippman-Hand and Fraser (1979) argue that, for women, it is not their risk that needs to be resolved but 'their existential state of being "at risk"'. It is this issue of the women's perceptions of risk in terms of carrier status that will be explored in the next section. Did the women define their carrier status in terms of a 'spoiled identity', and was that reflected in their information management?

Table 6.1 Women's self-ranking of carrier risk, compared with medically defined risk

	Women's self-ranking		
Carrier risk, per cent	*High*	*Low*	*Total*
<5	0	8	8
5–9.9	1	1	2
10–19.9	2	1	3
20–39.9	2	0	2
>40	21	0	21
Total number of women	26	10	36

Definitions of carrier risk status

Risk status, personal identity and information management

Carrier status in Duchenne only manifests itself at reproduction. This means that during the majority of their lives women do not exhibit any visible indicators which could stigmatise them to the outside world. There are no signs, or symptoms, which interfere with their everyday lives. This situation of 'being at risk' offers what Goffman (1968) describes as a 'discreditable stigma': something that can remain hidden in the majority of encounters. Scambler and Hopkins (1986), in their study of epilepsy, make the distinction between stigmas which are 'felt' and those which are 'enacted'; those which are based on the fear of being discriminated against because of an imputed stigma, and those where there is evidence of stigmatisation. They found that the 'felt' stigmas were more disruptive to individual lives and were based on personal definition rather than cited incidences.

Epilepsy is dormant between seizures, carrier status in Duchenne is dormant between reproductive episodes. Assessments of carrier status have the potential of being more closely related to definitions than they are to actualised stigmatisation. How did the women define their carrier status? Did they talk about it in terms of a spoiled identity, or was it referred to in the more limited terms of discreditable stigma with specific critical episodes? If the latter was the case, what were the events that triggered the disclosure of their latent stigma?

For Mrs Roper there was no question: her identity had been spoiled and she defined her carrier status as highly stigmatic. The condition may not be socially visible, and its significance evident only in reproduction, but for her it was something that had affected her total social identity. She said:

> MRS ROPER: It's when they tell you, like he – (referring to the doctor) – said – 'you're a carrier' that's horrible – (said with real anger in her voice) – I wish they would get some other word, you know, it sounds as if you have got some horrible disease. You do – it feels like a horrible disease – (near to tears) – horrible – horrible . . .

As a result of her definition Mrs Roper saw information management as an extremely sensitive matter. She took the conscious decision to leave telling her daughters that Duchenne was hereditary and that they were potential carriers until the last minute:

> MRS ROPER: I always waited until the very last minute, I didn't want it put on their backs too early, it isn't fair I don't think . . .

For her daughter the news of potential carrier risk had come as a major blow. Her mother said:

> MRS ROPER: She's taken it hard, she went very introvert, she is talking more now, but yes, she does, she thinks no-one will have her . . . (referring to boyfriends)

Camilla, Mrs Roper's daughter, said:

> CAMILLA: Well at first, the first time I know I cried . . .

Like her mother, she found information management difficult. She was in her late teens, and convinced that she was unable to establish a stable sexual relationship because of her carrier status:

> CAMILLA: I prefer when I have a boyfriend to tell him – I don't know, when I say like – um – that my brother can't walk, they do treat me like as if, you know, 'is there any thing wrong with you?' That gets me mad that does . . . I don't know, it's just I'm not right then, I'm different . . .

Camilla, like her mother, defined her carrier status in terms of spoilt social identity. Risk for the Ropers was not something latent that only became manifest at critical junctures, it was an experience which stigmatised them and brought into question their whole personhood. Scambler and Hopkins (1986) suggest that 'felt' stigmas come from a 'special view of the world' and that many parents act as 'stigma coaches'. The Ropers' definitions were of felt stigmatisation, which, as Scambler and Hopkins (1986) argue, is more disruptive than cited incidents.

Mrs White reacted in a similar way. She became quite agitated when asked if she knew what her carrier risk figure was:

> MRS WHITE: First of all I was very upset the way it was put that it was the mother's fault, you know as if you've done a crime, and then when all the tests were shown and they couldn't actually prove – couldn't prove one way or the other . . . Well they have never told me – they have never said, 'cause actually, when I went there you know and they said about the whaternames and they said – 'it's always the mother's fault' and I said 'What did my tests show?' and he said: 'Actually they don't really show anything as far as that goes.' He said in other words that it's something that has happened in the family and that once we lost David it's – as far as they are concerned in this family it's more or less dead.

Things were defined very differently in the Poole family. Mrs Poole and Victoria were interviewed together. Mrs Poole had been given a carrier risk of 92 per cent and her daughter, Victoria, one of 27 per cent. Mrs Poole had never defined her carrier status as a significant issue. She had always talked to her daughter about it, and when Victoria was asked about her reaction to the news she said:

> VICTORIA: I expected it I think . . . I think I was semi-told before and – um – I think it was just, I semi-expected it, but it was confirmed, but I didn't feel sad in any way because I think I was prepared for it, it wasn't a shock or anything like that.

She was engaged at the time of the interview and her fiancé had accepted her, and her potential carrier status, without question:

VICTORIA: He doesn't want boys – (loud laugh) he's quite happy not to have boys, he loves girls, he likes girls.

Risk for them was not a significant issue in terms of their identity and was relegated to a low zone of relevance. It was the same for Clare Clarke, one of the other daughters in the sample:

CLARE: I don't really think about it. I used to have these tests when I was young, I don't really think about anything, I don't, I'll think about it when it happens . . . I don't look any different or feel any different.

. . .

Risk perception and social interaction

It was possible from the women's stories to understand something of the temporal nature of their definitions of carrier status. Significant events and social encounters during the life course were factors which influenced the women's definitions of their potentially stigmatising condition.

Jessica's story illustrated how negative definitions of carrier status could be modified in social interaction. Like Mrs Roper she had initially defined herself as discredited:

JESSICA: It did sort of affect me earlier on, as I said, you feel there are going to be problems, you feel that there is something – something wrong with me you know, at the time that's what you feel – you think 'Nobody will ever want to marry me because I am a carrier – I won't ever be able to have children.' It's a very big thing at the time.

This definition of felt stigmatisation was negotiated in subsequent social interaction. A few years later she met her future husband who did not define her potential carrier status negatively. He did not see it as spoiling her social identity, or their relationship:

JESSICA: Well with my husband he knew about it when we were courting and things like that, we discussed it but it didn't make that much difference, you know, we said that we would have children eventually but we weren't sort of wanting them straight away. There were a lot of things we wanted to do and still want to do – (nervous laugh) – he said he still wanted to marry me, it wasn't as major as a lot of things.

Jessica's definition of her carrier status and its relevance were significantly altered as the result of establishing a permanent sexual relationship that was not dependent on successful reproduction. Her 'felt' stigmatisation was modified and she redefined risk in terms of its latency. She and her husband relegated her carrier risk to a low zone of relevance.

Laura Abbott had a similar experience to Jessica: her initial definition had been of a 'spoiled' identity. She recounted how fearful her mother had been about carrier risks:

LAURA: I think really my mother had this fear then and as far as my mother was concerned . . . I think she just had this fear that the easiest thing is – 'Don't have children . . . oh it would be better for you not to have children, you don't know, it could happen and it's best not to.'

Mrs Abbott defined carrier risk as a problem for her daughter, and Laura's initial reaction was very negative:

LAURA: I was frightened, I was first of all because . . . I thought it didn't matter what children I had, boy or girl, I thought that they'd be automatically have something wrong with them see . . . when I first found out I thought: 'Oh my God' – you know I thought I wouldn't be able to have any and all this but then it was explained to me . . . I was worried first of all.

More information and acceptance in a permanent sexual relationship changed Laura's definition:

LAURA: When I got a bit older then it all started coming clearer to me . . . he's (her boyfriend) been great, he's accepted it like he said – 'I know it's a problem but you're still the same person, you know, it's no difference to me, as long as you are willing it's your decision.'

It has been seen that there were very different reactions to carrier risk. For some women there was 'felt' stigmatisation and a spoiling of their social identity throughout their life course. They defined themselves as discreditable, if not discredited, and experienced problems in information management. For other women, there was a recognition of the latency of risk. There were certain critical junctures when it became significant but for the rest of their lives it was relegated to a low zone of relevance. For some women their first critical episode lay at the beginning of courtship, for others it did not come until they were in a stable relationship and wanting to family build. Assessments of carrier status and risk are often portrayed as having a high degree of consistency throughout the life course. The evidence from this study would challenge that assumption: definitions of carrier status were part of a continuous process of definition and redefinition as the women constructed and negotiated their everyday reality.

Conclusion

All social scientists are aware that they need to pay attention to the issue of 'levels of measurement'. It is not often that the interpretation of levels of measurement, and the translation of one level into another, is a problematic issue for the social actors who are the subject-matter of research. In the case of genetic risk, however, it is especially pertinent. As has been seen, for women in this study, specialists in medical genetics had generated risk values for Duchenne expressed in percentage terms. Each woman, at any given time, had a medically defined carrier risk value and a reproductive risk value. The first is an estimate of the likelihood of carrying the defective gene. The second is an estimate of her chances of having an affected male or a carrier female in a particular pregnancy.

It is clear that the women who were interviewed in this study frequently engaged in tasks of translating the percentage figures into *ordinal* or *categorical* measurements. The relative delicacy of the percentage risk figures was transposed into more elementary categories. In the process the inherently probabilistic notion of 'risk' was turned into definitive, descriptive categories. The women could still employ the vocabulary of percentages or ratios, but in simplified format (such as '50:50') or could express risk in ordinal terms (as 'high' or 'low'). There is a demonstrable relationship for most of the women between the medically defined level of risk and the lay use of 'high' or 'low' measures. It is equally clear, however, that a great deal of information about risk is lost in that translation process. Further, for many of the women carrier risk and reproductive risk were expressed as categorical recipes for knowledge and action. Risk was replaced with definitive proscriptions and prescriptions. The probabilistic was expressed as a matter of certainty.

The delicacy of 'risk' values may be of less relevance for many women than the effects on their identity. The revelation of a carrier risk for a genetically transmitted disorder may be felt as threatening and discreditable. For many of the women, their carrier status was a potentially stigmatising one – although the stigma was latent for many families for much of the time.

The genetic risks and the potential threats to the women's identity were expressed and defined primarily in terms of reproductive risk. For them, reproduction was the point when the latent became manifest. Awareness of being 'at risk' was therefore related to critical junctures in the life course. There were periods of time when the majority of women did not define themselves as being 'at risk', nor did they experience impaired identity. For much of the time carrier risk could be relegated to a low zone of relevance.

Kessler (1989) notes that for decision-making information to be useful it needs to be 'transformed into personally meaningful units'. The study of women who were potential carriers of the defective Duchenne gene shows how important such transformations can be. The majority of the women, even if they had retained some notion of mathematical probability, had translated their risk liability into everyday recipes for reproductive action that could be incorporated readily into their personal stocks of knowledge.

References

Goffman, E. (1968) *Stigma: Notes on the Management of Spoiled Identity*. Harmondsworth: Penguin Books.

Kessler, S. (1989) Psychological aspects of genetic counseling: A critical review of the literature dealing with education and reproduction. *American Journal of Medical Genetics*, 34, 340–53.

Lippman-Hand, A. and Fraser, F.C. (1979) Genetic counseling – the postcounseling period: Parents' perceptions of uncertainty. *American Journal of Medical Genetics*, 4, 51–71.

Parsons, E.P. (1990) Living With Duchenne Muscular Dystrophy: Women's Understandings of Disability and Risk. Unpublished Ph.D. thesis, University of Wales.

Rhona, R.J. *et al.* (1991) *The Resource Implications and Service Outcomes of Genetic Services in the Context of DNA Probes*, Report from the Department of Public Health Medicine, Guy's and St Thomas's Hospitals.

Scambler, G. and Hopkins, A. (1986) Being epileptic: Coming to terms with stigma, *Sociology of Health and Illness*, 8, 26–43.

Schutz, A. (1946) The well-informed citizen: An essay on the social distribution of knowledge, *Social Research*, 13, 463–78.

PART TWO

Inequalities and patterning of health and illness

IT HAS LONG BEEN ARGUED in medical sociology that health can be seen as a property of both individuals and societies. For those who believe that there is 'no such thing as society', or focus only on the individual, the social patterning of health must present particular difficulties. As we have seen in Part One of the Reader, beliefs and behaviour surrounding health reflect both scientific ideas about disease causation, and individual and collective experiences in specific communities, influenced in the latter case by the contours of modernity as a whole. In this sense beliefs reflect the fact that health and illness are not simply properties of individuals unconnected with each other. Cultural motifs of morality, responsibility and causation, and the influence of social structures can be glimpsed through the study of people's responses to the challenges of poor health, or attempts to maintain good health. Even notions of fate and chance are powerfully shaped by the cultures in which they exist.

Likewise, when we turn from beliefs to more objective indicators of health, such as rates of mortality and morbidity, we can see consistent variations within and between societies. Why this should be has been the focus of much argument. Differences in material circumstance and resources are an obvious starting point. In recent years, however, there has been much debate about how patterns of health, and especially inequalities between social groups, have come to be the way they are, and how social and material influences shape this patterning over time. In modern societies where there is a significant degree of social mobility, health may play a part in the shaping of social structures, as those with better health move up the social ladder and those with poorer health move down. Biological factors at birth, and later educational and occupational achievement, will interact with health to produce complex pathways. Medical sociology has made a major contribution to understanding some of these processes and we have selected material from articles that reflect this body of work.

The first extract, by Berkman *et al.*, sets out a comprehensive framework for understanding the impact of social relationships on health, especially those of social networks and social integration. In developing this framework, Berkman *et al.*, draw on Durkheim's ideas concerning the role of social integration and social change, and on Bowlby's attachment theory which stresses the need for developing close bonds in infancy and in later periods of the lifecourse, for example through marriage. Berkman *et al.*'s framework for understanding the patterning of health, therefore, begins with macro influences concerning socio-economic factors, cultural and political factors and the nature of social change. It then moves to 'mezzo' level processes which deal with network characteristics and social interactions, through to micro psychosocial factors such as social support and self-esteem. This framework for understanding health patterning provides a means of locating much of the diverse body of work currently being carried out on its social determinants.

One of the most controversial aspects of the debate about social determinants of health concerns the relative importance of material factors. The second extract by Wilkinson tackles this issue head on. Wilkinson's argument is that, historically, improvements in income levels have been one of the major forces for change in the health of populations, seen especially in a reduction in mortality. However, Wilkinson argues that today in the developed world, data show that it is not levels of income as such that matter, but the degree of income *inequality*. In societies where the income gradient is relatively flat then health inequalities are likewise less marked. In societies where income differentials are steep then health inequalities are similarly wide. Social and psychological factors linked to deprivation, rather than the direct effects of material scarcity, are particularly important in societies that have gone through an 'epidemiological transition', from being dominated by infectious diseases to the widespread experience of degenerative ones such as cancer and heart disease.

In the third extract, Vågerö and Illsley also challenge what they take to be the simplistic explanations of health inequalities provided by authors such as those of the Black Report. In the view of Vågerö and Illsley, approaches to health inequalities that rely on an appeal to 'material factors' need to specify what is meant by 'material'. Too often, they argue, assumptions about what goes to make up 'material factors' in relation to social class are left unexamined, as is how these translate into health outcomes. In addition, Vågerö and Illsley tackle another influential approach to health patterning, but this time stemming from medical and epidemiological research – that of David Barker and his colleagues. In Barker's view, health is strongly influenced if not programmed at birth. Patterns of health in adult life can be traced back to circumstances *in utero* and thus to maternal health. Poor health at birth – indicated for example, by low birth weight – correlates strongly with health disorders in later life, such as heart disease. Vågerö and Illsley argue against a biologically deterministic view based on such observations, as well as on an oversimplified sociological perspective, in favour of a view that recognises interaction between biological and social factors in different pathways to health and illness across the lifecourse.

The next extract by Wadsworth spells out in more detail what such a 'lifecourse' view of health comprises. Biological 'capital' at birth may well set parameters for health, but it does not 'programme' the rest of life. In Wadsworth's view social influences not only shape health at birth, but also influence its unfolding across the lifecourse. Longitudinal or 'follow-up' studies provide a clear view of the role of historical and social circumstances in shaping the health of groups of people as they age. Wadsworth shows that the effects of particular historical circumstances – for example, food rationing and air pollution in post Second World War Britain – can be seen in cohorts as they enter middle and late life. In turn, other social factors, such as educational achievement, can be seen to contribute to social mobility and thus to improved health. As with the three extracts already outlined in this Part of the Reader, Wadsworth illustrates how a more developed sociological research agenda can overcome reductionist views of either a biological or materialist nature in the study of health inequalities. His review of an extensive research base illustrates just how far medical sociology has moved on in developing this critique of earlier, 'cross-sectional' approaches.

One of the most important dimensions of current approaches to the social patterning of health lies in the study of ethnicity. In the next extract by Nazroo, the various influences on health – biological, cultural or material – are considered through the study of ethnic differences in health. Here, too, though material factors are important in explaining the pattern of health between and within minority ethnic groups, their reduction to 'class differences' does not take the argument very far. Nazroo shows that other dimensions of social experience, for example that of racism, or particular geographical locations can have their own independent effects. The extract shows that an overemphasis on 'cultural differences' in health among minority ethnic groups, focusing on such issues as dietary preferences or uptake in health promotion, can disguise the root causes of health in wider social inequalities. Work on the specific 'risk factors' that adhere to particular conditions can therefore deflect attention from these wider dynamics. Nazroo argues, instead, for a perspective that explores the relationships between culture, context and class and their influences on health – among minority ethnic groups, and in other populations.

The final extract in this Part tackles another major area of health inequalities research, namely that of gender. It is the case, of course, that some differences in health between men and women stem from inbuilt biological differences. However, it has long been held that as far as the influences of gender rather than sex differences on health are concerned, a consistent pattern exists where men have higher mortality rates than women, and women have higher morbidity rates than men. In other words, men die early but women get sick. Different explanations in terms of gender roles and relations have been advanced to help explain these apparent differences. However, in the extract included here from Macintyre *at al.*, when empirical data on a range of health conditions and symptoms are examined the situation becomes less clear-cut. Indeed, on some measures of morbidity higher rates in men are evident. One consistent finding reported by Macintyre *et al.*, though, is that higher rates of psychological distress in women are found in both of their data sets, focusing attention on gender inequalities in that particular area of concern.

Chapter 7

Lisa F. Berkman, Thomas Glass, Ian Brissette and Teresa E. Seeman

FROM SOCIAL INTEGRATION TO HEALTH
Durkheim in the new millennium

From *Social Science and Medicine,* 51, 2000:843–57 (Elsevier)

Introduction

OVER THE LAST 20 YEARS there have been dozens of articles and now books on issues related to social networks and social support. It is now widely recognized that social relationships and affiliation have powerful effects on physical and mental health for a number of reasons. However, at this juncture, almost 25 years after Cassel (1976) and Cobb (1976) suggested that networks might be critical and 20 years after first empirical studies illustrated effects on mortality (Berkman and Syme, 1979; Blazer, 1982: House *et al.*, 1982), it is worth evaluating this field with a critical and theoretical eye to see how we might move forward in the coming decade.

When investigators write about the impact of social relationships on health, many terms are used loosely and interchangeably including social networks, social support, social ties and social integration. The aim of this paper is to clarify these terms using a single framework. We will discuss: (1) theoretical orientations from diverse disciplines which we believe are fundamental to advancing research in this area; (2) a set of definitions accompanied by major assessment tools; and (3) an overarching model which integrates multilevel phenomena.

Theoretical orientations

There are several sets of theories that form the bedrock for the empirical investigation of social relationships and their influence on health. The earliest theories came from sociologists such as Émile Durkheim, as well as from psychoanalysts such as John Bowlby, a British psychoanalyst, who first formulated attachment theory. A major wave of conceptual development also came from anthropologists including Elizabeth Bott, John Barnes, and Clyde Mitchell as well as quantitative sociologists such as Claude Fischer, Edward Laumann, Barry Wellman and Peter Marsden who, along with others, have developed social network analysis. This eclectic mix of theoretical approaches coupled with the contributions of epidemiologists, Cassel and Cobb, form the foundation of research on social ties and health.

Émile Durkheim: social integration, alienation and anomie

Durkheim's contribution to the study of the relationship between society and health is immeasurable. Perhaps most important is the contribution he has made to the understanding of how social integration and cohesion influence mortality. Durkheim's primary aim was to explain how individual pathology was a function of social dynamics. In light of recent attention to "upstream" determinants of health (Link and Phelan, 1995), Durkheim's work reemerges with great relevance today.

In *Suicide*, Durkheim challenges us to understand how the patterning of one of the most psychological, intimate, and, on the surface, individual acts rests not upon psychological foundations but upon the patterning of "social facts." In *Suicide*, he shows how "social facts" can be used to explain changing patterns of aggregate tendency toward suicide. Durkheim starts his work with the observations that countries and other geographic units and social groups have very stable rates of suicide year after year. Once armed with the irrefutable social patterning of suicide, Durkheim goes on to theorize that the underlying reason for suicide relates, for the most part, to the level of social integration of the group.

Anomic suicide is of particular relevance. This type of suicide defined by Durkheim, is related to large-scale societal crises of an economic or political nature often occurring during times of rapid social change and turbulence. In these situations, social control and norms are weakened (e.g. the regulatory function of integration). Such rapid change serves to deregulate values, beliefs and general norms and fails to rein in or guide individual aspirations (Turner and Noh, 1983). Today crises in Russia and Eastern Europe might be classical situations leading to anomic suicide. Durkheim illustrates suicide is triggered by the erosion of society's capacity for integration. Durkheim's theories related not only to the patterning of suicide but easily extend to other major outcomes ranging from violence and homicides to cardiovascular disease.

John Bowlby: the architect of attachment theory

John Bowlby, one of the most important psychiatrists in the twentieth century (Storr, 1991), proposed theories suggesting that the environment, especially in early childhood, played a critical role in the genesis of neurosis. He believed that the separation of infants from their mothers was unhealthy and saw loss and separation as key issues for psychotherapy. Bowlby proposed that there is a universal human need to form close affectional bonds (Fonagy, 1996). Between 1964 and 1979, he wrote *Attachment* (Bowlby, 1969), *Separation* (Bowlby, 1973) and *Loss* (Bowlby, 1980) in which he lays out his theory of attachment and how it relates to both childhood and adult development.

Attachment theory contends that the attached figure, most often but not necessarily the mother, creates a secure base from which an infant or toddler can explore and venture forth. Bowlby argued with many psychoanalysts that attachment is a "primary motivational system" (e.g. not secondary to feeding or warmth) (Bowlby, 1969). "Secure attachment," he wrote, "provides an external ring of psychological protection which maintains the child's metabolism in a stable state, similar to internal homeostasis mechanism of blood pressure and temperature control" (Bowlby, 1969). These intimate bonds, created in childhood, form a secure base for solid attachment in adulthood and provide prototypes for later social relations (Fonagy, 1996). Secure attachment as opposed to avoidant, ambivalent, or disorganized attachment, allows the maintenance of affectional bonds and security in a larger system.

In adulthood, Bowlby saw marriage as the adult equivalent of attachment between infant and mother during childhood. If secure, marriage would provide a solid base from which to work and explore the world enmeshed in a "protective shell in times of need" (Holmes, 1993, p. 81).

The strength of Bowlby's theory lies in its articulation of an individual's need for secure attachment for its own sake, for the love and reliability it provides, and for its own "safe haven." Primary attachment promotes a sense of security and self-esteem that ultimately provides the basis on which the individual will form lasting, secure and loving relationships in adult life. The psychosocial environment in infancy and childhood paves the way for successful development that continues through adulthood. For Bowlby, the capacity for intimacy in adult life is not given, but is instead the result of complex dynamic forces involving attachment, loss, and reattachment. Early childhood emotional development is becoming widely recognized as a critical period of development not only for emotional and cognitive development but for health as well.

Social network theory: a new way of looking at social structure and community

During the mid-1950s, a number of British anthropologists found it increasingly difficult to understand the behavior of either individuals or groups on the basis of traditional categories such as kin groups, tribes, or villages. Barnes (1954) and Bott (1957) developed the concept of "social networks" to analyze ties that cut across traditional kinship, residential, and class groups to explain behaviors they observed such as access to jobs, political activity or marital roles. The development of social network models provided a way to view the structural properties of relationships among people with no constraints or expectations that these relationships occurred only among bounded groups defined "a priori."

Network analysis "focuses on the characteristic patterns of ties between actors in a social system rather than on characteristics of the individual actors themselves and uses these descriptions to study how these social structures constrain network members' behavior" (Hall and Wellman, 1985, p. 26). Network analysis focuses on the structure and composition of the network, and the contents or specific resources which flow through those networks. Social network analysis includes analyses of both egocentric networks with an individual at the center as well as entire networks of networks at the level of communities or workplaces.

The strength of social network theory rests on the testable assumption that the social structure of the network itself is largely responsible for determining individual behavior and attitudes by shaping the flow of resources which determine access to opportunities and constraints on behavior. Network theorists share many of the central assumptions of Durkheim and the structure functionalists. The central similarity is the view that the structural arrangement of social institutions shapes the resources available to the individual and hence that person's behavioral and emotional responses. Another contribution of network theory is the observation, initially made by Barnes and Bott, that the structure of networks may not always conform to preconceived notions of what constitutes "community" defined on the basis of geographic or kinship criteria. Thus, Wellman argues that the essence of community is its social structure, not its spatial structure (Wellman, 1988, p. 86). By assessing actual ties between network members, one can empirically test whether community exists and whether that community is defined on the basis of neighborhood, kinship, friendship, institutional affiliation, or other characteristics.

A conceptual model linking social networks to health: an overview

Throughout the 1970s and 1980s a series of studies appeared consistently showing that the lack of social ties or social networks predicted mortality from almost every cause of death (Cohen, 1988; House et al., 1988; Berkman, 1995). These studies most often captured numbers of close friends and relatives, marital status, and affiliation or membership in religious and voluntary associations. These measures were conceptualized in any number of ways as assessments of social networks or ties, social connectedness, integration, activity or embeddedness. Whatever they were named, they uniformly defined embeddedness or integration as involvement with ties spanning the range from intimate to extended. Most studies included measures of both "strong" and "weak" ties (Granovetter, 1973) (weak ties involve contacts with extended non-intimate ties who he found to be central to occupational mobility).

Although the power of these measures to predict health outcomes is indisputable, the interpretation of what the measures actually measure has been open to much debate. Hall and Wellman (1985) have appropriately commented that much of the work in social epidemiology has used the term social networks metaphorically since rarely have investigators conformed to more standard assessments used in network analysis. For instance, the existence of "weak ties" is not assessed directly but inferred from membership in voluntary and religious organizations. This criticism has been duly noted and several calls have gone out to develop a second generation of network measures (Berkman, 1986: House et al., 1988; Antonucci and Jackson, 1990) . . .

In order to have a comprehensive framework in which to explain these phenomena, we must move "upstream" and return to a more Durkheimian orientation to network structure and social context. Indeed, it is critical to maintain a view of social networks as lodged within those larger social and cultural contexts which shape the structure of networks. In fact, some of the most interesting work in the field today relates social affiliation to social status and social and economic inequality (Kawachi *et al.*, 1997; Wilkinson, 1999). Only then can we fully consider the multiple pathways by which social networks might so profoundly influence health outcomes.

Figure 7.1 presents a conceptual model of how social networks impact health. We envision a cascading causal process beginning with the macro-social to psycho-biological processes that are dynamically linked together to form the processes by which social integration affects health. As suggested above, we start by embedding social networks in a larger social and cultural context in which upstream forces are seen to condition network structure. Serious consideration of the larger macro-social context in which networks form and are sustained has been lacking in all but a small number of studies and is almost completely absent in studies of social network influences on health.

We then move downstream to understand the influences network structure and function have on social and interpersonal behavior. We argue that networks operate at the behavioral level through four primary pathways: (1) provision of social support; (2) social influence; (3) on social engagement and attachment; and (4) access to resources and material goods. These micro-psychosocial and behavioral processes, we argue, then influence even more proximate pathways to health status including (1) direct physiological stress responses, (2) psychological states and traits including self-esteem, self-efficacy, security, (3) health-damaging behaviors such as tobacco consumption or high-risk sexual activity, health promoting behavior such as appropriate health service utilization, medical adherence, and exercise, and finally to (4) exposure to infectious disease agents such as HIV, other sexually transmitted diseases (STDs) or tuberculosis.

By embedding social networks in this larger chain of causation, we can integrate "upstream" macro-social forces related to the political economy with social networks as mediating structures between the largest and smallest scale social forms. Thus, we can examine how labor markets, economic pressures and organizational relations influence the structure of networks (Luxton, 1980: Belle, 1982; Bodemann, 1988; Krause and Borawshi-Clark, 1995). We can examine specifically the role of culture, rapid social change, industrialization and urbanization on the structure of networks. Perhaps the most critical findings to date in this area relevant to social epidemiology are whether "community" is dead or dying in post-industrial American society. In fact, this question has been central to many social network analysts. See Wellman (1988) for an excellent discussion of this question.

The assessment of social networks

Next we come to identifying critical domains of social networks. Social networks might be defined as the web of social relationships that surround an individual and

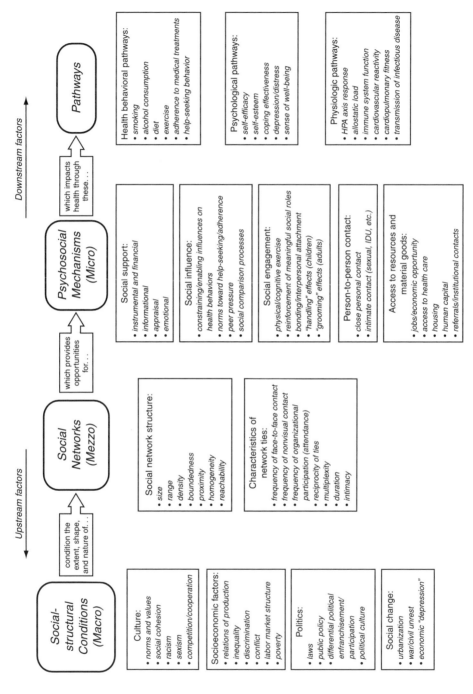

Figure 7.1 Network characterics.

the characteristics of those ties (Mitchell, 1969; Laumann, 1973; Fischer *et al.*, 1977; Fischer, 1982). Burt has defined network models as describing "the structure of one or more networks of relations within a system of actors" (Burt, 1982, p. 20). Thus, while we mainly have considered in this chapter egocentric networks (networks surrounding an individual) network analysis can easily examine networks of networks. Network characteristics (see Fig. 7.1) cover:

* *range* or *size* (number of network members);
* *density* (the extent to which the members are connected to each other);
* *boundedness* (the degree to which they are defined on the basis of traditional group structures such as kin, work, neighborhood);
* *homogeneity* (the extent to which individuals are similar to each other in a network).

Related to network structure, characteristics of individual ties include:

* *frequency of contact* (number of face-to-face contacts and/or contacts by phone or mail):
* *multiplexity* (the number of types of transactions or support flowing through a set of ties);
* *duration* (the length of time an individual knows another);
* *reciprocity* (the extent to which exchanges or transactions actions are even or reciprocal).

A number of researchers have developed measures to estimate network size and density. These measures may be particularly useful if they are employed in conjunction with standard social integration measures. This would enable one to test of whether social integration measures remain associated with positive health outcomes after controlling for network characteristics like the density of the participants' personal networks. . . .

Downstream social and behavioral pathways

Social support

Moving downstream, we now come to a discussion of the mediating pathways by which networks might influence health status. Most obviously the structure of network ties influences health via the provision of many kinds of support. This framework immediately acknowledges that *not all* ties are supportive and that there is variation in the type, frequency, intensity, and extent of support provided. For example, some ties provide several types of support while other ties are specialized and provide only one type. Social support is typically divided into subtypes which include emotional, instrumental, appraisal and informational support (Weiss, 1974). Emotional support is related to the amoung of "love and caring, sympathy and understanding and/or esteem or value available from others" (Thoits, 1995). Emotional support is most often provided by a confidant or intimate other, although less intimate ties can provide such support under circumscribed conditions.

Instrumental support refers to help, aid or assistance with tangible needs such as getting groceries, getting to appointments, phoning, cooking, cleaning or paying bills. House (1981) refers to instrumental support as aid in kind, money or labor. Appraisal support, often defined as the third type of support, relates to help in decision-making, giving appropriate feedback, or help deciding which course of action to take. Informational support is related to the provision of advice or informational in the service of particular needs. Emotional, appraisal and informational support are often difficult to disaggregate and have various other definitions (e.g. self-esteem support).

Perhaps even deeper than support are the ways in which social relationships provide a basis for intimacy and attachment. Intimacy and attachment have meaning not only for relationships that we traditionally think of as intimate (e.g. between partners, parents and children) but for more extended ties. For instance, when relationships are solid at a community level, individuals feel strong bonds and attachment to places (e.g. neighborhood) and organizations (e.g. voluntary and religious).

Social influence

Networks may influence health via several other pathways. One pathway that is often ignored is based on *social influence*. Marsden asserts that the "proximity of two actors in social networks is associated with the occurrence of interpersonal influence between the actors" (Marsden and Friedkin, 1994, p. 3). As the term is used, influence need be neither associated with face-to-face contact, nor does it require deliberate or conscious attempts to modify behavior (p. 4). Marsden refers to work by Erickson (1988) suggesting that under conditions of ambiguity "people obtain normative guidance by comparing their attitudes with those of a reference group of similar others. Attitudes are confirmed and reinforced when they are shared with the comparison group but altered when they are discrepant" (Marsden and Friedkin, 1994, p. 5). Shared norms around health behaviors (e.g. alcohol, and cigarette consumption, health care utilization, treatment adherence or dietary patterns) might be powerful sources of social influence with direct consequences for the behaviors of network members. These processes of mutual influence might occur quite apart from the provision of social support taking place within the network concurrently. For instance, cigarette smoking by peers is among the best predictors of smoking for adolescents (Landrine *et al.*, 1994). The social influence which extends from the network's values and norms constitutes an important and under-appreciated pathway through which networks impact health.

Social engagement

A third and more difficult to define pathway by which networks may influence health status is by promoting social participation and social engagement. Participation and engagement result from the enactment of potential ties in real life activity. Getting together with friends, attending social functions, participating in occupational or social roles, group recreation, church attendance — these are all instances of social engagement. Thus, through opportunities for engagement, social networks define and reinforce meaningful social roles including parental, familial, occupational, and community roles, which in turn, provides a sense of value, belonging, and attachment. Those roles that provide each individual with a coherent and consistent sense of identity are only possible because of the network context which provides the theater in which role performance takes place.

In addition, network participation provides opportunities for companionship and sociability. We, as well as others (Rook, 1990b), argue that these behaviors and attitudes are not the result of the provision of support per se, but are the consequence of participation in a meaningful social context in and of itself. We hypothesize that part of the reason measures of social integration or "connectedness" have been such powerful predictors of mortality for long periods of follow-up is that these ties give meaning to an individual's life by virtue of enabling him or her to participate in it fully, to be obligated (in fact, often to be the provider of support) and to feel attached to one's community.

Person-to-person contact

Another behavioral pathway by which networks influence disease is by restricting or promoting exposure to infectious disease agents. In this regard the methodological links between epidemiology and networks are striking. What is perhaps most remarkable is that the same network characteristics that can be health-promoting can at the same time be health-damaging if they serve as vectors for the spread of infectious disease. Efforts to link mathematical modeling applying network approaches to epidemiology are in their infancy and have started to appear over the last 10 years (Kloudahl, 1985; Laumann et al., 1989; Morris et al., 1991; Morris, 1994; Friedman, 1995).

The contribution of social network analysis to the modeling of disease transmission is the understanding that in many, if not most cases, disease transmission is not spread randomly throughout a population. Social network analysis is well suited to the development of models in which exposure between individuals is not random but rather is based on geographic location, sociodemographic characteristics (age, race, gender) or other important characteristics of the individual such as socioeconomic position, occupation, sexual-orientation (Laumann et al., 1989). Furthermore, because social network analysis focuses on characteristics of the network rather than on characteristics of the individual, it is ideally suited to the study of diffusion of transmissible diseases through populations via bridging ties between networks, or uncovering characteristics of ego-centered networks that promote the spread of disease.

Access to material resources

Surprisingly little research has sought to examine differential access to material goods, resources and services as a mechanism through which social networks might operate. This, in our view, is unfortunate given the work of sociologists showing that social networks operate by regulating an individual's access to life-opportunities by virtue of the extent to which networks overlap with other networks. In this way networks operate to provide access or to restrict opportunities in much the same way the social status works. Perhaps the most important among studies exploring this tie is Granovetter's classic study of the power of "weak ties" that, on the one hand lack intimacy, but on the other hand facilitate the diffusion of influence and information, and provide opportunities for mobility (Granovetter, 1973). . . .

The social environment in adulthood

. . . The impact of social attachments made in early years on health outcomes remains an intriguing and understudied area; however, the vast body of epidemio-logic evidence produced to date indicates that it is adult social circumstances that are linked to poor health outcomes. Debates in which we pitch continuity (the effect of early development/environment) against discontinuity (the effect of recent events) are not likely to be fruitful since both have consequences for health out-comes. Furthermore, we know that large scale social upheavals and transitions profoundly disrupt patterns of social organizations established in earlier life. Geographical relocation related to urbanization, housing policy, or employment opportunities, large scale social change or depression as seen in Russia or Eastern Europe, job stress and corporate policies that are not "family" friendly represent environmental challenges that tear at the fabric of social networks which in turn have deleterious consequences on health. . . .

Conclusion

Our aim in this review was to integrate some classical theoretical work in sociology, anthropology and psychiatry with the empirical research currently underway on social networks, social integration and social support. Rather than review the vast amount of work on health outcomes which is the subject of several excellent recent papers, we hoped to develop a conceptual framework that would guide work in the future.

With the development of this framework, we are struck by two issues of profound importance. The first is the "upstream" question of identifying those conditions which influence the development and structure of social networks. Such questions have been the substantive focus of much of social network research especially in relationship to urbanization, social stratification and culture change. Yet little of this work becomes integrated with health issues in a way that might guide us in the development of policies or intervention to improve the health of the public. Recent work relating social cohesion to economic inequality begins to help us decipher the complex interrelationships between these social experiences (Kawachi et al., 1997; Wilkinson, 1999) but much more multilevel work is needed in this area. Of particular interest, would be more cross-cultural work comparing countries with different values regarding social relationships, community, sense of obligation. The same might be true to specific areas within countries or specific cultural or ethnic groups with clearly defined values.

The second major issue relates to the "downstream" question. Many investigators have assumed that networks influence health via social support functions. Our framework makes clear that this is but one pathway linking networks to health outcomes. Furthermore, the work on conflicts and stress points out that not only are not all relationships positive in valence (Rook, 1990a) but that some of the most powerful impacts on health that social relationships may have are through acts of abuse, violence, and trauma. Fully elucidating these downstream experiences and how they are linked to health via which biological mechanisms remains a major challenge in the field.

References

Antonucci, T. C., and Jackson, J. S. (1990). The role of reciprocity in social support. In B. R. Sarason, I. G. Sarason, and G. R. Pierce, *Social support: an interactional view* (pp. 173–198). New York: John Wiley.

Barnes, J. A. (1954). Class and committees in a Norwegian island parish. *Human Relations*, 7, 39–58.

Belle, D. E. (1982). The impact of poverty on social networks and supports. *Marriage and the Family Rev.*, 5, 89–103.

Berkman, L. (1986). Social networks, support and health: Taking the next step forward. *AJE*, 123(4), 559–562.

Berkman, L. (1995). The role of social relations in health promotion. *Psychosom. Med.*, 57, 245–254.

Berkman, L., and Syme, S. (1979). Social networks, host resistance, and mortality: A nine-year follow-up of Alameda County residents. *AJE*, 109, 186–204.

Blazer, D. (1982). Social support and mortality in an elderly community population. *AJE*, 115, 684–694.

Bodemann, Y. M. (1988). Relations of product and class rule: the basis of patron/clientage. In B. Wellman, and S. D. Berkowitz. *Social structures: a network approach*. Cambridge, UK: Cambridge University Press.

Bott, E. (1957). *Family and social network*. London: Tavistock Press.

Bowlby, J. (1969). *Attachment and loss*. London: Hogarth Press.

Bowlby, J. (1973). *Attachment and loss*. London: Hogarth Press.

Bowlby, J. (1980). *Attachment and loss*. London: Hogarth Press.

Burt, R. S. (1982). *Toward a structural theory of action*. New York: Academic Press.

Cassel, J. (1976). The contribution of the social environment to host resistance. *AJE*, 104, 107–123.

Cobb, S. (1976). Social support as a moderator of life stress. *Psych. Med.*, 38, 300–314.

Cohen, S. (1988). Psychosocial models of the role of social support in the etiology of physical disease. *Health Psychology*, 7, 269–297.

Erickson, B. H. (1988). The relational basis of attitudes. In B. Wellman and S. D. Berkowitz. *Social structures: a network approach* (pp. 99–121). New York: Cambridge University Press.

Fischer, C. S. (1982). *To dwell among friends: personal networks in town and city*. Chicago: University of Chicago Press.

Fischer, C. S., Jackson, R. M., Steuve, C. A., Gerson, K., Jones, L. M., and Baldassare, M. (1977). *Networks and places*. New York: Free Press.

Fonagy, P. (1996). Patterns of attachment, interpersonal relationships and health. In D. Blane, E. Brunner, and R. Wilkinson. *Health and social organization: towards health policy for the twenty-first century* (pp. 125–151). New York/London: Routledge.

Friedman, S. R. (1995). Promising social network results and suggestions for a research agenda. *NIDA Research Monograph*, 151, 196–215.

Granovetter, M. (1973). The strength of weak ties. *Am. J. Sociol.*, 78, 1360–1380.

Hall, A., and Wellman, B. (1985). Social networks and social support. In S. Cohen, and S. L. Syme, *Social support and health* (pp. 23–41). Orlando: Academic Press.

Holmes, J. (1993). *John Bowlby and the attachment theory*. London: Routledge.

House, J. S. (1981). *Work, stress and social support*. Reading, MA: Addison Wesley.

House, J., Robbins, C., and Metzner, H. (1982). The association of social relationships and activities with mortality: Prospective evidence from the Tecumsch Community Health Study. *AJE*, 116, 123–140.

House, J. S., Landis, K. R., and Umberson, D. (1988). Social relationships and health. *Science*, 241, 540–545.

Kawachi, I., Kennedy, B., Lochner, K., and Prothrow-Stith, D. (1997). Social capital, income inequality, and mortality. *Am. J. Public Health*, 87, 1491–1498.

Kloudahl, A. S. (1985). Social networks and the spread of infectious diseases: the AIDS example. *Soc. Sci. Med.*, 21, 1203–1216.

Krause, N., and Borawshi-Clark, E. (1995). Social class differences in social support among older adults. *Gerontologist*, 35, 498–508.

Landrine, H., Richardson, J. K., Klondoff, E. A., and Flay, B. (1994). Cultural diversity in the predictors of adolescent cigarette smoking: the relative influence of peers. *J. Behav. Med.*, 17, 331–336.

Laumann, E. O. (1973). *Bonds of pluralism*. New York: Wiley.

Laumann, E. O., Gagnon, J. H., Michaels, S., Michael, R. T., and Coleman, J. S. (1989). Monitoring the AIDS epidemic in the U.S.: a network approach. *Science*, 244, 1186–1189.

Link, B., and Phelan, J. (1995). Social conditions as fundamental causes of disease. *Journal of Health and Social Behavior, extra issue*, 80–94.

Luxton, M. (1980). *More than a labor of love*. Toronto: Women's Press.

Marsden. P. V., and Friedkin, N. E. (1994). Network studies of social influence. In S. Wasserman and J. Galaskiewicz. *Advances in social network analysis: research in the social and behavioral sciences* (pp. 3–25). Thousand Oaks, CA: Sage.

Mitchell, J. C. (1969). *The concept and use of social networks*. Manchester, UK: Manchester University Press.

Morris, M. (1994). Epidemiology and social networks: modeling structured diffusion. In S. Wasserman and J. Galaskiewicz. *Advances in social network analysis: research in the social and behavioral sciences* (pp. 26–52). Thousand Oaks, CA: Sage.

Morris, P. L., Robinson, R. G., Raphael, B., and Bishop, D. (1991). The relationship between the perception of social support and post-stroke depression in hospitalized patients. *Psychiatry*, 54, 306–316.

Rook, K. (1990a). Stressful aspects of older adults' social relationships: current theory and research. In A. P. Stephens, J. H. Crowther, S. E. Hobfoll, and D. L. Tennenbaum. *Stress and coping in later-life families* (pp. 173–192). New York: Hemisphere.

Rook, K. (1990b). Social relationships as a source of companionship: implications for older adults' psychological well being. In B. R. Sarason, T. G. Sarason, and G. R. Pierce. *Social support: an interactional view* (pp. 221–250). New York: Wiley.

Storr, A. (1991). *"John Bowlby", Monks Roll*. London: Royal College of Physicians.

Thoits. P. (1983). Multiple identities and psychological well-being: a reformulation of the social isolation hypothesis. *American Sociological Review*, 48, 174–187.

Thoits, P. (1995). Stress, coping, and social support processes: where are we? What next? *Journal of Health and Social Behavior*, extra issue, 53–79.

Turner. R., and Noh. S. (1983). Class and psychological vulnerability among women: The significance of social support and personal control. *J. Health Soc. Behav.*, 24, 2–15.

Weiss, R. S. (1974). The provisions of social relationships. In Z. Rubin. *Doing unto others*. Englewood Cliffs. NJ: Prentice Hall.

Wellman, B. (1988). The community questions re-evaluated. In M. P. Smith. *Power, community and the city* (pp. 81–107). New Brunswick, NJ: Transaction.

Wilkinson, R. G. (1999). Income inequality, social cohesion and health: clarifying the theory. A reply to Muntaner and Lynch. *International Journal of Health Services*, 29(3), 525–543.

Chapter 8

Richard G. Wilkinson

THE EPIDEMIOLOGICAL TRANSITION
From material scarcity to social disadvantage?

From *Daedalus* (Journal of the American Academy of Arts and Sciences), 123(4) 1994: 61–77

Introduction

HEALTH AND WEALTH HAVE ALWAYS appeared to be closely related. But within that relationship there is an important historical discontinuity which not only tells us about the changing determinants of health, but also marks a fundamental change in the limiting constraints on the quality of life in modern societies. Mortality rates in the developed world are no longer related to per capita economic growth, but are related instead to the scale of income inequality in each society. This represents a transition from the primacy of material constraints to social constraints as the limiting condition on the quality of human life.[1]

The implications of this change are not confined to health. Health can be viewed as a general indicator of welfare and the effects of social and economic change. If health is influenced more by income distribution than by economic growth, then the same is likely to be true of other aspects of human welfare. Furthermore, if increases in the quality of life now depend primarily on improving the social fabric of society rather than on general rises in prosperity, then we must ask whether further *undifferentiated* economic growth is worth the environmental risks.

Life expectancy and Gross National Product per capita

Rising living standards were the basis of the historical decline of mortality in the developed world. While it is possible to argue the relative historical contributions of better nutrition, sewers, clean water supplies, improved housing, and eventually, immunization to the long decline in mortality rates in the developed world, there can be no doubt that the enabling and sustaining power of economic growth was behind them all.

Evidence of the broad relationship between economic growth and increasing life expectancy can be found not only in the history of the developed countries, but also in the Third World today. Figure 8.1 shows the relationship between Gross National Product per capita (GNPpc) and life expectancy at birth in rich and poor countries in 1970 and in 1990.

Although it is clear that life expectancy rises steeply with increased GNPpc among the poorer countries, the data in Figure 8.1 also suggests that the relationship between GNPpc and mortality peters out in the developed world. Apparently, there is some minimum level of income (around $5,000 per capita in 1990) above which the absolute standard of living ceases to have much impact on health.

Putting income on a log scale, as in Figure 8.2, it appears more accurate to think in terms of radically diminishing health returns to increasing income. However, as the curve in Figure 8.2 indicates, as countries get richer even equally large *proportional* changes in incomes produce diminishing absolute returns in life expectancy.

Figure 8.3 shows that between 1970 and 1990 there was very little correspondence between changes in the Gross Domestic Product per capita (GDPpc) and life

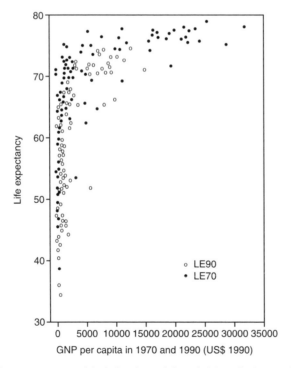

Figure 8.1 Life expectancy at birth (male and female) in relation to GNP per capita, 1970 and 1990

Source: World Bank, World Tables 1992

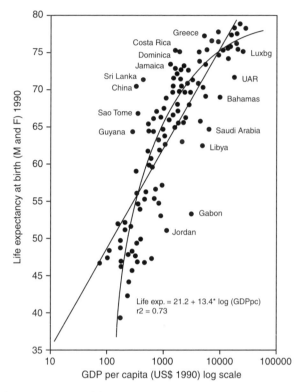

Figure 8.2 Life expectancy and GDP per capita, 1990

Source: World Bank, World Tables 1992

expectancy in the developed countries. In this example, GDPpc is converted at purchasing power parities to provide more accurate comparisons of the real material standard of living.

Figures 8.1, 8.2, and 8.3 show that regardless of whether one looks at Organization for Economic Cooperation and Development (OECD) countries at a single point in time or over several decades, there is no strong relationship between income and health among the developed countries.[2] People in one country can be twice as well-off on average as those in another without benefit to their mortality rates. As Figure 8.3 shows, one country's economy can grow twice as fast as another's for twenty years without having an effect on life expectancy.

Approaching limits of human life expectancy?

One obvious explanation for the virtual disappearance of a relationship between GNPpc and life expectancy is that it reflects the approaching limits of human life expectancy. However, this fails to explain why the rate of improvement in life expectancy is not slowing down where longevity is already high. Life expectancy continues to increase at 2 to 2.5 years per decade among the rich countries, as it has during most of this century (wartime excluded). In addition, it appears that in

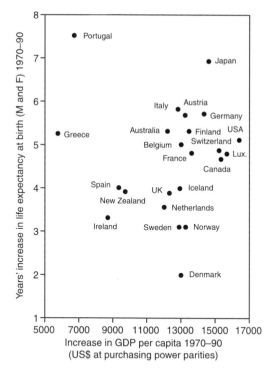

Figure 8.3 Increases in life expectancy related to increases in GDP per capita in OECD countries, 1970–90

Source: OECD National Accounts (Paris 1992) and World Bank, World Tables 1992

several developed countries the fastest improvements are coming from those sections of the population where life expectancy is highest. For these reasons, we must assume that the leveling of the curve of rising life expectancy with GNPpc (shown in Figure 8.1) indicates the declining health benefits of further increases in the standard of living in the developed world.

The epidemiological transition

The "epidemiological transition" is the shift in the main causes of death—from infectious diseases to degenerative cardiovascular diseases and cancers. It marks a fundamental change in the main determinants of health and seems to indicate the point in economic development at which the vast majority of the population gained reliable access to the basic material necessities of life.

The impact of medical science is not reflected in the epidemiological transition. In fact, the transition would have happened (and largely did happen) without it. The great infectious diseases of the nineteenth and early twentieth centuries dwindled to a fraction of what they had been long before immunization or effective medical treatment became available. Strongly associated with poverty, in the past as in the

Third World today, the decline of the great infections reflected improved living standards and conditions.

The effect of economic development is also illustrated by the way in which the epidemiological transition saw the so-called "diseases of affluence" transformed into the diseases of the poor. No longer primarily "businessmen's diseases," coronary heart disease, stroke, and obesity have all become more common among the less well-off.[3] That this transition was associated with the attainment of a certain level of material wealth is shown by the associated reversal in the social gradient in smoking and in the consumption of refined foods such as white bread and sugar. In all but a few countries the evidence on cardiovascular diseases is fragmentary, but it seems likely that many developed countries went through the same transition and experienced the same change in the class distribution of these diseases, although at different times.

The change in the social class distribution of obesity is much more widely recognized. Throughout most of history obesity was a condition which affected only the privileged, and in many cultures was a status symbol—embodied proof of prosperity. The rich were fat and the poor were thin. This remained true in the developed world well into the present century when rising living standards began to enable the poor to be fat, and is still true in some parts of the Third World.

In Britain the change appears to have been accelerated by nutritional changes during World War II.[4] The Chief Medical Officer in the British Ministry of Education commented on the increasing incidence of obesity in schoolchildren in his annual reports of 1956–1957 and 1960–1961.[5] As if to confirm Pierre Bourdieu's thesis of the importance of the desire to express social distinction in aesthetic judgments, as soon as the poor became able to be fat, obesity ceased to be a status symbol.[6]

A further indication of the widespread attainment of adequate material standards for the populations of developed countries comes from trends in the proportion of babies with birth weights below 2,500 grams. Although perinatal and infant mortality rates have continued to decline rapidly, since the 1950s in England and Wales there has been no further marked decline in the proportion of low birth weight babies: between 6 and 7 percent of babies have weighed less than 2,500 grams ever since.[7] This proportion of low birth weight babies seems to represent a residual core which is unaffected by improvements in average prosperity.

Thus, it seems that in the later stages of industrial development countries go through a health climacteric after which the health of the vast majority of the population is no longer substantially affected by the absolute material standard of living.

Income distribution

After the epidemiological transition, health remains closely associated with deprivation, but the relationship now is with relative rather than absolute deprivation. Health within developed countries continues to show a clear gradient with measures

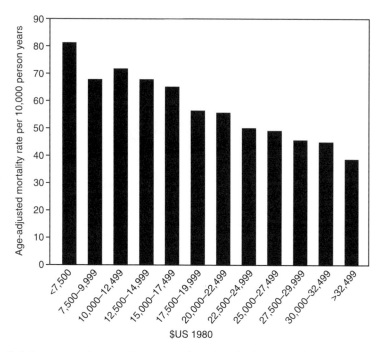

Figure 8.4 Income and mortality among three hundred thousand white US men

Source: MRFIT data from G. Davey Smith, J. D. Neaton and J. Stamler, *Income differentials in mortality risk among 305,099 white men* (1994)

of socioeconomic status.[8] Figure 8.4 shows how death rates vary according to income group in the United States. Evidence from Britain, covering most of the present century, suggests that the social class differences in death rates have increased or decreased as the proportion of the population living in *relative* poverty has increased or decreased.[9]

There is, however, a marked contrast between the well-ordered relationship between socioeconomic status and health within a country (as shown in Figure 8.4) and the lack of any clear relationship between socioeconomic status and health between countries (as shown in Figures 8.1 and 8.3). This contrast is extremely important. Given that the points in Figures 8.1 and 8.3 are whole nations, the fact that they do not even begin to line up like those for income groups within the United States cannot be chalked up to sampling error or the like. Something quite different is going on. Health is affected by differences in *relative* income (differences between groups of people within the same society), not by the absolute level of average incomes for each society as a whole. This is confirmed by the surprisingly strong relationship between income distribution and mortality rates in developed countries.[10]

The countries with the longest life expectancy are not the wealthiest but those with the smallest spread of incomes and the smallest proportion of the population in relative poverty. Using a standard measure of income distribution, Figure 8.5 shows that in 1970 the countries with the smallest income differences were also

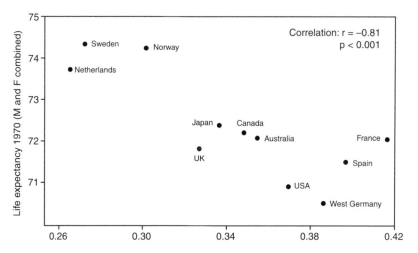

Figure 8.5 Life expectancy and income distribution in OECD countries

Sources: Sawyer (1976), Table 11; World Bank (1983) (Reproduced from R. G. Wilkinson 1986)

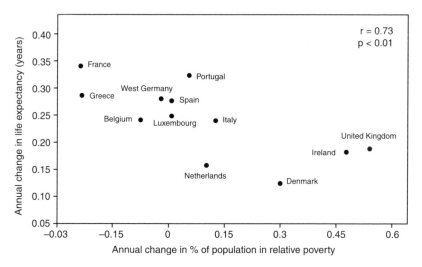

Figure 8.6 The annual rate of change of life expectancy in twelve EC countries 1975–1985 (with the rate of change in the percentage of the population in relative poverty)

Source: M. O'Higgins and S. P. Jenkins "Poverty in the EC", in R. Teekens and B. M. S. van Praag (eds) *Analyzing poverty in the European Community*, Luxembourg: EURO-STAT, 1990

the countries where average life expectancy was longest. Since then the rate of growth of average life expectancy has been closely related to changes in income distribution. Figure 8.6 shows that in the twelve member states of the European Community (EC), average life expectancy between 1975 and 1985 has grown fastest in those countries where relative poverty decreased fastest (or increased slowest). . . . .

Psychosocial interpretation

The fact that health seems to be influenced more by differences in income than by average level of income suggests that cognitive processes of social comparison are involved. The importance of relative income to health suggests that psychosocial factors related to deprivation and disadvantage are involved. That is to say, it is less a matter of the immediate physical effects of inferior material conditions than of the social meanings attached to those conditions and how people feel about their circumstances and about themselves.

The need to develop a psychosocial understanding of the impact of material differences on health is indicated by three other aspects of the relationship between health and socioeconomic status. (1) The socioeconomic gradient in health does not distinguish merely between the poor and the rest of society, but affects every rung of the social ladder. Thus, people who own houses and have two cars are healthier than those who rent houses and have one car,[11] administrative civil servants are healthier than executives,[12] and people in the highest income group are healthier than those only slightly less well-off (see Figure 8.4). (2) Despite rising real incomes, which have undoubtedly reduced the incidence during the second half of this century of absolute material deprivation, the mortality disadvantage of blue collar workers and their families appears to have increased in several countries. (3) In Britain, now one of the poorer developed countries, absolute living standards among the *poorest* 20 percent of the population are remarkably high. In 1992, some 72 percent had central heating, almost all had televisions and refrigerators, 72 percent had telephones, and almost 60 percent had video-cassette recorders.[13]

The socioeconomic gradient in mortality (Figure 8.4) could only be attributed to the direct effects of material factors if it is assumed that increasing standards of comfort higher up the income scale have as great an effect as material improvements further down the scale. However, if this were so, there would be a closer association between changes in GDPpc and mortality than is shown in Figure 8.3. . . .

Some wider implications of income distribution

If the psychological consequences of wider differences in income are powerful enough to exert a major influence on death rates, it is implausible that they do not also have other social implications. Although no one doubts that poorer areas suffer disproportionately from a wide range of social problems (including drugs, crime, violence, poor educational performance, and ill health), proving causality is not easy. . . .

If the relationship between health and income distribution is evidence of a powerful psychosocial effect of relative income, could it be said that each individual's desire for more income is more a desire to improve his relative standing in society than it is a desire for a higher level of material consumption? Such a desire would not be well served by general increases in prosperity, which leave relativities essentially unchanged. Indeed, it would mean that it is not legitimate to sum individual desires for more income into an aggregate societal demand for economic growth.

Beyond that, however, the psychosocial effect of relative income suggests that the quality of life is better served by reducing relative poverty and narrowing income distribution than it is by further haphazard economic growth. Because health is sensitive to the quantitative as well as qualitative aspects of both material and social change, it could be claimed that it is a better guide to the quality of life than is any mix of economic indicators. Economic indices can only reflect change by reducing qualitative change to quantitative increase, thereby ignoring the social dimension of life. In this context, the fact that in the developed world the predominant position of material factors as determinants of health has given way to social factors has profound implications.

At a time when the environmental impact of economic development is causing increasing concern, it is particularly important to know whether its advantages outweigh its disadvantages. In the developed world the answer to this question can no longer be taken for granted.[14] Clearly there are substantial reasons for thinking we need to be more selective about the direction and form which economic growth takes. We continue to think of it as desirable largely because of the short-term discomfort of recession and the need to keep unemployment down and profits up. This is not to suggest that it is time for the industrialized world to bring to a close its two hundred year involvement with economic development. But, rather than seeing innovation as serving the single goal of increasing per capita incomes, we should see it as a means of resolving growing environmental and social problems.

The environment cannot be safeguarded without major technical innovation, just as relative deprivation cannot be diminished except through income growth among the least well-off. Somehow growth has to be put into a new harness. Fortunately, there is increasing evidence that, in addition to the contribution it makes to welfare, income redistribution is also beneficial to productivity and growth. Among OECD countries, those with the fastest increases in productivity tend to be those with narrower income differences.[15] Among seventy rich and poor countries, investment was higher where income differences were narrower. In addition, eight of the rapidly growing East Asian economies narrowed their income differences between 1960 and 1980,[16] and Japan has the narrowest income differentials in the developed world.

This suggests that the pursuit of narrower income differentials may be complementary to growth. Social environments which are less divisive, less undermining of self-confidence, less productive of social antagonism, and which put greater resources into developing skills and abilities, may well turn out to be more innovative and better able to adapt to the environmental problems we face. The health data suggests that the quality of the social fabric, rather than increases in average wealth, may now be the primary determinant of the real subjective quality of human life. With this knowledge let us create high quality social environments where we will be less dependent on the destructive quick fix of indiscriminate economic growth.

Notes

1   This change was also marked by the decline of mortality from infectious diseases which had been associated with absolute poverty and by the reversal of the social class distribution of heart disease when the so-called "diseases of affluence" became the diseases of the relatively poor in affluent societies.

2   Richard G. Wilkinson, "The Impact of Income Inequality on Life Expectancy," in Stephen Platt, H. Thomas, S. Scott, and G. Williams, eds, *Locating Health: Sociological and Historical Explorations* (Aldershot: Avebury, 1993).

3   Michael G. Marmot, Abe Adelstein, Nicola Robinson, and Geoffrey Rose, "Changing Social Class Distribution of Heart Disease," *British Medical Journal* II (1978): 1109–12. Steve Wing, "Social Inequalities in the Decline of Coronary Mortality," *American Journal of Public Health* 78 (1988): 1415–16. Aaron Antonovsky, "Social Class and the Major Cardiovascular Diseases," *Journal of Chronic Diseases* 21 (1968): 65–106.

4   British Medical Association, *Report of the Committee on Nutrition* (London: BMA, 1950).

5   Ministry of Education, *The Health of the School Child, 1956–7 and 1960–1*, Report of the Chief Medical Officer (London: HMSO, 1958 and 1962).

6   Pierre Bourdieu, *Distinction: A Social Critique of the Judgement of Taste* (London: Routledge, 1984).

7   Alison Macfarlane and Miranda Mugford, *Birth Counts: Statistics of Pregnancy and Childbirth* (London: HMSO, 1984). Chris Power, "National Trends in Birthweight and Future Adult Disease," *British Medical Journal* (forthcoming).

8   John Fox, ed., *Health Inequalities in European Countries* (London: Gower, 1989).

9   Richard G. Wilkinson, "Class Mortality Differentials, Income Distribution and Trends in Poverty 1921–1981," *Journal of Social Policy* 18(3) (1989): 307–35.

10   Richard G. Wilkinson, "Income Distribution and Life Expectancy," *British Medical Journal* (1992): 165–68, 304. Irene Wennemo, "Infant Mortality, Public Policy and Inequality—A Comparison of 18 Industrialised Countries, 1950–85," *Sociology of Health and Illness* 15 (1993): 429–46.

11   Peter Goldblatt, ed., 1971–81 *Longitudinal Study: Mortality and Social Organisation*, OPCS Series LS 6 (London: HMSO, 1990).

12   George Davey Smith, Martin J. Shipley, and Geoffrey Rose, "Magnitude and Causes of Socioeconomic Differentials in Mortality: Further Evidence from the Whitehall Study," *Journal of Epidemiology and Community Health* 44 (1990): 265–70.

13   Department of Social Security, *Households Below Average Income, 1979–1990/1* (London: HMSO, 1993).

14   The various attempts to adjust GNPpc to produce better measures of economic welfare have also cast doubt on the benefits of undifferentiated economic growth. In Britain and the United States economic welfare has been declining despite increases in GNPpc. Herman E. Daley and John B. Cobb, *For the Common Good* (London: Green Print, 1990). Tim Jackson and Nic Marks, *U.K. Index of Sustainable Economic Welfare* (Sweden: Stockholm Environment Institute in cooperation with the New Economic Foundation, 1994).

15   Andrew Glyn and David Miliband, eds, *Paying for Inequality* (London: Rivers Oram, 1994).

16   The World Bank, *The East Asian Miracle* (Oxford: Oxford University Press, 1993).

Chapter 9

Denny Vågerö and Raymond Illsley

EXPLAINING HEALTH INEQUALITIES: BEYOND BLACK AND BARKER
A discussion of some issues emerging in the decade following the Black Report

From *European Sociological Review*, 11, 1995: 219–41

Introduction

ANY POLICY DISCUSSION of how to improve public health in general or how to influence the social distribution of health will be strongly influenced by prevailing ideas about what generates health and health inequalities. The Working Group on Inequalities in Health, commissioned by the British government in 1977, chaired by Sir Douglas Black and including Peter Townsend, delivered its report in 1980. Despite a hostile reception from the British government of the time, it has had a big impact on thought, if not on policy, inside and outside Britain. Most academic writing on health inequalities has subsequently tended to adopt its agenda, questions, concepts, and definitions, and to debate its conclusions. It has been influential not only in the way it responds to the problems but more importantly in the way it poses the questions.

Inevitably, however, changing trends in health and illness, advances in aetiological understanding, and developments in scientific and social thinking, have begun to modify or challenge the Black Report's approach and findings. Most recently a new focus for debate has emerged out of the research of David Barker and his co-workers, who, in more than 30 scientific articles between 1986 and 1992, developed their theory of 'biological programming' of adult health. They regard such programming during foetal and infant life as the most important determinant of social differences in adult health. The theory has evoked an argument across the editorials of the *British Medical Journal* (*BMJ*) and the *Lancet* and produced powerful critiques in scientific journals. As in the Black Report, it is poverty, but this time in foetal or infant life, that is seen as the main cause of health inequalities. Its early timing in the life course has very different policy implications.

The discussion of the Black Report over more than a decade has resulted in something of a stalemate, which on balance has not moved beyond the questions and explanations provided by the report. A further sociological explanation of health inequalities is needed. The new challenge represented by Barker's work makes such explanation more necessary than before. In this paper we examine both Black and Barker, and we suggest some elements of an alternative and more sociological explanation.

The four explanations of the Black Report

Why does social class continue to exercise so significant an influence on health?' was the question posed by the Black Report (Townsend and Davidson, 1982:112). This was certainly an important question. Do the explanations provided by the Black Report answer it? Four 'theoretical explanations' were formulated, which have since come to dominate thinking, arguments, and reviews of the field (for instance Blane, 1985; Bloor *et al.*, 1987; Morris, 1990; Davey Smith *et al.*, 1990; Joshi and Macran, 1991; Blane *et al.*, 1993; Davey Smith *et al.*, 1994). In the terminology of the Black Report they were: (1) artefactual explanations (2) theories of natural or social selection (3) materialist or structuralist explanations, and (4) cultural/ behavioural explanations.

We shall pay little attention to the artefactual explanation, because it is almost universally agreed in the academic literature that social class differences in health are real, a property of social relations in all societies, and not the by-product of measurement errors or errors of definition. The nature of artefactual effects was aptly summed up by Bloor and colleagues: 'the measurement process may be concealing as well as generating inequalities of health' (Bloor *et al.*, 1987). This does not deny, but rather reinforces, the importance of measurement and of issues of definition. Measurement problems may affect the size and pattern of differences but do not cast doubt on their existence.

We therefore concentrate on the second, third, and fourth types of explanation. We are in particular interested in the rationale for, or hidden assumptions behind, the choice of these explanatory categories. The report contains no general discussion, or review of previous research which would logically result in this typology of theoretical explanations. It is introduced without discussion (Townsend and Davidson, 1982: 112).

A distinction that obscures

The distinction between 'materialist or structural' and 'cultural/behavioural' explanations (the third and fourth types of explanation) is introduced and then upheld with some passion. What is its particular relevance here? It has been likened (Strong, 1990) to the Marxist distinction between the 'economic base' and the 'ideological superstructure'. In that theory, the first ultimately determines the second. The authors of the Black Report similarly chose to believe in the primacy of 'the material': 'it is in some form or forms of the "materialist" approach that the best answer lies' (Townsend and Davidson, 1982: 122).

This best answer is not helpful, because the meaning of 'material' or 'materialist' is not clear. Sometimes it refers to commonly accepted components of material circumstance (e.g. nutrition and housing). But 'levels of self-fulfilment and job satisfaction, and physical or mental strain', are also seen as 'dimensions of material inequality' (p. 117). Are all aspects of work to be classified as material, and are all explanations that involve work 'materialist'? That seems to be the unspoken assumption. Similarly 'deprivation in its various forms', such as 'in education and the upbringing of children', is refered to as material (p. 134).

Use of the term material (or materialist) to describe very different situations (or explanations) inevitably brings confusion. It would be clearer to distinguish *poverty, working conditions, education,* and *upbringing* as different types of explanation in their own right. It is not just that the term 'materialist' is undefined—it is also used so broadly that it includes very different levels of explanation: the biological and the social; the direct and the contextual; the micro, the macro, and the historical. Can 'the material' really have primacy on all these levels?

Behind the all-inclusive term 'material' there often seems to be a narrower latent connotation in particular when we move down to describe the situations of individuals and families. In Peter Townsend's introduction to the Pelican edition of the Black Report this connotation emerges clearly. 'Material deprivation' is the key concept (Townsend and Davidson, 1982: 21).

In the light of these and other comments, Black's 'material', as related to health risks, should perhaps best be interpreted to mean poverty and material (physical) deprivation wherever and whenever they occur and whatever form they may take. It is therefore not the full range of material circumstances or material inequality that is in focus, but rather the lower end of their distribution, affecting those who are poorest and most deprived.

The 'material' factors are also, one must assume, to be seen as structural factors, since structural/materialist explanations are always grouped together as a single type of explanation. This is therefore one of the assumptions hidden in the typology of explanations. Is it justified to equate material with structural; and to equate cultural with individual behaviour? This seems to be the implication of the Black Report's division of explanations into structural/materialist and cultural/behavioural. We believe that two different distinctions are mixed here. Could cultural factors, perhaps, also be seen as structural? And material as individual? . . .

Cultural explanations, in our opinion, are no more and no less individual, no more and no less structural, than the so-called materialist explanations. Individual characteristics can influence whether or not you become a member of a certain sub-culture as well as whether or not you get a certain job and income. Cultural constraints can be as forceful and imposing on the individual as can material constraints.

Material circumstances (such as frequent episodes of unemployment), could interact with cultural traits (such as social disregard for the non-employed), so that the combined effect of both increases the risk of disease (for example ischaemic heart disease, depression, or suicide). If such interaction is common, which is very likely, it becomes clear that theoretical work on health inequalities must be directed towards integrating, within the same theory, 'cultural' and 'material' factors, and the relationship of each to individual behaviour, rather than seeing them as so many alternative explanations.

A mode of explanation different from the four provided by the Black Report, and based on integrating individual choice and material or cultural constraint in the same theoretical framework, has been suggested, for instance by LeGrand (1985: 18). Similarly, Haan, Kaplan, and Syme propose an alternative approach to those of the Black Report, which embraces the notion of demand and control *vis à vis* one's life situation and its interaction with individual behaviour (1989: 103–5). Having cultural resources (such as education) or material resources (such as income) represents being under fewer constraints. On the whole we would expect good health to be more common in life situations over which a person can exercise more control and in which he or she suffers fewer constraints, constraints could be material or cultural, none being, a priori, more important than the other.

Thus, explanations could well be classified as structural or individual, with the former focusing on constraints, which exist independently of, or prior to, the individual, and the latter on individual characteristics, such as personal behaviour, or individual choice, such as whether to smoke, or on genetic features, such as susceptibility to cancer. These types of explanation are not mutually exclusive. If one relies on structural explanations, which we prefer, it does not follow that one accepts material deprivation as the best explanation . . .

Poverty and health

Being poor relatively speaking

Poverty in adult life has been seen as the most likely cause of health differentials among adults not only by the Black Report but also by subsequent commentators, such as Blane in discussing the Black Report in 1985, as well as by Morris (1990) and Davey Smith *et al.* (1990) in their reviews of the literature in the first decade following the report. The last review however, rightly we think, points to the scarcity of research actually addressing that issue directly. Perhaps one reason for this negligence is the strong conviction of the Black Report that we already know that it is poverty that causes the higher morbidity and mortality of the lower classes? A closer look into the health inequalities debate also reveals that concepts such as poverty, deprivation, or material inequality are often used with little precision.

Morris wrote: 'It followed that poverty and deprivation were the principal causes of premature death and lesser life expectancy of the lowest classes' (Morris, 1990: 491). Davey Smith *et al.*, while being more cautious, nevertheless assumed that 'on the basis of the general tendency towards wider material inequality, the 1991 decennial supplement may be expected to show further widening of social class differences in mortality' (Davey Smith *et al.*, 1990: 376).

The views of the latter, publishing their review in the *BMJ*, were reinforced and taken further by an editorial in the same issue called 'Poverty and Health in the 1990s' (Smith, 1990). Here it was concluded that 'as the poverty gap in Britain has widened so have differences in health become more striking'. The *BMJ* editorial defined poverty as living on less than half the average income. It claimed that 'as the gap between the rich and poor in Britain has widened half of our children now live in poverty'. It is not surprising then that the public health strategy should become one of 'a determined effort to reverse the progressive impoverishment of the poorest people in Britain'. Had there been a 'progressive impoverishment'? What was the nature of this? Was this phenomenon the cause of health differences between social classes? Of their persistence over the decades? Of a potential future widening?

The income statistics (mis)quoted by the *BMJ* above refer to the 1980s (DHSS, 1990). It is generally accepted that income inequality did increase in that period. It is however quite likely that this represented a reversal of a long-term trend towards a gradual reduction in income inequality from the 1920s onwards (Kuznets, 1955; Atkinson, 1993). The Black Report's conclusions were based on mortality trends up to 1972, that is, across the period of decreasing income inequality. The same period also saw a decrease in the prevalence of absolute poverty (in Britain). Later work on mortality suggested a trend of widening mortality differences in the whole 1931–71 period (Koskinen, 1985) as well as in the 1971–80 period (Marmot and McDowell, 1986. Thus empirical evidence relates to the period before the Thatcher era.

It is difficult to reconcile the long-term trend towards income equality and greater wealth with the thesis of a gradual widening of class death rates during the 1931–80 period, if this widening is explained by progressive impoverishment. Progressive impoverishment is a term, we think, which leads most people to think that the proportion of people living in conditions of absolute poverty has increased steadily. If social class has exercised such an important influence on health and survival during all of this century it seems unlikely that this could be due to 'progressive impoverishment'.

The aetiological significance of absolute vs. relative poverty

The distinction between absolute and relative poverty is a crucial one in discussing causes of differential health. It should be obvious that if we are interested in the impact of poverty on the human body, it matters a great deal whether we talk about absolute or relative poverty. The distinction can be exemplified by reference to Rowntree and Townsend. Seebohm Rowntree (1901) defined poverty as having an income which was insufficient to obtain 'the minimum necessities of merely physical efficiency'. Townsend (1979) defines poverty as 'the lack of resources to obtain the types of diet, participate in the activities and have the living conditions and amenities which are customary, or at least widely encouraged or approved, in the society to which they belong.' What is customary or widely encouraged is obviously different from the minimum necessities for physical efficiency.

Their aetiological significance is very different. Poverty, in its absolute meaning, is known to cause and to contribute to many diseases, and specific disease mechanisms are also known. If poverty, in its relative meaning, endangers health it is via different pathways and with different disease outcomes. McKeown, for instance, attributed the steady fall in mortality between 1841 and 1971 largely to increased wealth and reduced (absolute) poverty (McKeown, 1989). Poverty is still a major killer, mainly, but not exclusively, in less developed countries. This is a question of absolute poverty, working through poor nutrition, decreased physical and mental resistance, retarded growth, and impaired immune competence. Relative poverty, in contrast, need not carry any of those risks, if the level of resources of those living in relative poverty is sufficiently high. The relatively poor of the developed world are in general much better off than the absolutely poor of developing countries.

Sen, in a very readable essay, took a critical look at various relativistic definitions of poverty. He concluded (1984: 332) that 'neither the various relativist views, nor seeing poverty as "an issue in inequality", nor using the so called "policy-definition", can therefore serve as an adequate theoretical basis for conceptualising poverty. There is, I would argue, an irreducible absolutist core in the idea of poverty.' The idea that poverty could be measured by indicators derived from half the average income (as in the *BMJ* editorial quoted above) or, worse, from the level of supplementary income benefits (as in the Black Report: 116) was questioned: 'The tendency of many of these measures to look plausible in situations of growth, ignoring the possibility of contraction, betrays the timing of birth of these measures in the balmy sixties, when the only possible direction seemed forward' (Sen, 1984: 330). Thus, when income falls across much of the social spectrum (as in many countries in Eastern Europe today), the number of relatively poor could well stay the same, despite rising levels of absolute poverty and of poverty-related disease and death.

Sen's conceptualization of poverty focuses on the 'capability' to meet absolute needs of food, shelter, and social esteem. Satisfaction of these needs might well require command of greater material resources today than in earlier periods, and thus there is inevitably a relative element to absolute poverty. However, these resources are always related to the capability to meet certain specific needs. They are not formulated as having a certain income relative to that of the average, or as being poor, relatively speaking. Not being able to meet such absolute needs is clearly also what matters in terms of a number of traditional poverty-linked diseases. Disease and death linked to this kind of poverty have gradually decreased in Western Europe.

Sen's view of poverty as having 'an irreducible absolutist core' is theoretically clear, but it is less clear how to define such poverty in specific terms, for instance in terms of the necessary food intake. Nutritional studies do not permit a precise estimate of what is needed since there is a rather broad range within which physical efficiency declines with falling intake of calories. Further, current medical knowledge is insufficient for specifying the nutrient requirements for the specific stages of individual development, from foetal life to old age. In spite of these ambiguities it is clear to us that the distinction between absolute and relative poverty is real and important. We need not share Sen's preference for one against the other. The point is they are conceptually different—and different in their consequences for the lives and health of individuals. . . .

The Barker hypothesis

Poverty and disadvantage in the past

The present levels of absolute poverty, in most countries in Europe, are unlikely to cause present geographical or social class differences in health and mortality, then perhaps they are the delayed result of the poverty of the past? This seems, intuitively, to be a reasonable proposition. Poverty, in an absolute sense, plagued large parts of Europe earlier in the century. Even if such poverty is now less frequent, the poverty experienced previously might have had long-term effects which are now being manifested in the adult population, particularly among older age groups.

We explore this possibility in some detail below. The theory that the poverty of the past is a major cause of ill health today has been embraced as 'one of Thomas Kuhn's paradigmatic shifts' by the editor of the *British Medical Journal* (Robinson, 1992). It is best described as a powerful new medical theory, influencing a number of medical subdisciplines, such as cardiology, paediatrics, and diabetology. We will try to examine some of its assumptions and implications and suggest alternative explanations.

There are two main routes, one biological, the other sociological, whereby such a latent or long-term influence of past poverty might affect present health. The biological alternative has been developed and advocated most strongly by David Barker, professor of epidemiology in Southampton, and his co-workers, in a long series of papers published after 1986. They claim that the effects of past poverty are mediated through its influence on maternal constitution and health and therefore also through the foetal and infant environment of babies. They postulate that an early biological imprint on the human body occurs in the foetal and infant period. Low birth-weight and growth retardation of the foetus signal such an influence. Blood pressure and lipid metabolism, for instance, are thought to be set *in utero* or in infancy, having been negatively influenced by sub-optimal growth. This is described as 'biological programming', a key concept in this theory. Low birth-weight will therefore indicate an elevated risk for many important causes of death, such as respiratory disease, diabetes, ischaemic heart disease, stroke, and cancer of the breast, ovary, and prostate. Adult disease in general is seen as having foetal origins (Barker *et al.*, 1989; Barker, 1990; 1991; 1992; Barker *et al.*, 1993). The claims of this new set of ideas are obviously far-reaching.

Foetal and infant origins of health inequalities?

In his 1991 paper on 'The Foetal and Infant Origins of Inequalities in Health in Britain' Barker proposes that both geographical and social differences in adult health are the result of biological programming *in utero*. It is perhaps surprising that Barker should intervene in a more than ten-year-long discussion, following the Black Report, with a paper that simply ignores most of the writings of that period, with the exception of the Black Report itself. He proposes that poor maternal physique and health, due either to past poverty, or to poverty during pregnancy, or both, creates an unfavourable intra-uterine environment, which then influences foetal growth and development and ultimately adult health. In addition, although it seems less important in this theory, experience during infancy contributes to the so-called biological programming, perhaps through the influence of breast-feeding. Thus there is a way by which 'biological programming' could influence the social and regional distribution of health. Let us look at ischaemic heart disease as a major cause of death and one for which Barker's empirical evidence is most explicit. Our main argument, however, applies equally to all the disease outcomes.

The direct empirical evidence presented in support of the foetal origins of cardiovascular death relates birth-weight data to adult mortality for the same individuals. There are two such studies by Barker, Winter *et al.* (1989) and Barker, Osmond *et al.* (1993). The suggested linking mechanism is stated as follows: 'These findings suggest that processes linked to growth and acting in prenatal or early postnatal life strongly influence risk of ischemic heart disease'. And 'surveys undertaken during the early years of the century described in detail the social conditions which led to poor maternal and infant health and in consequence, reduced life expectancy among the children who survived into adult life' (Barker, 1991:67).

In his 1993 study, linking birth-weight to mortality, he wrote: 'We suggest that maternal undernutrition, by constraining fetal growth, may programme cardiovascular disease' (Barker *et al.*, 1993: 425).

The surveys referred to by Barker as undertaken during the early years of the century probably include the one by Seebohm Rowntree, published 1901, where poverty was defined as having insufficient means to obtain 'the minimum necessities of merely physical efficiency'. It would seem very likely, against the background of these quotations and their implicit meaning, that Barker is talking about poverty in its absolute sense, i.e. about women deprived of the physical resources to provide a normal functioning of the intra-uterine environment and to support normal growth of the foetus, and later of the infant. Being poor, relatively speaking, would hardly seem to be enough to create such a condition.

But this is not at all clear in Barker's writing. Indeed, Barker himself never makes the distinction between absolute and relative poverty. The claim that there is a linear trend (Barker *et al.*, 1989; Barker *et al.*, 1993), between birth-weight and the most common cause of death, would imply that it is relative poverty that matters. An effect of absolute poverty would be easier to reconcile with a non-linear relation, where the effect was limited to those in the lowest birth-weight groups. Therefore, there seems to be a discrepancy between the proposed linear relationship and the interpretation that poverty in its absolute sense is what matters. The conclusion in Barker's 1991 paper is that social and regional differences in Britain have, and will continue to have, foetal or infant origins. But how can a variety of social conditions, only some of which can be characterized by absolute poverty or maternal undernutrition, give rise to 'biological programming' of the foetus?

Critical assessments of Barker's work

Barker's theory has been sharply criticized primarily on methodological grounds. The methodological critique is summarized in two papers by Elford *et al.* (1991; 1992). The critique relates not only to the relationship on which we focus in this paper, namely birth-weight and adult mortality, especially heart-disease mortality, but relates to the whole field of hypotheses, results, and conjectures triggered by, or propagated from, the Barker group's research. Elford *et al.* (1992: 841), in reviewing 29 such studies, concluded that conventional criteria for causality, such as specificity of causal relations, consistency across studies, and independence from confounding factors, were not met.

Of particular importance is the last of these three. To draw the conclusion that an observed association between a factor measured early in life (birth-weight) and a health outcome very late in life (death) is a causal one, without controlling for the effects of any events during the life course whatsoever would seem to qualify as a textbook example of confounding. This methodological observation has been made by many critics (Ben-Shlomo and Davey Smith, 1991). A more theoretical critique can also be formulated. The theme of the latter is the following: 'continued social disadvantage' may give rise to low birth-weight, as well as to adult ischaemic heart disease, without any necessary causal connection between the latter two. . . .

It should be clear that the potential for confounding from such 'continuity in social disadvantage' is particularly great if the purpose is not to explain adult health in general, but to explain social class or regional differences in adult health, as Barker indeed attempted in his 1991 paper, quoted above. . . .

Conclusion

In December 1993 Sir Douglas Black, writing in the *BMJ* about the Black Report, embraced Barker's theory, seeing it as support for the original work by him and his colleagues (Black, 1993: 1631). There is a certain logic in that, since Barker in his earlier work focused on poverty and maternal undernutrition as being those social conditions which gave rise to disease and early death, although the proposed mechanism of biological programming was unconventional and without precedent in the Black Report. Poverty was indeed the preferred explanation in the Black Report. The maintenance of social-class mortality differences over this century, when income and material resources have improved dramatically in absolute terms, and probably become more equal in relative terms, suggests to us that we must look beyond explanations based on absolute or relative poverty. A more systematic study of how health development and social achievement become linked over an individual's life course, or in the historical experience of a social class, is both empirically feasible and, we believe, theoretically rewarding. We suggest that the hypothesis of the co-evolution of health and social achievement is a viable alternative to both Black and Barker.

References

Anonymous (1992): 'Heart Disease: In the Beginning' (editorial), *Lancet*, 339: 1386–7.

Arber S. (1990): 'Opening the "Black" Box: Understanding Inequalities in Women's Health', in Abbot P., Payne G. (eds) *New Directions in the Sociology of Health*, Brighton: Falmer Press.

Atkinson A.B. (1993): *What is Happening to the Distribution of Income in the UK?* STICERD, Welfare State Programme discussion paper no. 87, London: London School of Economics and Political Science.

Baker D., Illsley R., Vågerö D. (1993): 'Today or in the Past? The Origins of Ischemic Heart Disease', *Journal of Public Health Medicine*, 15: 243–8.

Barker D. (1989): 'Rise and Fall of Western Diseases', *Nature*, 338: 371–2.

—— (1990): 'The Fetal and Infant Origins of Adult Disease: The Womb may be more Important than the Home', Editorial, *British Medical Journal*, 301: 1111.

— (1991): 'The Foetal and Infant Origins of Inequalities in Health in Britain', *Journal of Public Health Medicine*, 13: 64–8.

— (1992) (ed.): *The Fetal and Infant Origins of Adult Disease*, London: BMJ Publications.

—, Winter P. D., Osmond C., Margetts B., Simmonds S. J. (1989): 'Weight in Infancy and Death from Ischemic Heart Disease', *Lancet* 1989: ii: 577–80.

—, Osmond C., Law C. (1989): 'The Intra-Uterine and Early Postnatal Origins of Cardiovascular Disease and Chronic Bronchitis', *Journal of Epidemiology and Community Health*, 43: 237–40.

—, —, Simmonds S., Wield G. (1993): 'The Relations of Small Head Circumference and Thinness at Birth to Death from Cardiovascular Disease in Adult Life', *British Medical Journal*, 306: 422–6.

—, Gluckman P., Godfrey K., Harding J., Owens J., Robinson J. (1993): 'Fetal Nutrition and Cardio-vascular Disease in Adult Life', *Lancet*, 341:938–41.

Ben-Shlomo Y., Davey Smith G. (1991): 'Deprivation in Infancy or in Adult Life: Which is more Important for Mortality Risk?', *Lancet*, 337: 530–4.

Black Report (1980): *Inequalities in Health: Report of a Research Working Party*, London: Department of Health and Social Services.

— (1993): 'Deprivation and Health', *British Medical Journal*, 307: 1630–1.

Blane D. (1985): 'An Assessment of the Black Report's Explanation of Health Inequalities', *Sociology of Health and Illness*, 7: 423–45.

Blane D., Davey Smith G., Bartley M. (1993): 'Social Selection: What does it Contribute to Social Class Differences in Health', *Sociology of Health and Illness*, 15: 2–15.

Blaxter M. (1990), *Health and Lifestyle*, London: Tavistock/Routledge.

Bloor M., Samphier M., Prior L. (1987) 'Artefact Explanations of Inequalities in Health: An Assessment of the Evidence', *Sociology of Health and Illness*, 9: 231–64.

Carstairs V., Morris R. (1989): 'Deprivation and Health', *British Medical Journal*, 299: 1462.

Davey Smith G., Bartley M., Blane D. (1990): 'The Black Report on Socio-Economic Inequalities in Health 10 Years on', *British Medical Journal*, 301: 373–7.

—, Blane D., Bartley M. (1994): 'Explanations for Socio-Economic Differentials in Mortality: Evidence from Britain and Elsewhere', *European Journal of Public Health*, 4: 131–44.

DHSS (1990): *Households below Average Income: A Statistical Analysis 1981–1987*, London: DHSS.

Elford J., Whincup P., Shaper A. (1991): 'Early Life Experience and Adult Cardiovascular Disease: Longitudinal Studies and Case-Control Studies', *International Journal of Epidemiology*, 20: 833–44.

—, Shaper A., Whincup P. (1992): 'Early Life Experience and Cardiovascular Disease: Ecological Studies', *Journal of Epidemiology and Community Health*, 46: 1–11.

Haan M. N., Kaplan G. A., Syme S. L. (1989): 'Socio-Economic Status and Health: Old Observations and New Thoughts', in Bunker J. P., Gomby D. S., Kehrer B. H. (eds), *Pathways to Health: The Role of Social Factors*, Menlo Park, Calif.: The Henry Kaiser Family Foundation.

Harvard University, School of Public Health (1985): *Hunger in America: The Growing Epidemic*, Cambridge, Mass.: Harvard University.

Illsley R. (1986): 'Occupational Class, Selection and the Production of Inequalities in Health', *Quarterly Journal of Social Affairs*, 2: 151–65.

Joshi H., Macran S. (1991): 'Work, Gender and Health', *Work, Employment and Society*, 5: 451–68.

Koskinen S. (1985): 'Time Trends in Cause-Specific Mortality by Occupational Class in England and Wales', International Union for the Scientific Study of the Population Conference, Florence.

Kuznets S. (1955): 'Economic Growth and Income Inequality', *American Economic Review*, 45: 1–28.

LeGrand J. (1985): *Inequalities in Health: The Human Capital Approach*, SunTory Toyota International Centre for Economics and Related Disciplines: Welfare State Project discussion paper no. 1, London: London School of Economics and Political Science.

—— (1991): *Equity and Choice: An Essay in Economics and Applied Philosophy*, London: Harper Collins Academic.

Macintyre S. (1986): 'The Patterning of Health by Social Position in Contemporary Britain: Directions for Sociological Research', *Social Science and Medicine*, 23: 394–415.

McKeown T. (1989): *The Role of Medicine: Dream, Mirage or Nemesis?* 2nd edn., Oxford: Basil Blackwell.

Marmot M., McDowell M. (1986): 'Mortality Decline and Widening Social Inequalities', *Lancet*, ii: 274–6.

Morris J. (1979): 'Social Inequalities Undiminished', *Lancet* i: 87–90.

—— (1990): 'Inequalities in Health: Ten Years and a Little Further on', *Lancet*, 336: 303–4.

Pahl R. (1993): 'Does class analysis without class theory have a promising future? A reply to Goldthorpe and Marshall', *Sociology*, 27: 253–258.

Ringen S. (1987): 'Poverty in the Welfare State?' in Erikson R., Hansen E., Ringen S., Uusitalo H. (eds), *The Scandinavian Model: Welfare States and Welfare Research*, New York and London: M. E. Sharpe Inc.

Robinson R. J. (1992): 'Is the Child the Father of the Man?' (editorial), *British Medical Journal*, 304: 789–90.

Rowntree S. (1901): *Poverty. A Study of Town Life*, London: Macmillan.

Sen A. (1984): 'Poor, Relatively Speaking', in Sen A. (1984), *Resources, Values and Development*, Oxford: Basil Blackwell; ong. pub. in *Oxford Economic Papers*, 35: 153–69.

—— (1992): *Inequality Reexamined*, Oxford: Clarendon Press.

Shiell A. (1991): *Poverty and Inequalities in Health*, York Centre for Health Economics, University of York, discussion paper no. 86.

Smith R. (1990): 'Poverty in the 1990s', editorial, *British Medical Journal*, 301: 349–50.

Stefansson C., Wicks S. (1991): 'Health Care Occupations and Suicide in Sweden 1961–1985', *Social Psychiatry and Psychiatric Epidemiology*, 26: 259–64.

Stern J. (1983): 'Social Mobility and the Interpretation of Social Class Mortality Differentials', *Journal of Social Policy*, 12: 27–49.

Strong P. (1990): 'Black on Class and Mortality: Theory, Method and History', *Journal of Public Health Medicine*, 12: 168–80.

Szreter S. (1984): 'The Genesis of the Registrar-General's Social Classification of Occupations', *British Journal of Sociology*, 356: 522–46.

—— (1988): *The Importance of Social Intervention in Britain's Mortality Decline c.1850–1914: A Re-interpretation of the Role of Public Health*, The Society for the Social History of Medicine. Vol X: 1–37.

Townsend P. (1987): 'Deprivation', *Journal of Social Policy*, 16: 125–46.

—— (1979): *Poverty in Britain*, Harmondsworth: Penguin Book.

——, Davidson N. (1982): *Inequalities in Health: The Black Report*, Harmondsworth: Penguin Books.

Vågerö D., Lundberg O. (1995): 'Socio-Economic Differentials among adults in Sweden—Towards an Explanation', in Lopez, Valonen and Casselli (eds), *Premature Adult Mortality in Developed Countries*, Oxford: Oxford University Press.

Chapter 10

M. E. J. Wadsworth

HEALTH INEQUALITIES IN THE LIFE COURSE PERSPECTIVE

From *Social Science and Medicine,* 44 (6) 1997: 859–69

Introduction

ALTHOUGH IMPROVEMENTS IN HEALTH since the Second World War have been considerable, particularly in terms of survival, social class differences in chances of good health have persisted.[1-3] The Black Report, referring to the period which ended in 1980, noted that "perhaps the most important general finding is the lack of improvement, and in some respects deterioration, of the health experience of *both* class V and IV relative to class I".[1] Social class differences in use of services, particularly preventive services, were persistently large during that same period.[1] Since then, according to many indicators, the extent of poverty has also increased in Britain over the last decade,[4] and inequalities in health have continued to be found.[2] Since mortality risk and other indicators of health problems are apparently associated with income distribution[5] and with disadvantaged social circumstances,[6-10] it is tempting to think about causes of health inequalities largely in terms of demographic scale factors and allocation of care resources. But the problem remains of how to begin to reduce inequalities. In recent years life history studies in health have begun to show the possibility that the roots of health inequalities lie in biological and social experience at the earliest times of life. . . .

Age related vulnerability

Biological factors

During the last 10 years there has been an increasing tendency to take a lifetime view of the natural history of some common serious illnesses which usually begin in middle or later life. Before this new approach, conditions such as raised blood pressure and chronic obstructive airways disease (COAD) were commonly believed to be associated with sources of risk which began only in middle adulthood, and most research was concentrated on that stage in life. This change and progression in perspective can be illustrated with the example of research into COAD.

Before the Second World War there was an urgent need for a solution to the problem of lower respiratory illness in working men; this was a time of heavy industry and a predominantly male work-force. Research concentrated then on the stage at which the problem began, in middle life, and where it was most trouble, in the labour force.[11] The effect of atmospheric pollution on the whole population was also acknowledged, but not resolved until well after the Second World War, in the Clean Air Act of 1956.[12] Although the mass of research on working men in middle life brought great improvements in working conditions and health in midlife,[13] and eventually a reduction in atmospheric pollution from coal burning, it did not greatly reduce the mortality rate from chronic bronchitis.[14] Reid,[15] and later Barker,[14] took a longer-term view, and using data on migration and on time and regional trends in mortality, concluded that biological risk of COAD was likely to be established in early life. Studies of long time periods in the lives of the same individuals added confirmation of this view by showing three things. First that respiratory function tracks during childhood, so that those who have poor function in early life have a strong tendency to continue to have poor function.[16] Second that those who have lower respiratory illness in early childhood are at greatest risk of respiratory illness later in childhood[17–19], and in adult life.[20,21] Third that low birth weight, an indicator of poor growth before birth, was associated with a significantly increased risk of COAD and poor respiratory function in adult life[14,21]. Barker[22] concluded that poor maternal nutrition during pregnancy, and other adverse influences on the developing foetus, such as mothers' smoking, reduced the opportunity for optimal development of organs associated with respiratory function, and the developmental process was still also at risk in the final stages of the baby's respiratory development during the first year of life. Thereafter, it is hypothesised, the individual can function only within the parameters set during this unique developmental opportunity. Barker[14,22] describes this process as biological programming.

Comparable hypotheses on the development of the kidney, the cardiovascular system, and glucose tolerance in adult life have been developed by Barker *et al.*,[14,22] and similar suggestions of factors affecting children in early life, during a uniquely occurring period of development, have been put forward in neurological studies.[23] However, since early life effects on biological development are hypothesised to determine the operational parameters of a biological system, then when demands on the system become too great problems would be expected. It is suggested, for instance, that kidney development that is less than optimal may not become a problem unless "the system is stressed, for example by high salt intake and thereby becomes unable to maintain the volume and composition of bodily fluids".[22] Hales and others argued that

> diabetes is a consequence of poor nutrition during critical periods of fetal life and infancy with consequent impaired development of beta cell function. If poor nutrition continues reduced ability to produce insulin is not a disadvantage. It becomes so only if nutrition becomes abundant, when increased demand for insulin outstrips the capacity for production.[24]

Much work remains to be done to validate the proposed biological programming hypotheses. It is not yet known whether such biological risk, apparently established early in life, is a source of vulnerability which necessarily requires a later life trigger, other than ageing, to activate its effects. Nor is it known how such early life effects interact with processes of ageing, nor with genetically defined risk. It may be that it is possible to escape from the apparent determinism of biological programming, through environmental or genetic means. Current work in a number of centres is exploring such questions, and biological and clinical researchers are investigating the process by which the proposed programming is established, so that it may be better measured. In terms of COAD the programming hypothesis continues to receive support from laboratory studies in humans and from animal research.[25]

Age related social factors

Socio-economic circumstance is a collective term for a wide range of factors which include not only occupational status and security, and at an earlier age educational attainment, but also housing environment and tenure, and family circumstances. Each of these factors seems likely to act differently to affect health at each stage in life. In this section evidence is presented of the range of social factors found to be associated with current health and future health potential in early life, infancy, childhood, adolescence and adulthood. Then the possible processes that may account for such associations are discussed.

Poor social circumstances at birth have long been shown to be associated with an increased risk of perinatal death. Originally this was thought to be the result of variation in quality of medical care, and time at which such care in pregnancy first began.[26] But risk of perinatal death was associated also with social class of family of origin, so that in risk terms "each mobile group carried with it, into marriage, the imprint of its class of origin",[26] and it was therefore hypothesised that this showed the effect of poor growth of the mother during her childhood. Short maternal stature was another powerful risk factor for perinatal death[26] and this effect, which was much greater in lower social classes, was thought likely to have been the result of poor maternal and child nutrition in the previous generation, and associated probably also with parental smoking.[27] Perinatal risk was much higher among single mothers, and this was thought to be because, at that time, the social unacceptability of single parenting tended to delay attendance at antenatal clinics.[26] More recently, the Barker hypotheses,[14,22] described in the previous section, implicate

poor socio-economic circumstances before birth as risks to intrauterine development that were incurred in the mother's own generation. Here again parental
smoking, maternal alcohol consumption and levels of nutrition are all known risk
factors, and each varies with socio-economic circumstances.

In infancy, socio-economically differentiated factors continue to act on
children's health. Parental smoking, poor housing, and nutrition habits continue to
have direct effects on the child's risk of current illness,[28] and on future respiratory
capacity.[21,22] Rates of growth are faster in those whose families are in higher socio-
economic circumstances.[29] Poor nutrition at this time has, like parental smoking,
both a current and a long-term effect. Another long-term effect begins at this time,
which is also strongly differentiated by current socio-economic circumstances,
namely opportunities for educational attainment. Children in poorer home circumstances, and with parents with low educational attainment, have reduced chances of
preschool experience,[30,31] which provides a disadvantaged beginning to the school
years,[30,32] and a consequent long-term health disadvantage, since, in adult life, little
or no educational attainment is associated with poor health related habits and
health.[33] Findings on family circumstances, in terms of parental relationships and
physical health in infancy, have shown associations between quality of maternal care
and health,[34] that infants and children in poor socio-economic circumstances are at
greater risk of injury,[35,36] and that those in families experiencing chronic parental
emotional disruption are at greater risk of disturbed behaviour,[37] and intentional
injury.[36]

During childhood the most consistent socio-economic difference in health is the
variation in height growth,[38] which in due course becomes associated with adult
health risks. This continuation of socio-economic differences in speed of growth and
in achieved height seems to be the result of continuing socio-economic differences in
nutrition and possibly also exercise.[39,40] Data from a longitudinal study showed that
poor home physical environment, low levels of parental education, and large family
size were also associated with height growth.[38,41] Since upward paternal (in the past,
and probably now parental) social mobility is associated with accelerated growth,[38]
this general indicator of improved circumstances within the family emphasises the
importance of socio-economic circumstances for growth. Also in childhood there
are significant social class differences in morbidity, with a greater illness burden
falling on children in the lower socio-economic groups.[42] Poor health during childhood is associated with reduced educational attainment.[32] Health associated habits of
parents and children also have long-term implications in that, for example, children
who begin to smoke, and those who live with parents who smoke, have significantly
reduced development of respiratory capacity.[43]

In adolescence, whilst there is little apparent socio-economic variation in many
aspects of health,[44] there is such variation still in the differences in growth already
evident at earlier ages,[38] and therefore in potential for health in adult life. For
example, although there is little social patterning in respiratory function at this
stage, the potential for the significant adult social variation in respiratory health is
already present in terms of the effects of smoking by individuals and by their parents
on adolescent respiratory capacity,[43] and in the influential early life factors of birth
weight, socio-economic circumstances and lower respiratory illness.[21,22] Similarly
the ground work for socio-economic variation in adult height has already been

prepared,[38] and the social variation in educational attainment is continued at this stage in the socio-economic differences in age at school leaving, and in going on to further and higher education.[45] Within the family, during adolescence, parental concern for educational attainment continues to be a powerful predictor of attainment and of occupational status,[46] and family disruption caused by parental divorce and separation increases the risk of the child not continuing into further and higher education.[47,48] Sweeting and West[49] have shown family conflict to be associated with a somewhat raised risk of physical health problems in young women adolescents, and confirm the association of family functioning with later occupational opportunity.

By early adulthood growth is completed, not only in height but also in all other aspects of development.[22] The patterns and extent of growth carry the imprint of the social environment of the previous generation, via the mother, as well as of the time *in utero*, and in childhood. Educational attainment makes its mark in adulthood in a number of ways, most evidently in occupational and socio-economic status; and these in turn are strongly associated with health. Health related habits of smoking,[50,51] nutrition,[33] exercise,[51,52] and alcohol consumption,[33,51] all have a strong socio-economic bias; they are also each associated with education, which generally has the effect of reducing adverse health habit practices. Consequently, it is unsurprising to find that biological risk factors associated with these health related habits, in particular overweight and obesity, are also significantly differentiated by social class.[51,53,54] Findings from a longitudinal study showed that women who came from manual social class families and held non-manual social class occupations in adulthood (at 36 years) tended significantly to show the prevalence of low obesity, as in the class they had joined, compared with the class they had left.[53] Unemployment is also commonly found to be associated with ill health[55–57] and premature death,[58] and a life history approach to this subject shows the importance of pre-existing vulnerability.[59] Longitudinal studies have shown that unemployment is a greater risk for young adults from less favourable family circumstances, with low or no educational attainment, and with early signs of vulnerability to ill health in adulthood.[59] Experience of divorce and separation is associated with raised risk of self-reported ill health[51] and with psychiatric morbidity,[56] but little work has been reported on its association with physical health. It seems an important area for new work,[49] particularly since it is an experience which in childhood affects mental health, and increases vulnerability to adult mental health problems,[60–62] and since parental divorce or separation is associated with raised risk of offspring's divorce or separation in the following generation.[63]

While most life history research on social factors and health has concentrated on the association of childhood factors with adult health, there has been less work, although some hypothesising in retrospect from studies of the elderly, on the relationship of adult midlife experience with later life health, and even less on the relationship of childhood factors with old age. Research on these areas will be increasingly reported, as current studies of cohorts begun in mid-life and at birth continue into later life, for example the 1946 and 1958 national birth cohort studies,[46,64] and the British Regional Heart Study.[59] There are a number of psychological studies of middle life[65] and of ageing and cognitive change with age,[66] which include new concern with social factors and ageing; of particular interest in life history research is the measurement in longitudinal studies of ageing of biological and psychological latent reserves, and adaptability or plasticity of individuals.[66] Some medical studies of ageing have generated hypotheses about associations between mid-life health related habits and, for instance, later life skeletal state and risk of damage,[67] in which social habits play a part, through their influence on health related habits.[33]

Such a range of social factors is implicated in the life history studies of health, that it is difficult to categorise their possible processes of operation. Unlike the processes suggested by the biological programming hypotheses, the social hypotheses do not propose that their effects operate solely or mainly at critical developmental periods. From the life history studies of childhood and adolescence it may be concluded that social factors probably operate in a cumulative fashion. Children of families in favourable socio-economic circumstances have what is, in effect, a stock of social capital, which is enhanced if one or both parents have further or higher educational attainment,[46,68] and still further by strong parental concern for their child's education.[32,69] These beginnings predispose children to higher educational attainment which is, in turn, associated with better health in adulthood.[70] Conversely, vulnerability to physical ill health in childhood and later adult life is associated with poor parental socio-economic circumstances, and low levels of parental education and concern,[46,21] and consequent lower levels of educational attainment with changes of lower occupational status, greater vulnerability to unemployment, risk of more adverse health related behaviour in adulthood, and poorer health.

But how may these social factors have their effects?

In childhood, for instance, do poor home circumstances affect health in a bio-social fashion, because of the concomitant increased chances of poor nutrition, the greater likelihood of parental smoking, the slower rate of growth, and the greater risk of childhood infection and other illnesses, which strike the child at biologically vulnerable times, particularly since children in these poor circumstances are those who are likely to have had a less than optimal development before birth? Are there also psychosocial processes of importance? Do the higher levels and chronic persistence of anxiety about money in poor families, and the poor nutritional. Smoking, and exercise habits provide the growing child with poor examples in coping styles and health associated habits which may be difficult to change later? It is possible to argue for a dynamic model of a childhood acquisition of a stock of socially related potentiating factors for later health, susceptible to change from parental social mobility and from education, which seem to make it possible to escape from the adverse health related aspects of early life social factors since, for example, upward parental social mobility is associated with raised chances in education[32] and in height growth.[38] The psychosocial processes seem less easy to escape,[71] although here too education is likely to be a key factor. It is worth noting, in terms of assessment of pre-crises psychological functioning, that life history studies in psychophysiology and deviant behaviour suggest that early acquisition of styles of stress management and of behaviour seem to be remarkably stable in the long term.[71,72]

Much of the work on how social factors may operate in adult life comes from studies of social factors and health in relation to crises experienced by individuals, such as divorce and unemployment. This work is beginning to ask how far earlier, pre-crises, social, psychological, and biological states mediate the effect on health of such crises.[55,60,73] Conclusions for physical health are most often in terms of psychological stress leading to biochemical and immunological change,[55] but such processes have yet to be fully explored.

Studies of the association of social factors with adult health, not associated with crises, have been greatly concerned with poverty. Findings about the effects of poor housing, chronic anxiety about money, and adverse health related habits need now to be supported with studies of how such social factors have their effects on the health of individuals. Life history approaches will be necessary in such new work on processes, in order to take account of earlier life established vulnerability and protective factors, already known, such as parental social class and own educational attainment[21,33,53] as well as more recent attributes and experiences. . . .

Conclusions

Life history studies offer new opportunities to examine processes that generate health inequalities for the individual. New methods for undertaking such studies show that it is not always necessary to use long-term prospective methods.

Biologically it seems arguable that in some important respects early life health and development delineate the parameters of health possibilities for adulthood. In that case the adverse social factors that affect infant health and development would be important originating aspects of social differences in health and health potential during adulthood. Social factors experienced in childhood encompass also many important aspects of the potential for later educational attainment, and for the socio-economic circumstances of adult life. These factors make it possible for children born in poor socio-economic circumstances to experience upward social mobility, and they are associated also with improved chances in health. So although biological programming may have a deterministic effect on the range of adult health parameters, the social and family circumstances of childhood are the beginnings of pathways which will be protective to health or increase vulnerability to ill health. The social factors that affect both biological programming and the social and educational pathways from childhood to adult socio-economic circumstances, vary with historical time, and so the extent of health inequality in actuality and in potential in a cohort of a given age is likely to be different from that of a cohort of another age.

So far, life history contributions to the study of inequalities in health show that health is a lifelong development for the individual. The implication of these findings is that chances of reduction of inequalities for any given generation will be greater, the earlier that attempts at reduction are begun. It is unlikely that health inequalities can be easily or rapidly reduced, increasingly so as the individual ages, since individuals carry an accumulation of health potential which is hard to change.

References

1 Townsend, P. and Davidson, N. (1982) *Inequalities in Health: The Black Report*. Penguin, London.
2 Davey Smith, G. and Morris, J. (1994) Increasing inequalities in the health of the nation. *British Medical Journal* **309**, 1453.
3 McLoone, P. and Boddy, F. A. (1994) Deprivation and mortality in Scotland. *British Medical Journal* **309**, 1465.
4 Joseph Rowntree Foundation (1995) *Inquiry into Income and Wealth* (2 volumes). Joseph Rowntree Foundation, York.
5 Wilkinson, R. J. (1992) Income distribution and life expectancy. *British Medical Journal* **304**, 165.
6 Blaxter M. (1990) *Health and Lifestyles*. Tavistock/ Routledge, London.
7 Power, C., Manor, O. and Fox, J. (1991) *Health and Class: The Early Years*. Chapman and Hall, London.
8 Blane, D., Davey Smith, G. and Bartley, M. (1993) Social selection: what does it contribute to social class differences in health? *Sociology of Health and Illness* **15**, 1.
9 Lahelma, E. and Arber, S. (1994) Health inequalities among men and women in contrasting welfare states: Britain and three Nordic countries compared. *European Journal of Public Health* **4**, 213.
10 Mackenbach, J. P. (1994) Socioeconomic inequalities in health in the Netherlands: impact of a five year research programme. *British Medical Journal*, **309**, 1487.
11 Medical Research Council (1943) Chronic pulmonary disease in South Wales Coalminers. *Special Report Series*, no. 244.
12 Hall, P. L. H., Parker, R. and Webb, A. (1975) *Change, Choice and Conflict in Social Policy*. Heinemann, London.
13 Hunter, D. (1959) *Health in Industry*. Penguin, London.
14 Barker, D. J. P. (1991) *Fetal and Infant Origins of Adult Disease. British Medical Journal*, London.
15 Reid, D. D. (1969) The beginnings of bronchitis. *Proceedings of the Royal Society of Medicine* **62**, 311.
16 Hibbert, M. E., Hudson, I. L., Lanigan, A., Landau, L. I. and Phelan, P. D. (1990) Tracking of lung function in healthy children and adolescents. *Pediatrics Pul.* **8**, 172.
17 Holland, W. W., Halil, T., Bennett, A. E. and Elliott, A. (1969) Factors influencing the onset of chronic respiratory disease. *British Medical Journal* **ii**, 205.
18 Mok, J. Y. Q. and Simpson, H. (1984) Outcome for acute bronchitis, bronchiolitis, and pneumonia in infancy. *Archives of Disease in Childhood* **59**, 306.
19 Strope, G. L., Stewart, P. L., Henderson, F. W., Ivins, S. S., Steadman, H. C. and Henry, M. M. (1991) Lung function in school age children who had mild lower respiratory illness in early childhood. *American Review of Respiratory Disease* **144**, 655.
20 Strachan, D. P., Anderson, H. R., Bland, J. M. and Peckham, C. (1988) Asthma as a link between chest illness in childhood and chronic cough and phlegm in young adults. *British Medical Journal* **296**, 890.
21 Mann, S. L., Wadsworth, M. E. J. and Colley, J. R. T. (1992) Accumulation of factors influencing respiratory illness in members of a national birth cohort and their offspring. *Journal of Epidemiology and Community Health* **46**, 286.
22 Barker, D. J. P. (1994) *Mothers, Babies, and Disease in Later Life. British Medical Journal*, London.

23   Lucas, A., Morley, R., Cole, T. J., Lister, G. and Leeson-Payne, C. (1992) Breast milk and subsequent intelligence quotient in children born preterm. *Lancet* **339**, 261.

24   Hales, C. N., Barker, D. J. P., Clark, P. M. S., Cox, L. J., Fall, C., Osmond, C. and Winter, P. (1991) Fetal and infant growth and impaired glucose tolerance at age 64. In *Fetal and Infant Origins of Adult Disease*, ed. D. J. P. Barker. British Medical Journal, London.

25   Shaheen, S. O., Barker, D. J. P., Shiell, A. W., Crocker, F. J., Wield, G. A. and Holgate, S. T. (1994) The relationship between pneumonia in early childhood and impaired lung function in late adult life. *American Journal of Respiratory Critical Care Medicine* **149**, 616.

26   Illsley, R. and Kincaid, J. C. (1963) Social correlations of perinatal mortality. In *Perinatal Mortality*. eds N. R. Butler and D. G. Bonham. Livingstone, Edinburgh.

27   Butler, N. R. and Alberman, E. D. (eds) (1969) *Perinatal Problems*. Livingstone, Edinburgh.

28   Pless, I. B. (1994) *The Epidemiology of Childhood Illness*. Oxford University Press, New York.

29   Douglas, J. W. B. and Mogford, C. (1953) The results of a national inquiry into the growth of premature children from birth to 4 years. *Archive of Diseases in Childhood* **28**, 436.

30   Wadsworth, M. E. J. (1981) Social class and generation differences in pre-school education. *British Journal of Sociology* **32**, 560.

31   Osborn, A. F. and Milbank, J. E. (1989) *The Effects of Early Education*. Clarendon Press, Oxford.

32   Douglas, J. W. B. (1964) *The Home and the School*. MacGibbon and Kee, London.

33   Braddon, F. E. M., Wadsworth, M. E. J., Davies, J. M. C. and Cripps, H. A. (1988) Social and regional differences in food and alcohol consumption and their measurement in a national birth cohort. *Journal of Epidemiology and Community Health* **42**, 341.

34   Douglas, J. W. B. and Blomfield, J. M. (1958) *Children Under Five*, Allen and Unwin, London.

35   Rivara, F. P. (1994) Unintentional injuries. In *The Epidemiology of Childhood Disorders*, ed. I. B. Pless. Oxford University Press, New York.

36   Christoffel, K. K. (1994) Intentional injuries: homicide and violence. In *The Epidemiology of Childhood Disorders*, ed. I. B. Pless. Oxford University Press, New York.

37   Wadsworth, M., Maclean, M., Kuh, D. and Rodgers, B. (1990) Children of divorced and separated parents: summary and review of findings from a long-term follow-up study in the UK. *Family Practice*, **7**, 104.

38   Kuh, D. and Wadsworth, M. E. J. (1989) Parental height: childhood environment and subsequent adult height in a national birth cohort. *International Journal of Epidemiology* **18**, 663.

39   Johnston, F. E. (1986) Somatic growth of the infant and preschool child. In *Human Growth*. eds F. Faulkner and J. M. Tanner. Plenum Press, London.

40   Bailey, D. A., Malina, R. M. and Mirwald, R. L. (1986) Physical activity and growth of the child. In *Human Growth*, eds F. Faulkner and J. M. Tanner. Plenum Press, London.

41   Douglas, J. W. B. (1969) Effects of early environment on later development. *Journal of the Royal College of Physicians* 3, 359.

42   Woodroffe, C., Glickman, M., Barker, M. and Power, C. (1993) *Children, Teenagers, and Health*. Open University, Buckingham.

43   Tager, I. B., Weiss, S. T., Munoz, A., Rosner, B. Speizer, F. E. (1983) Longitudinal study of the effects of maternal smoking on pulmonary function in children. *New England Journal of Medicine* **309**, 699.

44   West, P. (1988) Inequalities? Social class differentials in health in British youth. *Social Science & Medicine* 27, 291.

45   Halsey, A. H. (1988) *British Social Trends Since* 1900, Macmillan, London.

46   Wadsworth, M. E. J. (1991) *The Imprint of Time: Childhood, History and Adult Life*. Oxford University Press, Oxford.

47   Lundberg, O. (1993) The impact of childhood living conditions on illness and mortality in adulthood. *Social Science & Medicine*, **36**, 1047.

48   Wadsworth, M. E. J. and Maclean, M. (1986) Parents' divorce and children's life chances. *Children and Youth Serv. Rev.* **8**, 145.

49   Sweeting, H. and West, P. (1995) Family life and health in adolescence: a role for culture in the health inequalities debate? *Social Science & Medicine* **40**, 163.

50   Graham, H. (1984) *Women, Health and the Family*. Wheatsheaf Books, Brighton.

51   Cox, B. D., Huppert, F. A. and Whichelow, M. J. (1993) *The Health and Lifestyle Survey: Seven Years On*. Dartmouth, Aldershot.

52   Kuh, D. J. L. and Cooper, C. (1992) Physical activity at 36 years: patterns and childhood predictors in a longitudinal study. *Journal of Epidemiology in Community Health*. **46**, 114.

53   Braddon, F. M., Rodgers, B., Wadsworth, M. E. J. and Davies, J. M. C. (1986) Onset of obesity in a 36 year birth cohort study. *British Medical Journal* **293**, 299.

54   Bennett, N., Dodd, T., Flatley, J., Freeth, S. and Bolling, K. (1995) *Health Survey for England 1993*. HMSO, London.

55   Bartley, M. (1994) Unemployment and ill health: understanding the relationship. *Journal of Epidemiology in Community Health*. **48**, 333.

56   Meltzer, H., Gill, B., Petticrew, M. and Hinds, K. (1995) *The Prevalence of Psychiatric Morbidity Among Adults Living in Private Households*. HMSO, London.

57   Moylan, S., Millar, J. and Davies, R. (1984) *For Richer For Poorer: DHSS Cohort Study of Unemployed Men*. HMSO, London.

58   Morris, J. K., Cook, D. G. and Shaper, A. G. (1994) Loss of unemployment and mortality. *British Medical Journal* **308**, 1135.

59   Montgomery, S. M., Bartley, M. J., Cook, D. G. and Wadsworth, M. E. J. (in press) Health and social precursors of unemployment in young men. *Journal of Epidemiology in Community Health*.

60   Rodgers, B. (1994) Pathways between parental divorce and adult depression. *Journal of Child Psychology and Psychiatry* **35**, 1289.

61   Rodgers, B. (1996) Reported parental behaviour and adult affective symptoms 1: associations and moderating factors. *Psychology and Medicine* **26**, 51–61.

62   Rodgers, B. (1996) Reported parental behaviour and adult affective symptoms 2: mediating factors. *Psychology and Medicine* **26**, 63–77.

63   Kiernan, K. E. (1986) Teenage marriage and marital breakdown: a longitudinal study. *Population Studies* **40**, 35.

64   Ferri, E. (ed.) (1993) *Life at 33*. Longmans, London.

65   Eichorn, D. H., Clausen, J. A., Haan, N., Honzik, M. P., and Mussen, P. H. (eds) (1981) *Present and Past in Middle Life*. Academic Press, New York.

66   Baltes, P. B. and Baltes, M. M. (eds) (1990) *Successful Aging: Perspectives from the Behavioural Sciences*. Cambridge University Press, Cambridge.

67   Kane, R. L., Evans, J. G. and MacFadyen, D. (eds) (1990) *Improving the Health of Older People*. Oxford University Press, Oxford.

68   Kuh, D. and Wadsworth, M. (1991) Childhood influences on adult male earnings in a longitudinal study. *British Journal of Sociology* **42**, 537.

69   Essen, J. and Wedge, P. (1982) *Continuities in Childhood Disadvantage*. Heinemann, London.

70   Kuh, D. J. L. and Wadsworth, M. E. J. (1993) Physical health status at 36 years in a British national birth cohort. *Social Science & Medicine* **37**, 905.

71   Farrington, D. (1995) The development of offending and antisocial behaviour from childhood: key findings from the Cambridge study of delinquent behaviour. *Journal of Child Psychology and Psychiatry* 36, 929.

72   Caspi, A. and Silva, P. A. (1995) Temperamental qualities at age 3 predict personality traits in young adulthood: longitudinal evidence from a birth cohort. *Child Development* **66**, 486.

73   Robins, L. N. and Rutter, M. (eds) (1990) *Straight and Devious Pathways from Childhood to Adulthood*. Cambridge University Press, Cambridge.

Chapter 11

James Y. Nazroo

GENETIC, CULTURAL OR SOCIO-ECONOMIC VULNERABILITY?
Explaining ethnic inequalities in health

From *Sociology of Health and Illness*, 20(5) 1998: 710–30

Introduction

OVER THE LAST THREE decades there has been considerable interest in both class inequalities in health and the health of ethnic minority populations. A relatively early, but key, publication in both of these fields has influenced the direction they took – the Black Report (Townsend and Davidson 1982) on class inequalities in health and Marmot *et al.*'s (1984) study of immigrant mortality. Importantly, these two pieces of work came to quite different conclusions. The Black Report placed emphasis on material explanations for class inequalities in health, which, given the class locations of ethnic minority people at that time (Brown 1984), would suggest that such issues might also be relevant to ethnic inequalities in health. However, the data published on immigrant mortality rates, a few years after the Black Report, indicated that class and, consequently, material explanations were unrelated to mortality rates for most migrant groups, and made no contribution to the higher mortality rates found among those who had migrated to Britain (Marmot *et al.* 1984). Indeed, for one group, those born in the 'Caribbean Commonwealth', the relationship between class and overall mortality rates was the opposite of that for the general population. Marmot *et al.* concluded:

> (a) that differences in social class distribution are not the explanation of the overall different mortality of migrants; and (b) the relation of social class (as usually defined) to mortality is different among immigrant groups from the England and Wales pattern. (1984: 21)

The two fields have subsequently taken quite different directions. Those interested in class inequalities have, on the whole, concentrated on providing additional evidence for a material explanation and on unpacking the mechanisms that might link material disadvantage with a greater risk of poor health (e.g. Macintyre 1997, Vågerö and Illsley 1995, Davey Smith et al. 1994, Lundeberg 1991). While, with a few notable exceptions (Ahmad et al. 1989, Fenton et al. 1995, Smaje 1995, Harding and Maxwell 1997), class has largely disappeared from investigations into the relationship between ethnicity and health, particularly in the UK. For example, in an overview of existing data produced for the NHS Executive and NHS Ethnic Health Unit, there is no mention of class, even though there is some discussion of other demographic features of the ethnic minority population of Britain (Balarajan and Soni Raleigh 1995).

In contrast to Marmot et al.'s (1984) data, work in the US (Rogers 1992, Sterling et al. 1993, Davey Smith et al. 1996, 1997a) and recent work in the UK has suggested both that material factors are relevant to the health of ethnic minority people and that they make the key contribution to differences in health between different ethnic groups (Nazroo 1997a). The work undertaken in the UK was based on a nationally representative survey of ethnic minority and white people living in England and Wales (the Fourth National Survey of Ethnic Minorities) that was identified through a process of focused enumeration (Brown and Ritchie 1981, Smith and Prior 1997). One or two adults in the identified households underwent a structured face-to-face interview conducted by an ethnically matched interviewer in the language of the respondents' choice. In addition to physical (Nazroo 1997a) and mental health (Nazroo 1997b), the questionnaire covered a comprehensive range of information on both ethnicity and other aspects of the lives of ethnic minority people, including demographic and socio-economic factors (see Modood et al. 1997 for a full report on these data). Its novel findings were, at least in part, a reflection of its methodological strengths and the depth of the data collected.

In some ways, findings suggesting a material base for ethnic inequalities in health run counter to the wider sociological literature on ethnicity and 'race'. Although, within this work there appears to be complete agreement that 'race' is a concept without scientific validity (see, for example, the collected works of Barot 1996) – an artificial construct, used to justify the hierarchical ordering of groups of people and the exploitation of 'inferior races' – in contrast, most writers give credence to a notion of ethnicity, which reflects self-identification with cultural traditions that both provide strength and meaning, and boundaries (perhaps fluid) between groups. So, although socio-economic disadvantage might contribute to health differences, it is suggested that there remains an essential component to ethnicity that could make a major contribution to differences in health, that when explaining the relationship between ethnicity and health, ethnicity cannot be 'simply emptied into class disadvantage' (Smaje, 1996).

This paper sets out to explore in more detail these various approaches to understanding the relationship between ethnicity and health and some of the implications of these for policy. Data from the Fourth National Survey will be used to illustrate the points made.

Un-theorised ethnicity – epidemiological approaches

Researchers and commentators in the field of ethnicity and health seem divided over whether this work should be empirically or theoretically driven. Not surprisingly, those with a more epidemiological bent tend to argue for the former. If differences in rates of disease are present between groups that have been identified on the basis of an emergent 'ethnic' classification, these differences will provide a useful starting point for the identification and exploration of aetiological factors associated with those groups at higher risk. For example, Senior and Bhopal state:

> Epidemiology is the study of the distribution and determinants of disease. The main method of study, particularly for investigating the causes of disease, is to compare populations with different risks of disease. Ethnicity is a variable that is used increasingly to define populations for epidemiological studies. (1994:327)

A good example of this approach can be found in the work of McKeigue and colleagues (*e.g.* McKeigue *et al.* 1988, 1989 and 1991). This focuses on a particular disease (Coronary Heart Disease – CHD), rather than health *per se*, and uses the variation in the pattern of this disease across ethnic groups to provide clues for an understanding of its aetiology.

If the empirically driven approach of this work is accepted, criticism inevitably falls to the accuracy with which key variables are measured. Most epidemiological research on health and ethnicity has taken a crude approach to the allocation of individuals into ethnic groups. As might be expected, because country of birth is recorded on death certificates and in the census, much of the published data in this area have allocated ethnicity according to country of birth, a strategy that is clearly limited. In addition, many studies use 'ethnic' groupings with quite inappropriate boundaries, such as Black or South Asian. The data are then interpreted as though the individuals within them are ethnically (i.e. genetically and culturally) homogeneous, even though such categories are heterogeneous, containing ethnic groups with different cultures, religions, migration histories, and geographical and socio-economic locations (see Bagley's (1995) comments on a similar situation in the US).

Such criticisms lead to a focus on the technical problems with assigning individuals to ethnic categories during the research process, and a concern with such things as: collecting sufficiently detailed information to differentiate between distinct groups; recording ethnic background in a consistent way; and dealing with issues such as mixed parentage (see Chaturvedi and McKeigue's (1994) comments on the British data, and McKenney and Bennett's (1994) comments on the data provided by the US Bureau of the Census). Solutions proposed involve more sensitive strategies for collecting information on ethnicity, for example by allowing individuals to define their ethnic group in their own terms. It is argued that this reduces the use of groups which are artefactual and without 'real' meaning (Aspinall 1995) and avoids the construction of ethnic boundaries on the basis of the racist assumptions of researchers (Sheldon and Parker 1992). (Although in most research using this model respondents are offered only a limited number of categories to choose from.)

In apparent support of this position, recent work based on the *Fourth National Survey* (Nazroo, 1997a) has shown that a more detailed approach to the assignment of individuals into ethnic groups reveals important additional differences between them. In that survey, individual respondents could be allocated into particular ethnic groups on the basis of a number of criteria. Figure 11.1 uses a categorisation based on the respondents' replies to a question on the country of their family origin. It shows the relative risk compared with whites for reporting fair or poor general health for various ethnic minority groups. (Relative risk is the chance of the member of a group having a particular attribute compared with a member of a reference group – in this case whites. In Figure 11.1, and subsequent figures, the relative risk for each minority group is represented as the range within which there is a 95 per cent statistical probability of the true value lying, with the mid point of the range also indicated. If the range does not cross the solid line at the value of '1', the value for the comparison white group, differences are, of course, statistically significant.) If the first three groups are examined, the data show that the use of an overall ethnic minority group obscures important differences between Caribbeans and South Asians. And, if the final four groups are compared, the data show that the use of an overall South Asian group obscures important differences between Indians on the one hand and Pakistanis and Bangladeshis on the other.

Of course, the refining of our ethnic classification need not stop here. For example, those ethnic minority people with Indian family origins are ethnically very diverse. They can be broadly divided into at least three cultural/geographical groups: Hindus from the Gujarati region of India; Sikhs from the Punjabi region of India; and Muslims from a number of areas. Figure 11.2 shows how the rate of

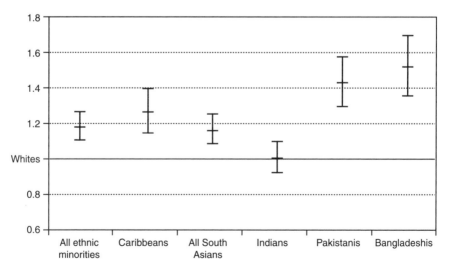

Figure 11.1 Relative risk of reporting fair or poor health compared with whites (age and gender standardised)

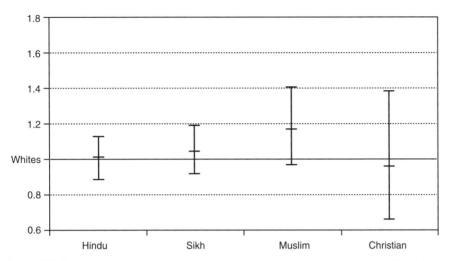

Figure 11.2 Relative risk of reporting fair or poor health compared with whites – Indians only (age and gender standardised)

reported fair or poor health compared with whites varied across these three groups, identified on the basis of their religion, and a fourth, Christian Indians. It suggests that the health experience of Indians also varies along religious/cultural lines, with Muslims appearing to have worse health than the other groups (although the differences shown are not statistically significant).

Similar refinements can be made for the other ethnic groups included in Figure 11.1, for example Caribbeans can be divided into African and Indian Caribbeans, and whites can be divided in many ways. The implication of these figures is that further refining the assessment of ethnicity used in epidemiological research will improve its power. More accurate assignments of ethnicity reveal additional differences and should allow a more careful generation of aetiological hypotheses and a more finely tuned programme for intervention.

It is here that the lack of theoretical work done by such researchers becomes important. Despite this lack, it is a mistake to assume that the process of identifying 'ethnic' groups is theoretically neutral (hence my use of the term 'un-theorised' rather than atheoretical). Take the example of Marmot et al.'s (1984) immigrant mortality study, which in some ways could be seen as opportunistic, being based on the combination of country of birth data that is recorded on death certificates and at the 1981 Census. When discussing the rationale for their analysis, Marmot et al. have in mind a clear notion of the significance of their 'country of birth' variable:

> Comparisons of disease rates between immigrants and non-immigrants in the 'old' country, between immigrants and residents of the 'new' country, and between different immigrant groups in the new country have helped elucidate the relative importance of genetic and environmental factors in many diseases. (1984: 4)

And, in his discussion of equivalent data relating to the period covered by the 1991 Census, Balarajan suggests that differences could be due to 'biological, cultural, religious, socio-economic or other environmental factors' (1995: 119).

However, in this work these explanatory factors are rarely assessed with any accuracy and the search for clues regarding aetiology is typically done with a focus on the *assumed* genetic or cultural characteristics of individuals within the ethnic group at greater risk. Consequently, explanations tend to fall to unmeasured genetic and cultural factors based on stereotypes, because such meanings are easily imposed on ethnic categorisations (see Bhopal (1997) for a critique of this 'Black Box' approach to epidemiology). Theory is brought in surreptitiously – ethnicity, how-ever measured, equals genetic or cultural heritage. This then leads to a form of victim blaming, where the *inherent* characteristics of the ethnic (minority) group are seen to be at fault and in need of rectifying (Sheldon and Parker 1992). It is the ways in which ethnic and racial groups are constructed during this process, and the kinds of attributes focused on, that raise a concern with racialisation.

An example of this can be found in the well publicised greater risk of 'South Asians' for CHD. A *British Medical Journal* editorial (Gupta *et al.* 1995) used research findings to attribute this problem to a combination of genetic (i.e. 'race') and cultural (i.e. ethnicity) factors that are apparently associated with being 'South Asian'. Concerning genetic factors, the suggestion was that 'South Asians' have a shared evolutionary history that involved adaptation 'to survive under conditions of periodic famine and low energy intake'. This resulted in the development of 'insulin resistance syndrome', which apparently underlies 'South Asians'' greater risk of CHD. From this perspective 'South Asians' can be viewed as a genetically distinct group with a unique evolutionary history – a 'race'. In terms of cultural factors, the use of ghee in cooking, a lack of physical exercise and a reluctance to use health services were all mentioned – even though ghee is not used by all of the ethnic groups that comprise 'South Asians', and evidence suggests that 'South Asians' do understand the importance of exercise (Beishon and Nazroo 1997) and do use medical services (Nazroo 1997a, Rudat 1994). It is important to note how the policy recommendations flowing from such an approach underline the extent to which the issue has become racialised. The authors of the editorial recommend that 'community leaders' and 'survivors' of heart attacks should spread the message among their communities and that 'South Asians' should be encouraged to under-take healthier lifestyles (Gupta *et al.* 1995). The problem is, apparently, viewed as something inherent to being 'South Asian', nothing to do with the context of the lives of 'South Asians' and as only solvable if 'South Asians' are encouraged to modify their behaviours to address their genetic and cultural weaknesses.

Given this risk of racialisation, it is not helpful to refine an ethnic classification scheme in a way that allows further assumptions to be made about the importance of culture and genetics when neither are measured, and environment continues to be ignored. For example, analysis of the *Fourth National Survey* showed that, while a South Asian group had a greater risk of indicators of CHD, once the group was broken down into constituent parts, this only applied to Pakistanis and Bangladeshis – Indians had the same rate as whites (Nazroo 1997a). In addition, within the Indian group Muslims had a high rate of indicators of CHD, while Hindus and Sikhs had low rates (producing very similar findings to those shown for reported general health in

Figures 11.1 and 11.2). While this approach was useful in uncovering the extent to which convenient assumptions of similarity within obviously heterogeneous groups were false, it could be suggested that these findings mean we can use the term 'Muslim heart disease', or 'Pakistani and Bangladeshi heart disease', rather than 'South Asian heart disease', to describe the situation. And explanations can be sought in assumptions about Muslim, Pakistani and Bangladeshi cultural practices or their shared evolutionary history. This potential results from the use of un-theorised and apparently emergent ethnic classifications that allow ethnicity to be treated as a *natural and fixed* division between social groups, and the *description* of ethnic variations in health to become their *explanation* (Sheldon and Parker, 1992). Explanations are, consequently, based on cultural stereotypes or suppositions about genetic differences, rather than attempting directly to assess the nature and importance of such factors, the contexts in which they operate and their association with health outcomes.

So, in addition to refining our measurement of ethnicity, in order to progress we need to examine the degree to which the indicator used (country of birth, country of family origin, self-assigned ethnic groups, etc.) reflects an underlying construct (Williams *et al.* 1994, Bagley 1995, McKenzie and Crowcroft 1996) – are we measuring genetics, biology, culture, lifestyle, the consequences of racialisation, socio-economic position etc., and are the indicators used appropriate to whichever of these we are concerned with?

Ethnicity as structure – socio-economic status

As implied in the introduction, one of the key contexts relevant to the relationship between ethnicity and health should be socio-economic position. Indeed, findings from the *Fourth National Survey*, shown in Table 11.1, suggest important differences between different ethnic groups in socio-economic positions. Overall, there were few differences between the white and Indian groups, but Caribbeans, Pakistanis and Bangladeshis were, to varying degrees, worse off than the other two groups. Interestingly, these differences mirror those for health shown in Figure 11.1.

However, following Marmot *et al.*'s (1984) analysis, rather than puzzling over why such an important explanation for inequalities in health among the general

Table 11.1 Ethnic differences in socio-economic position

	White %	Caribbean	Indian	Pakistani	Bangladeshi
Registrar General's Class					
I/II	35	22	32	20	11
IIIn	15	18	20	15	18
IIIm	31	30	22	32	32
IV/V	20	30	26	33	40
Unemployed	11	24	15	38	42

population did not apply to ethnic minorities, researchers have ignored class and simply accepted that different sets of explanations for poor health apply to the ethnic minority and majority populations. In fact, there are a number of reasons why class effects might be suppressed in immigrant mortality data. Most important is that Marmot *et al.* (1984) had to use occupation as recorded on death certificates to define social class. The inflating of occupational status (where, according to Townsend and Davidson (1982), occupation is recorded on death certificates as the 'skilled' job held for most of the individual's life rather than the 'unskilled' job held for the last few years of life) will be particularly significant for immigrant mortality data if migration to Britain were associated with downward social mobility for members of ethnic minority groups, a process that both Smith (1977) and Health and Ridge (1983) have documented. So, the occupation recorded on the death certificates of migrants may well be an inaccurate reflection of their experience in Britain prior to death. In addition, given the socio-economic profile of ethnic minority groups in Britain, this inflation of occupational status would only need to happen in relatively few cases for the figures representing the small population in higher classes to be distorted upwards. For example, Table 3.7 in Marmot *et al.* (1984) reports only 212 deaths occurring in the class I group to those born in the Indian sub-continent in 1970–72, and only 37 for those born in the Caribbean.

In fact, data from the *Fourth National Survey* suggest that class effects are similar for ethnic minority and white people. Figure 11.3 shows the relationship between class and reporting fair or poor health for different ethnic groups. (Here a distinction has been drawn between households that are manual and those that are non-manual, according to the Registrar General's criteria, and a third group of respondents from households containing no full-time worker has also been identified. Those aged 65 or older have not been included in any of the socio-economic analyses.) There was a clear and strong relationship between class and health for all the ethnic groups covered.

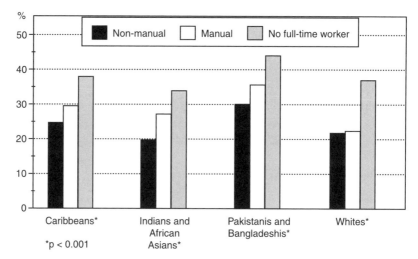

Figure 11.3 Reported fair or poor health by ethnic group and class (age and gender standardised)

Others have presented similar findings, both in smaller scale regional studies (e.g. Fenton *et al.* 1995) and in the most recent analysis of immigrant mortality data (Harding and Maxwell 1997). The implication of this is clear, the second conclusion drawn by Marmot *et al.* (1984), that social class has a different relationship to health for ethnic minority compared to majority people, is not supported. However, a closer examination of the Figure suggests that their first conclusion, that differences in social class distribution do not explain ethnic differences in health, is supported. For example, within each class group Pakistanis and Bangladeshis (who Figure 11.1 suggests have the poorest health) were more likely than equivalent whites to report fair or poor health, and the same is true for non-manual and manual Caribbeans (who overall also had poorer health than whites). Similarly, the most recent analysis of immigrant mortality data found that adjustments for occupational class made little change to the differences between groups, despite finding a class gradient within country of birth groups, leading the authors to conclude that: 'social class is not an adequate explanation for the patterns of excess mortality observed [among migrant groups]' (Harding and Maxwell 1997: 120). The implication of both sets of data is that there remains some unidentified component of ethnicity that increases (some) ethnic minority groups' risk of poor health. It is tempting to reduce this unexplained variance to assumed cultural or genetic factors.

However, this interpretation is misleading. There has been an increasing recognition of the limitations of traditional class groupings, which are far from internally homogeneous. A number of studies have drawn attention to variations in income levels and death rates among occupations that comprise particular occupational classes (*e.g.* Davey Smith *et al.* 1990). And within an occupational group, ethnic minorities may be more likely to be found in lower or less prestigious occupational grades, to have poorer job security, to endure more stressful working conditions and to be more likely to work unsocial hours. Evidence from the *Fourth National Survey* illustrates this point clearly. Table 5.2 in Nazroo (1997a) showed that ethnic minority people had a lower income than white people in the same class, that unemployed ethnic minority people had been unemployed for longer than equivalent white people, and that some ethnic minority groups had poorer quality housing than whites regardless of tenure. Similar findings have been reported in the US (Lillie-Blanton and Laveist 1996, Williams *et al.* 1994). The conclusion to be drawn is that, while standard indicators of socio-economic status have some use for making comparisons *within* ethnic groups, they are of little use for 'controlling out' the impact of socio-economic differences when attempting to reveal a pure 'ethnic/race' effect . . . .

Here it is also important to remember that, as well as being imperfect, socio-economic indicators do not account for other forms of disadvantage that might play some role in ethnic variations in health. That is, the structural context of ethnicity needs to cover a number of additional issues, including:

1   A lifetime perspective – differences are likely to be a consequence of a lifetime accumulation of disadvantage (Davey Smith *et al.* 1997b), which may be particularly important for migrants who will have been through a number of lifecourse transitions, and whose childhood might have involved significant deprivation.

2   Living in a racist society – in addition to being directly discriminated against, ethnic minority people know that they are disadvantaged and excluded compared with others, and hence have a clear perception of their relative disadvantage, which, as Wilkinson (1996) has argued, may well have a significant impact on health.

3   Ecological effects – ethnic minority people are concentrated in particular geographical locations that are quite different from those populated by the white majority (Owen 1994) and there is a growing body of work suggesting that the environmental circumstances may have a direct impact on health over and above individual circumstances (Townsend et al. 1988. Macintyre et al. 1993).

One possible interpretation of the *Fourth National Survey* findings on socio-economic effects is that ethnic inequalities in health can be reduced to socio-economic disadvantage, a position that has been supported by a number of commentators in the field and that raises questions about the legitimacy of using ethnicity as an explanatory variable (Navarro 1990, Sheldon and Parker 1992). This potentially reduces ethnicity to class, and shifts the focus to a concern with how racism leads to the disadvantaged socio-economic positions of 'ethnic minority' groups (see Miles's (1989) comments on this in relation to 'race'), a position that needs additional empirical support. Indeed, as I pointed out in the introduction, others have suggested that regardless of any socio-economic contribution, ethnic inequalities in health cannot be reduced to class, because ethnicity involves far more than this. And, of course, a similar debate is present in the wider literature on ethnicity. Consequently, it is worth considering how ethnicity might be brought back into the picture.

Ethnicity as identity

Smaje (1996) has commented that ethnicity needs to be considered both as identity and as structure. Insofar as ethnic minority status can be equated with various forms of disadvantage, ethnicity is perhaps best viewed as an 'external definition' imposed on ethnic minority people by the majority (Jenkins 1996). In this sense 'ethnicity' is used to signify the 'other', allowing the construction and maintenance of boundaries of exclusion and hierarchical relationships. Although most commentators on such a process of signification have emphasised the role of physical characteristics and the ideological notion of 'race', they recognise that this process also involves cultural characteristics (e.g. Miles 1989: 40, Mason 1996: 201). So, although the biological and cultural can be analytically separated, the ideological representations of 'race' and 'ethnicity' overlap, both representing notions of the inherent, inevitable and inferior biological and cultural characteristics of signified groups (Miles 1996). Indeed such a relationship between these two concepts is clearly present in the health field, as the example on CHD previously cited illustrates (Gupta et al. 1995). In terms of understanding ethnic inequalities in health, this leads to a focus on the process and origins of 'ethnic' signification (perhaps located in the wider demands of capitalism (Miles 1989)), how this leads to the disadvantaged position of ethnic minority groups, and the links between that (material) disadvantage and poor health.

In terms of ethnic identity, however, others have argued that underlying the 'racist categorisation' imposed on ethnic minority groups lie 'real collectivities, common and distinctive forms of thinking and behaviour, of language, custom, religion and so on; not just modes of oppression but modes of being' (Modood 1996: 95). This is the 'internal definition' where individuals and groups establish their own identity (Jenkins 1996). To emphasise this point, some have attempted to draw a distinction between the notions of 'race' and 'ethnicity'. While the former is a boundary of exclusion imposed on a minority group, the latter is a boundary of inclusion, providing a sense of identity and access to social resources. So relations between ethnic groups 'are not necessarily hierarchical, exploitative and conflictual' (Jenkins 1996: 71). In addition, Modood argues, in the context of his analysis and interpretation of data from the *Fourth National Survey*, that ethnic identity provides a political resource:

> Ethnic identity, like gender and sexuality, has become politicised and for some people has become a primary focus of their politics. There is an ethnic assertiveness, arising out of the feelings of not being respected or lacking access to public space, consisting of counterposing 'positive' images against traditional or dominant stereotypes. It is a politics of projecting identities in order to challenge existing power relations; of seeking not just toleration for ethnic difference but also public acknowledgement, resources and representation. (1997: 290)

In this sense a politicised and mobilised ethnic identity can be construed as a new social movement (Scott 1990) occurring in a vacuum provided by the disappearance of a class-based politics (Gilroy 1987).

It is important to recognise that this notion of ethnicity is also some considerable distance from the immutable and reified elements of 'race'. Ethnic identity cannot be considered as fixed, because culture is not an autonomous and static feature in an individual's life. Cultural traditions are historically located, they occur within particular contexts and change over time, place and person. In addition, ethnicity is only one element of identity, whose significance depends on the context within which the individual finds him/herself. For example, gender and class are also important and in certain situations may be more important. The implication is that there are a range of identities that come into play in different contexts and that identity should be regarded as neither secure nor coherent (Hall 1992).

This conception of ethnic identity promises exciting new avenues to follow in the exploration of the relationship between ethnicity and health. Ethnic identity as a source of pride and political power provides an interesting contrast to ethnicity as a sense of discrimination and relative disadvantage, a contrast which could be of great relevance to Wilkinson's (1996) arguments on the relationship between relative deprivation and health. Indeed, there is evidence to suggest that the concentration of ethnic minority groups in particular locations is protective of health (Smaje 1995), perhaps because this allows the development of a community with a strong ethnic identity that enhances social support and reduces the sense of alienation. Such a conception of ethnic identity also allows a contextualised culture to be brought into view. Identification with cultural traditions that may be both harmful and, now we can separate ethnicity from the outsiders' negative definition, beneficial to health, are of obvious importance to health promotion. . . .

Conclusion

Following Smaje (1996), I have suggested that to understand the relationship between ethnicity and health we need to theorise ethnicity adequately. This involves recognising ethnicity as both structure and identity; hence the unresolved answer to this paper's title – although current evidence provides more support for a structural-material explanation (Nazroo 1997a). Insofar as ethnic differences in health can be seen as a consequence of class inequalities, the discussion so far indicates that work on the relationship between ethnicity and health has the potential to be at the leading edge of inequalities in health research.

In terms of the cluster of competing and complementary explanations for inequalities in health, ethnic background is strongly related to most of them. There is variation in the class position of different ethnic minority and majority groups, and this is reflected in differing levels and types of material disadvantage. Ethnic minority groups are discriminated against, and recognise themselves as disadvantaged. This disadvantage not only occurs in the form of a failure to achieve the full potential of economic success, but also in everyday exclusion from elements of white, mainstream, society. Consequently, there is the potential to explore the psychological, as well as material, consequences of disadvantage. Ethnic minority people are concentrated in particular geographical locations and these locations have specific attributes that should allow us to explore both the extent and the nature of an ecological contribution to inequalities in health. Migrant ethnic minority people have been through a number of life-course transitions, some of which would be related to changes in material resources, others to changes in social networks and position in the social hierarchy. Exploring ethnicity also has the potential to allow an examination of the relationship between lifestyle and health and how this might contribute to inequalities. In particular it should allow a dynamic exploration of culture and the relationship between culture, context and class. There are important differences in the social position and expectations of women in different ethnic groups, allowing us to explore issues relating to gender inequalities. And, of course, there are purported differences in the genetic make-up of different ethnic groups.

In terms of methodological issues, exploring ethnic inequalities in health could help resolve a number of problems. Such work relies on indicators of health that are valid across different ethnic groups. Exposing the extent to which the validity of health assessments might vary across ethnic groups raises questions that are applicable to other forms of comparison, such as class and gender. The difficulties of finding indicators of socio-economic status that operate consistently across ethnic groups provides an impetus to be clear about what we mean by the concepts of 'class' and 'material disadvantage' in this research, and how these might apply to other forms of social division, such as gender. And operationalising a concept of ethnicity should make us focus on what we mean by ethnicity and which dimensions of ethnicity might be relevant to inequalities in health.

However, it is worth stepping back for a moment (at least) to reconsider our motives for undertaking work on inequalities in health. In terms of ethnic inequalities in health, I have suggested that motives for the work are related to competing desires to expose the extent and consequences of wider social inequalities, and to uncover aetiological processes, and I have argued that the latter approach has great potential for racialising inequalities in health (Nazroo 1997c). Although at first sight it seems that inequalities in health research are very much concerned with the former, a reconsideration of the preceding sections of this conclusion might suggest otherwise. The tight focus on the pathways that lead from disadvantage to poor health should contribute greatly to our understanding of aetiology, particularly if we meet the requirement that material causes of inequalities in health must be biologically plausible. And there is no reason why such pathways should be identical for different health outcomes. This focus produces an exclusive concern with inequalities in health as an adverse outcome, and how the complex pathways leading to this outcome can be understood and broken. The root cause, wider social inequalities, becomes obscured from view. The policy implications of this are clear, the more difficult and dramatic interventions to address social inequalities can continue to be avoided and health promotion can focus on improving our understanding of pathways and designing interventions along them. Inequalities in health become a problem requiring technical interventions tailored to individual diseases and individual circumstances, they become a problem for individuals rather than a reflection of social malaise. Williams *et al.*'s comments in this regard are worth citing:

> There is a temptation to focus on identified risk factors as the focal point for intervention efforts. In contrast, we indicate that the macrosocial factors and racism are the basic causes of racial differences in health. The risk factors and resources are the surface causes, the current intervening mechanisms. These may change, but as long as the basic causes remain operative, the modification of surface causes alone will only lead to the emergence of new intervening mechanisms to maintain the same outcome. (1994: 36)

We need to remember that we are concerned with (ethnic) inequalities in health because they are a component and a consequence of an inequitable capitalist society, and it is this that needs to be directly addressed.

References

Ahmad, W.I.U., Kernohan, E.E.M. and Baker, M.R. (1989) Influence of ethnicity and unemployment on the perceived health of a sample of general practice attenders, *Community Medicine*, 11, 2, 148–56.

Aspinall, P. (1995) Department of Health's requirement for mandatory collection of data on ethnic group inpatients, *British Medical Journal*, 311, 1006–9.

Bagley, C. (1995) A plea for ignoring race and including insured status in American research reports on social science and medicine, *Social Science and Medicine*, 40, 8, 1017–19.

Balarajan, R. (1995) Ethnicity and variations in the nation's health, *Health Trends*, 27, 4, 114–19.

Balarajan, R. and Soni Raleigh, V. (1995) *Ethnicity and Health in England*. London: HMSO.

Barot, R. (ed.) (1996) *The Racism Problematic: Contemporary Sociological Debates on Race and Ethnicity*. Lewiston: The Edwin Mellen Press.

Beishon, S. and Nazroo, J.Y. (1997) *Coronary Heart Disease: Contrasting the Health Beliefs and Behaviours of South Asian Communities in the UK*. London: Health Education Authority.

Bhopal, R.S. (1997) Is research into ethnicity and health racist, unsound, or important science? *British Medical Journal*, 314, 1751–6.

Brown, C. (1984) *Black and White Britain: the Third PSI Survey*. London: Heinemann.

Brown, C. and Ritchie, J. (1981) *Focussed Enumeration: the Development of a Method for Sampling Ethnic Minority Groups*. London: Policy Studies Institute/SCPR.

Chaturvedi, N. and McKeigue, P. (1994) Methods for epidemiological surveys of ethnic minority groups, *Journal of Epidemiology and Community Health*, 48, 107–11.

Davey Smith, G., Shipley, M.J. and Rose, G. (1990) Magnitude and causes of socioeconomic differentials in mortality: further evidence from the Whitehall study, *Journal of Epidemiology and Community Health*, 44, 265.

Davey Smith, G., Blane, D. and Bartley, M. (1994) Explanations for socio-economic differentials in mortality: evidence from Britain and elsewhere, *European Journal of Public Health*, 4, 131–44.

Davey Smith, G., Wentworth, D., Neaton, J., Stamler, R. and Stamler, J. (1996) Socioeconomic differentials in mortality risk among men screened for the Multiple Risk Factor Intervention Trial: II. Black Men, *American Journal of Public Health*, 86, 4, 497–504.

Davey Smith, G., Neaton, J., Wentworth, D., Stamler, R. and Stamler, J. (1997a) Cause-specific and all-cause mortality differentials between black and white men in the United States: men screened for the Multiple Risk Factor Intervention Trial (MRFIT), *Lancet*, 351, March 28, 934–9.

Davey Smith G., Hart, C., Blane, D., Gillis, C. and Hawthorne, V. (1997b) Lifetime socioeconomic position and mortality: prospective observational study, *British Medical Journal*, 314, 547–52.

Fenton, S., Hughes, A. and Hine, C. (1995) Self-assessed health, economic status and origin, *New Community*, 21, 1, 55–68.

Gilroy, P. (1987) *'There Ain't No Black in the Union Jack': the Cultural Politics of Race and Nation*. London: Hutchinson.

Gupta, S., de Belder, A. and O'Hughes, L. (1995) Avoiding premature coronary deaths in Asians in Britain: spend now on prevention or pay later for treatment, *British Medical Journal*, 311, 1035–6.

Hall, S. (1992) The question of cultural identity. In Hall, S., Held, D. and McGrew, T. (eds) *Modernity and its Futures*. Cambridge: Polity Press.

Harding, S. and Maxwell, R. (1977) Differences in mortality of migrants. In Drever, F. and Whitehead, M. (eds) *Health Inequalities: Decennial Supplement No. 15*. London: The Stationery Office.

Heath, A. and Ridge, J. (1983) Social mobility of ethnic minorities, *Journal of Biosocial Science*, supplement, 8, 169–84.

Jenkins, R. (1996) 'Us' and 'Them': ethnicity, racism and ideology. In Barot, R. (ed.) *The Racism Problematic: Contemporary Sociological Debates on Race and Ethnicity*. Lewiston: The Edwin Mellen Press.

Lillie-Blanton, M. and Laveist, T. (1996) Race/ethnicity, the social environment, and health, *Social Science and Medicine*, 43, 1, 83–91.

Lundeberg, O. (1991) Causal explanations for class inequality in health – an empirical analysis, *Social Science and Medicine*, 32, 4, 385–93.

Macintyre, S. (1997) The Black Report and beyond: what are the issues? *Social Science and Medicine*, 44, 6, 723–45.

Macintyre, S., Maciver, S. and Soomans, A. (1993) Area, class and health: should we be focusing on places or people? *Journal of Social Policy*, 22, 2, 213–34.

McKeigue, P., Marmot, M., Syndercombe Court, Y., Cottier, D., Rahman, S. and Riermersma, R. (1988) Diabetes, hyperinsulinaemia, and coronary risk factors in Bangladeshis in East London, *British Heart Journal*, 60, 390–6.

McKeigue, P., Miller, G. and Marmot, M. (1989) Coronary heart disease in South Asians overseas: a review, *Journal of Clinical Epidemiology*, 42, 7, 597–609.

McKeigue, P., Shah, B. and Marmot, M. (1991) Relation of central obesity and insulin resistance with high diabetes prevalence and cardiovascular risk in South Asians, *Lancet*, 337, 382–6.

McKenney, N.R. and Bennett, C.E. (1994) Issues regarding data on race and ethnicity: the Census Bureau experience, *Public Health Reports*, 109, 1, 16–25.

McKenzie, K. and Crowcroft, N.S. (1996) Describing race, ethnicity, and culture in medical research, *British Medical Journal*, 312, 1054.

Marmot, M.G., Adelstein, A.M., Bulusu, L. and OPCS (1984) *Immigrant Mortality in England and Wales 1970–78: Causes of Death by Country of Birth*. London: HMSO.

Mason, D. (1996) Some reflections on the sociology of race and racism. In Barot, R. (ed.) *The Racism Problematic: Contemporary Sociological Debates on Race and Ethnicity*. Lewiston: The Edwin Mellen Press.

Miles, R. (1989) *Racism*. London: Routledge.

Miles, R. (1996) Racism and nationalism in the United Kingdom: a view from the periphery. In Barot, R. (ed.) *The Racism Problematic: Contemporary Sociological Debates on Race and Ethnicity*, Lewiston: The Edwin Mellen Press.

Modood, T. (1996) If races don't exist, then what does? Racial categorisation and ethnic realities. In Barot, R. (ed.) *The Racism Problematic: Contemporary Sociological Debates on Race and Ethnicity*. Lewiston: The Edwin Mellen Press.

Modood, T. (1997) Culture and identity. In Modood, T., Berthoud, R., Lakey, J., Nazroo, J., Smith, P., Virdee, S. and Beishon, S. *Ethnic Minorities in Britain: Diversity and Disadvantage*. London: Policy Studies Institute.

Modood, T., Berthoud, R., Lakey, J., Nazroo, J., Smith, P., Virdee, S. and Beishon, S. (1997) *Ethnic Minorities in Britain: Diversity and Disadvantage*. London: Policy Studies Institute.

Navarro, V. (1990) Race or class versus race and class: mortality differentials in the United States, *Lancet*, Nov. 17, 1238–40.

Nazroo, J.Y. (1997a) *The Health of Britain's Ethnic Minorities: Findings from a National Survey*. London: Policy Studies Institute.

Nazroo, J.Y. (1997b) *Mental Health and Ethnicity: Findings from a National Community Survey*. London: Policy Studies Institute.

Nazroo, N. (1997c) Why do research on ethnicity and health? *Share*, 18, 5–8.

Owen, D. (1994) Spatial variations in ethnic minority groups populations in Great Britain, *Population Trends*, 78, 23–33.

Rogers, R.G. (1992) Living and dying in the USA: socio-demographic determinants of death among blacks and whites, *Demography*, 29, 287–303.

Rudat, K. (1994) *Black and Minority Ethnic Groups in England: Health and Lifestyles*. London: Health Education Authority.

Scott, A. (1990) *Ideology and the New Social Movements*. London: Unwin Hyman.

Senior, P.A. and Bhopal, R. (1994) Ethnicity as a variable in epidemiological research, *British Medical Journal*, 309, 327–30.

Sheldon, T.A. and Parker, H. (1992) Race and ethnicity in health research, *Journal of Public Health Medicine*, 14, 2, 104–10.

Smaje, C. (1995) Ethnic residential concentration and health: evidence for a positive effect? *Policy and Politics*, 23, 3, 251–69.

Smaje, C. (1996) The ethnic patterning of health: new directions for theory and research, *Sociology of Health and Illness*, 18, 2, 139–71.

Smith, D. (1977) *Racial Disadvantage in Britain*. Harmondsworth: Penguin.

Smith, P. and Prior, G. (1997) *The Fourth National Survey of Ethnic Minorities: Technical Report*. London: Social and Community Planning Research.

Sterling, T., Rosenbaum, W. and Weinkam, J. (1993) Income, race and mortality, *Journal of National Medical Association*, 85, 12, 906–11.

Townsend, P. and Davidson, N. (1982) *Inequalities in Health (the Black Report)*. Middlesex: Penguin.

Townsend, P., Phillimore, P. and Beattie, A. (1988) *Health and Deprivation: Inequality and the North*. London: Routledge.

Vågerö, D. and Illsley, R. (1995) Explaining health inequalities: beyond Black and Barker, *European Sociological Review*, 11, 3, 219–39.

Wilkinson, R.G. (1996) *Unhealthy Societies: the Afflictions of Inequality*. London: Routledge.

Williams, D.R., Lavizzo-Mourey, R. and Warren, R.C. (1994) The concept of race and health status in America, *Public Health Reports*, 109, 1, 26–41.

Chapter 12

Sally Macintyre, Kate Hunt and Helen Sweeting

GENDER DIFFERENCES IN HEALTH

Are things really as simple as they seem?

From *Social Science and Medicine,* 42, 1996: 617–24

Introduction

ONE OF THE MOST FREQUENTLY made observations in medical sociology or social epidemiology is that in industrialized countries males tend to die earlier than females but that females tend to have higher rates of morbidity. The following quotations from the authors of the present paper are typical of statements commonly made about such differences:

> It has consistently been reported from developed countries that although male death rates are higher than women's at all ages, women report more symptoms, disability days, use of medications and contacts with the medical profession[1] (p. 15).

> The excess of female over male morbidity in adulthood has been one of the most consistent findings in social science research on health and illness[2] (p. 24).

> Differences in morbidity between men and women are well known . . . females give poorer self evaluation of health, show higher rates of acute illness, have more (but less severe) chronic conditions, use more out-patient services and consume greater amounts of both prescription and non prescription drugs[3] (p. 77).

Very similar summary statements are found in more general discussions of health. For example

> At all ages women experienced, or were more ready to describe, more illness and higher rates of psychosocial malaise than men. This is, of course, an invariable finding in health surveys[4] (p. 50).

> As elsewhere, the findings showed that women reported higher rates of illness at all ages[5] (p. 7).

They are also used to introduce many of the recent articles which examine more specific aspects of gender differences in health, such as amongst older ages,[6,7] at younger ages,[3] in developing countries,[8] amongst people with a specific diagnosis,[9] when seeking to pursue particular explanations for these apparent differences, or when the focus is on structural inequalities amongst women.[10,11] The existence of these gender differences in health is so taken for granted in medical sociology and social epidemiology that it has become

> Standard good practice to present and analyse data separately for men and women . . . this separate treatment of men and women can become routinised to such an extent that all curiosity about differences between men and women seems to disappear[12] (p. 57).

But is the literature on gender differences in health in the developed world really so clear cut? Can we assume that gender differences described in one decade and in one culture are generalizable to other decades and other cultures? Is there any virtue in further descriptive accounts of gender differences in health, or should we be concentrating on explanations for well-established differences? Our original intention in preparing this paper was to further the work on explanations for gender differences, in particular by examining the effect of role occupancy on gender differences by controlling for social class, domestic circumstances and age. However, in examining our own and other recent British data we were struck not by the consistency of a female excess in reported ill health, but by the lack of the pre-dicted female excess, and by the complexity and subtlety of the pattern of gender differences across different measures of health and across the life course.

For example, the British General Household Survey annually asks approxi-mately 25,000 individuals a range of questions, including some about health. Although it is widely believed in Britain that this shows a marked female excess of self-reported longstanding and limiting longstanding illness,[13] this is not the case if one examines the data by age. Table 12.1, for example, shows that in 1992 males were reported as having more longstanding illness in early childhood, and that thereafter up to the age of 74 there was little difference in reported prevalence between males and females; it was only after 75 that there was a female excess of more than 1 per cent. Similarly, Table 12.2 shows, for the same year, a male excess of limiting longstanding illness in childhood, and a small female excess (of 3 per cent) in only two age groups (16–44, the childbearing years, and 75 plus). Given the very large sample size of this study, such 3 per cent differences in reported prevalence may be *statistically* significant, but it is doubtful whether Tables 12.1 and 12.2 can legitimately be interpreted as showing a large, and socially or biologically significant, consistent female excess as is often described. (Table 3.1 in the 1992

Table 12.1 Percentage of males and females reporting longstanding illness by age group. British General Household Survey 1992

| | *Age group* | | | | | | |
	0–4	5–15	16–44	45–64	65–74	75+	Total
Males	15	19	23	42	60	64	31
Females	10	18	24	43	58	67	33

Source: Thomas M., Goddard E., Hickman M. and Hunter P. (1994) *General Household Survey 1992*. Office of Population Censuses and Surveys, HMSO, London.

Table 12.2 Percentage of males and females reporting limiting longstanding illness by age group. British General Household Survey 1992

| | *Age group* | | | | | | |
	0–4	5–15	16–44	45–64	65–74	75+	Total
Males	5	8	10	26	40	49	18
Females	2	7	13	26	38	52	20

Source: Thomas M., Goddard E., Hickman M. and Hunter P. (1994) *General Household Survey 1992*. Office of Population Censuses and Surveys, HMSO, London.

GHS report shows rates by sex and age group since 1972, and although this demonstrates a rising prevalence over time in longstanding and limiting longstanding illness, it does not show variation over time in the male/female differences[14]).

In this paper we therefore address the question: what is the direction and magnitude of gender differences in health, using a variety of measures of health, at different points in the life course in contemporary Britain?

Data and methods

We use two main data sources, the West of Scotland Twenty-07 study (hereafter called Twenty-07), and the Health and Lifestyles Survey (hereafter called HALS).

The Twenty-07 study is a longitudinal study of three age cohorts, aged 15, 35 and 55 when first studied in 1987/8, resident in the Central Clydeside Conurbation, a socially varied but mainly urban area centred on Glasgow in the West of Scotland. The initial sample sizes were around 1000 per cohort. Participants are interviewed in their own homes by nurses trained in interviewing techniques. A wide range of measures of self-reported health, of physical development and functioning, and of personal and social circumstances, has been collected (for further details see[15,16,17]). Thus far the youngest cohort has been re-contacted for interview at 18, and by postal survey at 16 and 21; the older two cohorts were re-interviewed at 39 and 58.

HALS was a national survey of health and lifestyles among adults in Britain, first undertaken in 1984/5. The achieved sample size was 9000 with an age range from 18 upwards. Respondents were interviewed in their own homes, using a similarly wide range of measures of health and social circumstances as the Twenty-07 study (though some of the measures differ slightly between the two studies; for further details see Refs 18 and 4).

In this paper we present data from both studies to check for the consistency (or otherwise) between them in observed relationships between gender, age and a variety of health measures. Because the Twenty-07 study consists of three single age cohorts twenty years apart, and the youngest subjects in HALS are 18, we examine the Twenty-07 subjects at the time of their second interviews (i.e. at 18, 39 and 58), and compare them with HALS subjects in five year age groups (to get sufficient numbers) as close as possible to the Twenty-07 cohorts, i.e. 18–22, 36–40 and 56–60. The numbers in the Twenty-07 cohorts at these ages were: 430 males and 478 females in the youngest, 379 males and 473 females in the middle, and 399 males and 459 females in the oldest cohort. The numbers in the three HALS 'synthetic cohorts' were 364 males and 445 females in the youngest, 423 males and 548 females in the middle, and 312 males and 367 females in the oldest. In order to look in more detail at trends over the life span, we have also looked at the HALS data decade by decade (i.e. teenagers, twenties, thirties etc.) . . .

Results

We first present results for the measures of general health. As Table 12.3 shows, although in both studies the proportions reporting their health as being 'fair' or 'poor' for their age are higher among women in most age groups, these differences do not reach statistical significance except among the 18 year olds in Twenty-07. There were no significant gender differences in the percentages reporting any long-standing nor any limiting longstanding illness at any age for either study.

Turning now to the experience of particular symptoms in the past month, as Table 12.4 demonstrates, if we simply compare mean number of symptoms, we find that in both data sets there is a consistent and significant female excess at all ages examined. However, when the symptoms are categorized as either 'malaise' or 'physical' a different picture emerges: a female excess in total 'malaise' symptoms at all ages in both studies ($P < 0.001$), but in 'physical' symptoms only at 39 years in Twenty-07 ($P < 0.05$) and at 56–60 years in HALS ($P < 0.001$).

This is demonstrated in more detail in Table 12.5 which shows the patterns of sex differences for each of the 18 symptoms reported. 'Worrying', 'nerves', 'always tired', 'headaches', 'constipation' and 'fainting or dizziness' show the most consistent female excess, followed by 'difficulty concentrating', 'sleeping problems' and 'bladder or kidney problems'. Two symptoms show a significant female excess in only one study at a single age: 'sickness, nausea or stomach trouble' (among 18 year olds in Twenty-07) and 'trouble with eyes' (among 56–60 year olds in HALS). In

Table 12.3 Percentage of men and women at three ages reporting (a) health as 'fair' or 'poor' for own age, (b) any longstanding illness and (c) limiting longstanding illness. Twenty-07 Study and Health and Lifestyles Survey

	Twenty-07				Health and Lifestyles			
	Age	Males, %	Females, %	Sig.	Age	Males, %	Females, %	Sig.
Health 'fair' or 'poor'	18	35.9	43.6	*	18–22	28.8	34.0	
	39	20.1	24.1		36–40	19.7	20.7	
	58	33.1	29.5		56–60	35.3	37.1	
Any longstanding illness	18	17.4	17.4		18–22	19.2	14.6	
	39	46.4	44.8		36–40	21.7	22.4	
	58	70.2	71.7		56–60	46.0	40.5	
Limiting longstanding illness	18	10.7	11.9		18–22	8.0	7.0	
	39	29.3	30.9		36–40	8.7	9.3	
	58	53.1	50.3		56–60	25.9	27.2	

Note: * $P < 0.05$.

Table 12.4 Mean number of symptoms reported at three ages. Twenty-07 Study and Health and Lifestyles Survey

		Twenty-07				Health and Lifestyles			
	Age	Males, %	Females, %	Sig.	Age	Males, %	Females, %	Sig.
All symptoms	18	2.80	3.56	***	18–22	1.98	2.64	***
	39	2.07	2.62	***	36–40	2.04	2.81	***
	58	2.77	3.40	***	56–60	2.61	3.86	***
'Malaise' symptoms	18	0.72	1.02	***	18–22	1.06	1.30	***
	39	0.65	0.92	***	36–40	0.56	1.02	***
	58	0.80	1.16	***	56–60	0.73	1.30	***
'Physical' symptoms	18	1.33	1.43		18–22	1.02	1.09	
	39	0.69	0.83	*	36–40	0.88	0.95	
	58	1.09	1.17		56–60	1.07	1.42	***

Note: *** $p < 0,001$; *P 0.05.

contrast, two symptoms, 'palpitations' and 'trouble with ears' show a male excess among 58 year olds in Twenty-07, while in both studies the excess reporting 'stiff or painful joints' shifts from males at younger ages to females at older ages. Finally, 'back trouble', 'colds or flu', 'sinus, catarrh or blocked nose' and 'persistent cough' show no significant gender differences at any age in either study. . . .

Table 12.5 Patterns of sex differences for 'malaise' and 'physical' symptoms reported at three ages. Twenty-07 Study and Health and Lifestyles Survey

		Twenty-07				Health and Lifestyles		
	Age	Males, %	Females, %	Sig.	Age	Males, %	Females, %	Sig.
'Malaise' symptoms								
Worrying	18	8.4	18.8	***	18–22	13.7	24.3	***
	39	7.4	14.8	**	36–40	10.2	24.8	***
	58	10.8	20.7	***	56–60	16.2	30.7	***
Nerves	18	6.8	12.6	**	18–22	6.3	10.6	*
	39	13.2	21.1	**	36–40	2.8	11.9	***
	58	15.8	22.7	*	56–60	8.3	16.3	**
Difficulty	18	13.0	14.2		18–22	11.5	12.4	
concentrating	39	7.4	12.5	*	36–40	9.0	15.0	**
	58	9.5	13.7		56–60	9.3	18.2	**
Always tired	18	23.5	33.3	**	18–22	20.9	32.6	***
	39	15.0	22.6	**	36–40	18.4	31.2	***
	58	20.6	23.1		56–60	19.5	26.6	*
Sleeping	18	20.9	22.8		18–22	16.5	23.1	*
problems	39	21.6	20.5		36–40	16.5	19.0	
	58	23.1	35.5	***	56–60	19.2	37.8	***
'Physical' symptoms								
Headaches	18	26.3	45.4	***	18–22	24.7	40.0	***
	39	25.9	43.3	***	36–40	26.5	38.7	***
	58	17.3	33.1	***	56–60	17.6	31.5	***
Constipation	18	0.9	11.1	***	18–22	3.6	9.2	**
	39	3.2	14.2	***	36–40	2.4	10.4	***
	58	6.8	11.5	*	56–60	3.8	12.8	***
Fainting or	18	4.9	10.9	**	18–22	5.5	10.1	*
dizziness	39	2.1	6.1	**	36–40	1.7	7.3	***
	58	5.8	8.3		56–60	6.7	8.4	
Bladder or	18	0.0	3.1	***	18–22	0.8	4.7	**
kidney	39	1.8	5.1	*	36–40	1.7	2.9	
problems	58	8.0	7.8		56–60	3.8	5.2	
Sickness/nausea/	18	13.7	24.1	***	18–22	9.6	9.7	
stomach	39	3.2	4.2		36–40	17.7	14.6	
trouble	58	3.0	5.4		56–60	19.8	20.4	
Trouble with	18	13.5	15.7		18–22	11.0	14.8	
eyes	39	8.7	5.9		36–40	9.0	11.3	
	58	10.0	9.8		56–60	9.9	22.3	***
Palpitations	18	4.7	6.9		18–22	5.8	6.1	
	39	5.5	7.8		36–40	6.9	8.8	
	58	16.8	11.8	*	56–60	18.8	21.7	

Trouble with	18	7.7	10.0		18–22	5.2	5.8	
ears	39	6.6	7.0		36–40	6.4	5.7	
	58	16.5	9.6	**	56–60	12.5	13.0	
Stiff/painful	18	28.1	20.5	**	18–22	9.1	6.5	
joints	39	16.6	16.3		36–40	13.7	15.0	
	58	33.8	43.1	**	56–60	31.6	39.1	*
Back trouble	18	15.6	15.9		18–22	12.4	14.2	
	39	20.3	17.8		36–40	15.6	18.1	
	58	20.3	25.5		56–60	18.8	24.5	
Colds or flu	18	45.0	48.1		18–22	43.1	45.2	
	39	14.2	15.9		36–40	34.0	30.3	
	58	14.8	14.2		56–60	31.3	29.6	
Sinus, catarrh/	18	37.5	34.3		18–22	21.2	16.0	
blocked nose	39	17.9	18.4		36–40	21.3	19.7	
	58	19.3	20.7		56–60	14.1	19.8	
Persistent	18	9.1	11.1		18–22	8.0	10.3	
cough	39	6.9	5.5		36–40	8.3	8.8	
	58	12.0	10.0		56–60	12.1	12.8	

Note: Significance of male–female difference, *P <0.05, **P <0.01, ***P <0.001.

Discussion

Although like many other medical sociologists all three authors of this paper are on record as stating as a matter of known fact that females consistently report higher levels of ill health than men, we have found on more detailed inspection of two recent British data sets that the pattern is in fact more complicated than this. The direction and magnitude of sex differences in health vary according to the particular symptom or condition in question, and according to the phase of the life cycle. Female excess is only consistently found across the life span for the more psychological manifestations of distress, and is far less apparent, or reversed, for a number of physical symptoms and conditions.

This finding might not surprise members of the general public, or clinicians dealing with more specific diseases, who might expect sex differences in exposure to health risks to vary between different types of risk and between different parts of the life cycle, problems relating to reproduction to show a female excess in the childbearing years, and hormonal differences to show different effects before and after the menopause. What is perhaps surprising is the predominance for so long within medical sociology and social epidemiology of a relatively undifferentiated model of sex differences, with the hypothesis of female over-reporting or willingness to accept the sick role usually being assumed to apply across most or all conditions.

We wish to suggest that, even when one focuses on commonly used measures (such as self-assessed health, aspects of mental health, or use of health services), the 'story' about gender differences in health as presented in much recent sociological and epidemiological literature has become oversimplified, and that overgeneralization has become the norm, with inconsistencies and complexities in patterns of gender differences in health being overlooked. In the face of an apparently clear pattern, there has been a tendency to downplay (or maybe not even report) data that conflict with rather than confirm the general pattern (thus fitting Thomas Kuhn's model of scientific development, in which anomalies can be accommodated for a considerable period of time without disturbing the dominant scientific paradigm.[19]

We do not deny that there is substantial evidence of gender differences in a wide range of health outcomes during much of adult life in industrialized countries. Verbrugge, for example, has reported that of 67 different measures of health status and behaviour amongst a sample of white adults in Detroit, U.S.A., 60 demonstrated higher morbidity and health care use among women ($P < 0.10$), with 42 of these differences significant at conventional levels of significance ($P < 0.05$). One of those to show a difference was self-ratings of health, with women rating their health as poorer than men's[20] (p. 286). Haavio-Manila has reported a female excess of longstanding illness and anxiety in Denmark, Norway and Sweden,[21] and Wingard et al. have reported a female excess of functional disability and heart disease morbidity among the Alameda County population in California.[22] Such findings fit the conventional wisdom. However, inspection of other research during the last decade reveals much that does not fit the dominant paradigm, and much that is consistent with our own data. . . .

We suggest that, given the data we have presented above which indicate that the picture of 'female excess' in ill health is more complex than it is sometimes described, the whole topic of gender differences in health warrants periodic re-examination. The research which has accumulated over the last decade or so seems increasingly to support the view that gender differences in health are rooted in social roles, against the backdrop of some male biological disadvantages.[23] There have been many changes in gender roles in the last few decades, and some of these may produce changes in men's and women's experiences of health and illness; but the predominance of the 'women's higher morbidity' paradigm may have prevented people from noticing the 'anomalies', such as those cited above, which might provide evidence about the consequences of such changes.

How can we account for the fact that our data show a more complex picture of gender differences, and a picture of less consistent female excess in illness, than is often suggested in the literature? One possibility is that female/male differences in health have changed over time (in the same way that male/female differences in life expectancy may have changed over time[12]), so that whereas there was once a female excess, there is now less of one. Certainly in Finland women's excess reporting of restricted activity declined between 1964 and 1976,[21] and in the U.S.A. women's excess of reported chronic conditions decreased between 1957 and 1972.[24] There have been changes in the participation of men and women in education, employment, recreation and domestic life, and although it seems unlikely that changes in the gendered allocation of roles in Britain have already been sufficiently widespread to alter the expected pattern across all three age groups, it would be interesting to explore the ways in which gender differences in health vary across different historical periods and social settings within Britain.

Another possibility is that self-reported illness rates do not differ as much between men and women in Britain as they do elsewhere, but the data from Finland, the U.S.A. and Canada[21,25,26] suggest that our findings are not unique to Britain. Again, it would be interesting systematically to examine health survey findings from different societies; for example, from northern, southern and eastern Europe, north and south America, and various African and Asian cultures. Gender differences in health may vary, as do gender differences in life expectancy,[12] between societies at different stages of economic and industrial development and with differing religious or cultural attitudes towards appropriate gender roles. There are likely to be differences between more and less developed countries, given that in the latter health is still threatened by infectious disease and by unregulated environmental and occupational exposures, and the penalties of reproduction are higher because of pressures towards early and repeated childbearing;[27,28] there are also likely to be differences between developed countries depending on labour market and other conditions, as shown for the Nordic countries.[21]

Thus, in conclusion, we support those who have argued that summarizing the morbidity experiences of men and women is "exceedingly difficult",[29] and those who have shown that gender differences in health vary by age, morbidity measure, and social context.[21,22,24] Despite their arguments and findings, the picture of near universal female excess morbidity has tended to persist in the general literature, taking on the characteristics of a dominant scientific paradigm with anomalous or inconsistent findings not being noticed or seriously discussed.[19] We believe that if we are to make progress . . . towards understanding the processes (whether social, psychological or biological) which produce or maintain gender differences in health, it is important to pay attention to the social and historical context of our observations, and to take a more differentiated age-specific and condition-specific view of 'health' when examining differences between the sexes. This is not a new recommendation[21,22,24] but seems worth repeating since previous suggestions to this effect do not seem to have had much impact on the general medical sociological or epidemiological literature.

References

1   Macintyre S. Gender differences in the perceptions of common cold symptoms. *Soc. Sci. Med.* **36**, 15, 1993.
2   Annandale E. and Hunt K. Masculinity, femininity and sex: an exploration of their relative contribution to explaining gender differences in health. *Soc. Hlth Illness* **12**, 24, 1990.
3   Sweeting H. Reversals of fortune? Sex differences in health in childhood and adolescence. *Soc. Sci. Med.* **40**, 77, 1994.
4   Blaxter M. *Health and Lifestyles.* Routledge, London, 1990.
5   Miles A. *Women, Health and Medicine.* Open University Press, Milton Keynes, 1991.
6   Johnson R. J. and Wolinsky F. D. Gender, race and health: the structure of health status among older adults. *Gerontologist* **34**, 24, 1994.
7   Rahman O., Strauss J., Gertler P., Ashley D. and Fox K. Gender differences in adult health: an international comparison. *Gerontologist* **34**, 463, 1994.
8   Fuller T. D., Edwards J. N., Sermsri S. and Vorakitphokatorn S. Gender and health: some Asian evidence. *J. Hlth Soc. Behav.* **34**, 252, 1993.

9   Anson O., Paran E., Neumann L. and Chernichovsky D. Gender differences in health perception and their predictors. *Soc. Sci. Med.* **36**, 419, 1993.

10   Arber S. Gender and class inequalities in health: understanding the differentials. In *Health Inequalities in European Countries* (Edited by Fox J.), pp. 250–279. Gower Company, Aldershot, 1989.

11   Macran S., Clarke L., Sloggett A. and Bethune A. Women's socio-economic status and self-assessed health: identifying some disadvantaged groups. *Soc. Hlth Illness* **16**, 182, 1994.

12   Macintyre S. Gender differences in longevity and health in Eastern and Western Europe. In *Locating Health: Sociological and Historial Explanations* (Edited by Platt S., Thomas H., Scott S. and Williams G.), pp. 57–74. Avebury, Aldershot, 1993.

13   Macintyre S. The patterning of health by social position in contemporary Britain: directions for sociological research. *Soc. Sci. Med.* **23**, 393, 1986.

14   Thomas M., Goddard E., Hickman M. and Hunter P. *General Household Survey, 1992.* Office of Population Censuses and Surveys, HMSO, London, 1994.

15   Macintyre S., Annandale E, Ecob R., Ford G., Hunt K., Jamieson B., Maciver S., West P. and Wyke S. The West of Scotland Twenty-07 Study: health in the community. In *Readings for a New Public Health* (Edited by Martin C. J. and McQueen D. V.), pp. 56–74. Edinburgh University Press, Edinburgh, 1989.

16   Ford G., Ecob R., Hunt K., Macintyre S. and West P. Patterns of class inequality in health through the lifespan: class gradients at 15, 35 and 55 years in the West of Scotland. *Soc. Sci. Med.* **39**, 1037, 1994.

17   West P., Ford G., Hunt K., Macintyre S. and Ecob R. How sick is the West of Scotland? Age specific comparisons with national datasets on a range of health measures. *Scottish Med. J.* **39**, 101, 1994.

18   Cox B. D., Blaxter M., Buckle A. L. J., Fenner, N. P., Golding J. F., Gore M., Huppert F. A., Nickson J., Roth M., Stark J., Wadsworth M. E. J. and Whichelow M. *The Health and Lifestyle Survey: Preliminary Report.* The Health Promotion Research Trust, London, 1987.

19   Kuhn T. S. *The Structure of Scientific Revolutions.* Chicago University Press, Chicago, 1970.

20   Verbrugge L. M. The twain meet: empirical explanations of sex differences in health and mortality. *J. Hlth Soc. Behav.* **30**, 282, 1989.

21   Haavio-Manila E. Inequalities in health and gender. *Soc. Sci. Med.* **22**, 141, 1986.

22   Wingard D. L., Cohn B. A., Kaplan G. A., Cirillo P. M. and Cohen R. D. Sex differentials in morbidity and mortality risks examined by age and cause in the same cohort. *Am. J. Epidemiol.* **130**, 601, 1989.

23   Verbrugge L. M. Unveiling higher morbidity for men. In *Social Structures and Human Lives. Volume I* (Edited by Riley M. W., Huber B. J. and Hess B. B.), pp. 138–160. Sage, London, 1988.

24   Verbrugge L. M. Females and illness: recent trends in the U.S.A. *J. Hlth Soc. Behav.* **17**, 387, 1976.

25   Seeman T. Personal communication. Department of Epidemiology and Public Health, Yale University, 1995.

26   Kandrack M. A., Grant K. R. and Segall A. Gender differences in health related behaviour: some unanswered questions. *Soc. Sci. Med.* **32**, 579, 1991.

27   Vlassof C. Gender inequalities in the Third World: uncharted ground. *Soc. Sci. Med.* **39**, 1249, 1994.

28   Okojie C. E. E. Gender inequalities in the Third World. *Soc. Sci. Med.* **39**, 1237, 1994.

29   Clarke J. N. Sexism, feminism and medicalism: a decade review of literature on gender and illness. *Soc. Hlth Illness* **5**, 63, 1983.

PART THREE

Professional and patient interaction

A S WE HAVE INDICATED IN our General Introduction, whatever the influences of social factors on health may be, the role of *health services* remains central to modern societies and to the experience of health. While many health problems are dealt with outside of the health sector, the consumption and use of health services means that medical sociology is bound to pay continued attention to their influence, both as the site of professional power and of key interactions. As with the first two Parts of the Reader, our selection reflects the changing sociological perspectives of research, as they confront changes in health care organisation and delivery.

However, the first extract is a necessary exception, taken as it is from one of the most influential books in medical sociology, namely Freidson's *Profession of Medicine*. In the extract reprinted here, Freidson outlines his approach to medical practice and to illness experience, in so far as it is shaped by interactions within the medical arena. Though the self-image of the medical profession is of a disinterested and benign social institution, with an accepted authority in society, Freidson shows that social control of illness and patients, as well as the defining and treatment of illness, lies at the heart of the medical encounter. Doctors define what the 'real' nature of illness is, whether or not it coincides with the views of the patient. Moreover, the medical view of illness becomes part of the established order, culturally sanctioned and, for Freidson, imposed on the patient. In his depiction of the negotiations between doctors and patients Freidson argues that though the conflict may not be overt, the 'clash of perspectives' between patients and doctors is an ever present potential. The different viewpoints between patients and doctors can 'never be synonymous' for Freidson. It is for this reason that Freidson argues for a critical view of the power of the medical profession and the need to limit its dominant position, whether in the clinic or in society as a whole.

Although the main thrust of Freidson's analysis remains relevant to the study of the medical profession, the position of doctors and other health care personnel has obviously changed considerably since Freidson first published *Profession of Medicine* in 1970 in the USA. One of the most important changes has been that of nurses. In Freidson's analysis nurses were seen to have lost their earlier autonomy, becoming increasingly subordinate to doctors. In the second extract in this part, Annandale identifies additional difficulties facing nurses in contemporary practice. During the 1990s in particular, nurses have had to deal with the growth of organisational pressures involving increasing accountability, as well as consumerist pressures coming from a more assertive patient body. Drawing on research in two UK hospital trusts, Annandale examines the strategies nurses employ in managing the 'risk culture' that these pressures create. Fears that current actions may be judged as inadequate if called to account at a later date have, according to Annandale, created an acutely contradictory climate for practice. As with other professional groups, successful moves to deal with such pressures may create forms of defensive practice that in the long term serve the interests of neither patients, nor the nurses themselves.

The issue of consumerism raised by Annandale, with respect to nursing practice, is dealt with in a more general context in the next extract by Lupton. Here, Lupton looks at the recent vogue for consumerism in health care as part of a more general cultural setting in which (lay) people are expected to be self-reflexive and sceptical of expert knowledge. Drawing on interview data with sixty people in Sydney, Australia, Lupton finds that consumerism and a more passive role (of the sort depicted by Freidson in his approach to patients in the medical encounter) are drawn upon variously and sometimes simultaneously by patients in their dealings with doctors. Emotional and bodily needs among patients, as much as asymmetry in knowledge, may cut across more rational and reflective consumerism in health care. From this viewpoint Lupton concludes that consumerism has limited applicability, at least in the doctor–patient relationship. Even where complementary therapies are 'consumed' by patients, Lupton shows that this does not necessarily mean a rejection of orthodox medical practice.

In the next extract another important feature of modern medical practice is examined – especially relevant, though often neglected in societies such as the UK where public provision of health care is dominant – that of doctor–patient interactions in private medicine. Though private medical care has been of minor significance in such systems, it is growing, and of course is of great importance in systems that are based on a fee for service or on private insurance. More importantly, the study of private practice in a social context such as that of the UK can throw important light on supposed absences in the public sector. Silverman's study of two oncology clinics set out to examine what it was that private patients were 'buying', in contrast to the 'standard, somewhat impersonal product with a minimum of choice' offered by systems such as the UK's National Health Service. Silverman concludes that patients buy a personalised service, where care is 'personally orchestrated' and where the best features of general practice are combined with high quality interventions for life-threatening conditions. However, such 'orchestration' may at times be used as a device that obscures the lack of resource available in a private setting – for example, the inability to sort out a patient's treatment programme rapidly. Private patients may also be cut off from 'peer group relations' that may be available in an NHS clinic and which may act as a resource for such patients.

The trade-offs between a 'tried and tested', if bureaucratic, form of doctor–patient encounter might also help to explain the growth and use of complementary medicine, the subject of the next extract. In studies drawn upon by Cant and Sharma, it is possible to assess the attractions of complementary therapy and what it reveals about health and health care in contemporary settings. In part it may be that 'consumers' feel – rightly or wrongly – that complementary medicine will, at the very least, do them no harm. But perhaps the most cited attraction of complementary medicine is that it holds out the prospect of offering more time and the opportunity to discuss problems in depth. Indeed, Cant and Sharma argue that many initial encounters with a UK complementary practitioner last for over an hour. In addition to this, the image of alternative medicine includes the possibility of being treated in a more 'holistic' manner and of being included as a partner in decisions about treatment. Such an expectation and its realisation in practice could in turn create ambiguities in the relationship, such that some patients expect to be treated in an overly personal manner or be contacted when they have been admitted to hospital. Cant and Sharma link such expectations, and thus the attractions of alternative medicine, to a culture which is more disillusioned with expertise and in which more 'reflexive selves' develop a wider set of ideas for dealing with bodily and emotional distress.

The question of partnership in the medical encounter and in decision making concerning treatment brings us to the final extract in this part of the Reader, that of Cathy Charles and her colleagues. In this article Charles *et al.* revisit their earlier work and develop a framework that covers different models of decision making: paternalistic, informed and shared. Each of these models contains different ways of dealing with information exchange, deliberating on the implications of information and the nature of treatment options, and deciding which treatment to choose. Paternalistic approaches reproduce Freidson's viewpoint of the active and dominant doctor. The informed model almost reverses this pattern by providing the patient with information and expecting the patient to make the final decision. The shared model comes closest to the current UK policy approach to 'partnership', where both doctor and patient share information and mutually agree on the option to be followed. Charles *et al.* make the point that much depends on the 'situated context' in which patients and their doctors are operating. In addition, it is clear that these different models are only analytically separate. They may operate interchangeably in any particular sequence of doctor–patient interaction, and patient preferences may not always be in the direction of partnership, now favoured by politicians. Nonetheless, Charles *et al.* show, as do authors of other articles in this part, that medical practice and the doctor–patient relationship have moved on to a more complex sociological terrain in recent years. Sociological research will undoubtedly thus retain its importance in addressing the issues involved.

Chapter 13

Eliot Freidson

THE SOCIAL ORGANIZATION
OF ILLNESS

From *Profession of Medicine: A Study of the Sociology of Applied Knowledge*, Chicago: University of Chicago Press (1970)

PREVIOUSLY I HAVE discussed the variables that seem to be important for predicting the likelihood that members of a population will enter the medical consulting room. Some of the variables are similar to those predicting the likelihood that members of a population will buy a new product or adopt a new innovation.[1] In spite of that similarity, though, there are essential differences between the use of a professionally controlled service or product and the use of a commercial product – differences that stem from the status of the profession. The status of the profession allows it to shape the official recognition of need for service as well as the way that need will be organized by the service it controls. It is in this sense that the social organization of treatment may be seen to create the conditions by which the experience of being ill, the relationships one has with others when ill, and the very life of the sick person become organized. It is these conditions and these consequences that I wish to focus on in this chapter. I wish to show how, once one enters the professional domain, that domain imposes organization on the experience and manifestation of illness . . . .

---

[1] For a summary of much of this material see Everett Rogers, *Diffusion of Innovation* (New York: The Free Press of Glencoe, 1962).

The institutional organization of responses to illness

. . . In the process whereby the treatment institution can impose its own organization on the social behavior connected with illness, two prominent characteristics
facilitate staff control. First, the patient may be isolated from the lay community
and those of his (sic) associates who are concerned with his welfare. Contact with the
lay world is carefully rationed where possible. While there may be medical reasons
for such isolation, it is frequently a matter of administrative convenience, minim-
izing "bother" for the staff more than protecting the patient from disturbance. The
social consequences are to isolate the patient from the sources of social leverage that
supported him while in ambulatory consultation and that could sustain his resistance
to the therapeutic routine in the institution. Second, and more important, is the
tendency of the staff of all such institutions to carefully avoid giving the patient or
his lay associates much information about the illness and what is supposed to be done
for it. Virtually every study of patients in hospital points out how ignorant of
condition, prognosis, and the medically prescribed regimen are both the patients
and their relatives and how reluctant is the staff to give such information.[2] In
Davis' words, describing staff behavior toward parents of children stricken with
poliomyelitis, the parents' questions were "hedged, evaded, rechannelled, or left
unanswered."[3]

As Davis noted in his analysis, the staff's reluctance to give information is often
explained as a desire to avoid an emotional scene with the parents. Sometimes, as
Glaser and Strauss note in the case of the dying patient, the staff withholds information in the belief, based on "clinical experience," that it will protect the patient
and his family from shock and excessive grief.[4] Sometimes this reluctance to give
information is explained by a genuine uncertainty, so that no really reliable information is available. However, as Davis has noted in detail, "in many illnesses . . .
'uncertainty' is to some extent feigned by the doctor for the purpose of gradually
getting the patient ultimately to accept or put up with a state-of-being that initially is
intolerable to him."[5] Whatever the reason, however, the net effect of the withholding of information is to minimize the possibility that the patient can exercise much
control over the way he is treated. If he does not know that he is supposed to have a
yellow pill every four hours, he cannot comment on the fact that it is sometimes
overlooked and insist on getting it regularly. And if he does not know that his
condition normally responds to a given treatment in a week, he cannot insist on

---

[2]   See the detailed analysis in Raymond S. Duff and August B. Hollingshead, *Sickness and Society* (New
      York: Hanpes and Row, 1968) Chapter 13.
[3]   Fred Davis, *Passage Through Crisis: Polio Victims and Their Families* (Indianapolis: Bobbs-Merrill Co.,
      1963), p. 64. For other observations on the extent to which patients are kept ignorant, see Ailon
      Shiloh, "Equalitarian and Hierarchal Patients," *Medical Care*, III (1965), 87–95.
[4]   Barney G. Glaser and Anselm L. Strauss, *Awareness of Dying* (Chicago: Aldine Publishing Co., 1965),
      pp. 29ff.
[5]   Davis, *op. cit.*, p. 67, and see Fred Davis, "Uncertainty in Medical Prognosis, Clinical and Func-
      tional," *American Journal of Sociology*, LXVI (1960), 41–47.

a consultation after several weeks have passed without change in condition or treatment.[6]

A great deal more can be said about the institutional shaping of illness, particularly in qualification of the point I have been trying to make here. Not all treatment institutions are the same, nor are all patients or treatment staffs. For example, the rehabilitation institution studied by Roth and Eddy[7] had a particularly powerful influence on the course of illness behavior because its patients were largely supported by public funds and lacked effective advocates from the community outside. They rarely, therefore, "got well enough" to leave. This helplessness is somewhat tempered by the fact that in rehabilitation, tuberculosis, and other institutions, many patients have similar illnesses and are in a position to socialize and organize each other. When these conditions exist, the patients are able to develop a common conception of the way their illness should be managed and to generate the influence required to impose some of their own conceptions on the staff.[8] Furthermore, institutions can be dominated by a staff ideology which specifies that the patient participate in his treatment. In fact, there are a number of patterns of interaction that reflect the degree of influence and activity allowed the patient in the course of his treatment and that express the meaning of his illness to himself and to those treating him.

Patterns of interaction in treatment

I have already suggested that when in treatment in a client-dependent practice, interaction will be fairly free between doctor and patient, the latter initiating and controlling some part of it. Conversely, when in treatment in a colleague-dependent practice, interaction will likely be lesser in quantity and less free, the physician initiating and controlling the greater part of it. By the time the patient reaches the latter practice, which often involves institutionalization, he has been rendered relatively helpless and dependent, perhaps, as Goffman suggests, already demoralized by a sense of having been stripped of some part of his normal identity.[9] In other cases he has been rendered helpless by his failure to find help on his own or by the way his physical illness has incapacitated him.

A second element that seems to be able to predict some part of the quality of the interaction between patient and physician lies in what physicians consider to be

[6] See James K. Skipper, Jr., "Communication and the Hospitalized Patient," in James K. Skipper, Jr., and Robert C. Leonard, eds, *Social Interaction and Patient Care* (Philadelphia: J. B. Lippincott Co., 1965), pp. 75–77.

[7] See Julius Roth and Elizabeth Eddy, *Rehabilitation for the Unwanted* (New York: Atherton Press, 1967).

[8] For a very useful discussion of the implications of such characteristics, see Stanton Wheeler, "The Structure of Formally Organized Socialization Settings," in O. G. Brim, Jr., and Stanton Wheeler, *Socialization After Childhood* (New York: John Wiley & Sons, 1966), pp. 53–116.

[9] See Erving Goffman, "The Moral Career of the Mental Patient," in his *Asylums* (New York: Anchor Books, 1961), pp. 125–161. In the context of the succeeding discussion of interaction, it is also appropriate to cite, in the same book, pp. 321–386, "The Medical Model and Mental Hospitalization."

the demands of proper treatment for a given illness. This is to say, all that doctors do is not the same and does not require the same type of interaction. Following Szasz and Hollander's typology of doctor–patient relationships[10] but reversing the direction of analysis, we may note that under some circumstances – as in surgery and electroconvulsive therapy – the patient must be thoroughly immobilized and passive, wholly submissive to the activity of the physician. The work itself requires such minimal interaction: attendants, straps, anesthesia, and other forms of restraint are employed to enforce the requirement of submission. This model for interaction Szasz and Hollander call *activity–passivity*. In it, the patient is a passive object.

The second treatment situation, discussed by most writers as *the* doctor–patient relationship, is one in which the patient's consent to accept advice and to follow it is necessary. Here, the patient "is conscious and has feelings and aspirations of his own. Since he suffers . . . he seeks help and is ready and willing to 'cooperate.' When he turns to the physician, he places [him] . . . in a position of power . . . The more powerful . . . will speak of guidance or leadership and will expect cooperation of the other."[11] The interaction is expected to follow the model of *guidance–cooperation*, the physician initiating more of the interaction than the patient. The patient is expected to do what he is told; he assumes a less passive role than if he were anesthetized but a passive role nonetheless, submissive to medical requirements.

Finally, there is the model of *mutual participation*, found where patients are able or are required to take care of themselves – as in the case of the management of some chronic illnesses like diabetes – and therefore where initiation of interaction comes close to being equal between the two. Here, "the physician does not profess to know exactly what is best for the patient. The search for this becomes the essence of the therapeutic interaction."[12] Obviously, some forms of psychotherapy fall here.

Szasz and Hollander's scheme, however, is defective logically and empirically, for their models represent a continuum of the degree to which the *patient* assumes an *active* role in interaction in treatment without being extended to the logical point where the *physician* assumes a *passive* role. Such a defect reflects the characteristically normative stance of the medical thinker: while the existence of situations where the practitioner more or less does what the patient asks him to do may not be denied, such situations are rejected out of hand as intolerably nonprofessional, non-therapeutic, and nondignified to be conceded for mere logic and dignified by the recognition of inclusion.[13] Logic and fact do, however, require recognition, and they

[10] See Thomas S. Szasz and Mark H. Hollander, "A Contribution to the Philosophy of Medicine," *A.M.A. Archives of Internal Medicine*, XCVII (1956), 585–592.

[11] *Ibid.*, pp. 586–587.

[12] *Ibid.*, p. 589.

[13] This lack of concern for being logically consistent and systematic is characteristic of virtually all writing about the doctor–patient relationship by medical men. Another interesting analysis of the doctor–patient relationship explores other facets to be found in nature but restricts itself to the "pathological." See F. W. Hanley and F. Grunberg, "Reflections on the Doctor–Patient Relationship," *Canadian Medical Association Journal*, LXXXVI (1962), 1022–1024, where nine "syndromes" are constructed out of three stereotypical patients and three stereotypical physicians. So long as medical writers persist in crippling their logic by normative considerations, they cannot expect serious intellectual consideration.

dictate the suggestion of two other patterns of interaction – one in which the patient guides and the physician cooperates, and one in which the patient is active and the physician passive. It is difficult to imagine an empirical instance of the latter possibility, which requires that the physician cease being a consultant, so we may label it "merely" a logical construct. For the former instance, however, we may find empirical examples in a fair number of the interactions in client-dependent practices, particularly where the practice is economically unstable and the clientele of high economic, political, and social status.[14]

As I have noted, what distinguishes Szasz and Hollander's models from those I have added is the fact that they represent patterns of relations with patients that medical practitioners *wish* to establish and maintain on various occasions for various illnesses and patients. Assuming one type of interaction pattern is necessary for the therapist's work to proceed successfully, what social circumstances are prerequisite to its existence and how are they established? When the *activity–passivity* model does not automatically exist by virtue of coma or the like, some of the physician's behavior must be devoted to soothing the patient in order to get him to submit to the straps, injections, face-masks or whatever. The basic prerequisite, however, is *power* as such – sustained by the a priori incapacity of the patient, or by *making* the patient incapacitated. Such power is created by the fact that the individual is, let us say, unconscious and in a coma. In other instances, the exercise of power to overcome resistance when the patient is not in a coma is legitimized by the social identity imputed to the patient: he is just an infant, a cat, a retardate, a psychotic, or in some other way not fully human and responsible and so cannot be allowed to exercise his own choice to withdraw from treatment. Aside from circumstances where the patient's identity legitimizes the exercise of force, this pattern of inter-action is most likely to be found where cultures diverge a great deal. There, few patients voluntarily enter medical consultation: their participation may be required by political power or may be facilitated by the incapacitating force of the disease itself.

The second pattern of interaction, *guidance–cooperation*, is essentially the one most people have in mind when they speak of the doctor–patient relationship. Obviously, its existence is contingent on a process that will bring people into interaction with the therapist in the first place, the process of seeking help that leads to the choice of utilizing one service rather than another. Here, the patient must exercise his own choice. Utilization is not merely something that facilitates establish-ing the relationship; it constitutes one-half of the battle in interaction: to actively choose to utilize a doctor in the first place requires that one in some degree concede his value and authority in advance[15] and that one in some degree already shares the doctor's perspective on illness and its treatment. The problem of interaction in treatment lies in the details of this acceptance, in the concrete areas in which lay and professional cultures converge. The doctor's tool for gaining acceptance is his

---

[14] See Freidson, *Patients' Views of Medical Practice* (New York: Russell Sage Foundation, 1961), pp. 171–191 for historical and contemporary examples of such relationships.
[15] See Theodore Caplow, *The Sociology of Work* (Minneapolis: University of Minnesota Press, 1954), p. 114.

"authority," which is not wholly binding by his incumbency in a formal legal position as expert.[16] Here, to the extent that the patient's culture is congruent with that of the professional, the authority of the latter is likely to be conceded in advance and reinforced in treatment by the fact that what the professional diagnoses and pre-scribes corresponds with what the patient expects and that communication between the two is relatively easy, so that confidence can be established when the professional must make new or unexpected demands on the patient. In this situation, what is problematic most of all is the physician's authority as such: it must be conceded before examination can begin and if treatment is to proceed. It is the *motive* for cooperation. Only secondarily problematic but problematic nonetheless is the capacity of the physician to make his desires for information and cooperation known and the capacity of the patient to understand the physician sufficiently to do as he is told. Essentially, then, faith and confidence on the part of the patient, and authority on the part of the physician, are the critical elements.

Finally, there is the pattern of *mutual participation*. Clearly, the interaction specified by this model requires characteristics on the part of the patient that facilitate communication. Communication is essential in order to determine what is to be done in therapy. Cultural congruence is thus obviously one necessary con-dition for such free interaction. According to Szasz and Hollander, the relationship "requires a more complex psychological and social organization on the part of both participants. Accordingly, it is rarely appropriate for children, or for those persons who are mentally deficient, very poorly educated, or profoundly immature. On the other hand, the greater the intellectual, educational and general experiential similarity between physician and patient the more appropriate and necessary this model of therapy becomes."[17] However, it is not only educational and experiential similarity but also a collaborative *status* that is required. Here the patient is not to merely accept the authority of the doctor; each must accept the other as an equal in the search for a solution to the problem. Deference on the part of either patient or physician is likely to destroy such mutual participation. Thus, status congruence is necessary to the relationship in order that the interaction of each *can* be fairly equal, and the influence of the doctor on the patient will hinge essentially not on physical power or professional authority but on his capacity to *persuade* the patient of the value of his views.[18]

These characterizations of different patterns of interaction may be used to distinguish (1) the needs of different kinds of medical work, (2) the way different kinds of illness are managed, and (3) the problems of practice that arise when the character of the lay community and particularly the lay referral system varies. (1) Veterinary medicine, pediatrics, and surgery are among those practices obviously prone to require the activity–passivity model, though the families of pets and pediatric patients are prone to interfere more than the model predicts. Internal medicine and general practice are among those prone to require the guidance–cooperation model. And verbal psychotherapy as well as rehabilitation and the

---

[16] See Eliot Freidson, *Professional Dominance* (New York: Atherton Press, 1970).

[17] Szasz and Hollander, *op. cit.*, p. 387.

[18] In this sense the influence of the expert rather than the authority of the professional is indicated.

treatment of the chronic diseases are all prone to need the mutual-participation model. (2) Stigmatized illnesses that spoil the identities of the sufferers are prone to be managed by the activity–passivity pattern, as are those with severe trauma, coma, and psychosis, and with patients who are extremely variant in culture or capacity: these characteristics prevent the patient *or* the physician from being socially responsive in treatment. In any single community, most "normal" – which is to say conditionally legitimate – illnesses are prone to be managed by the guidance–cooperation pattern; in those cases not clearly legitimized by lay culture (and so withholding authority from the physician), the mutual-participation pattern is likely to be common and the pattern where the patient guides and the physician cooperates is possible. (3) I might note that the activity–passivity pattern of interaction in treatment is most likely to be found where lay culture diverges greatly from professional culture and where the status of the layman is very low compared to the professional. Where these divergences are lesser, the guidance–cooperation pattern is likely to be found, whereas where both the lay culture and status of the patient are very much like that of the professional, the mutual-participation pattern is likely to be used often.

The conflict underlying interaction

In discussing interaction in treatment, I have adopted here, as elsewhere, a situational approach: I have attempted to discern whether some regularities in situations exist such that, by specifying the situation, we can predict the kinds of people likely to be in it, the kinds of illness, and the kinds and amount of interaction likely to take place. This seems to me to be an eminently useful approach, but we should not lose sight of the fact that it is merely an approach specifying regularities across arrays of individuals – statistical regularities. Furthermore, those regularities are defined as *relative*, not absolute. Nonetheless, it is unwise to assume too much regularity in the interaction in treatment settings. While the patient can be more or less excluded from assuming an active role in interaction, he can rarely be wholly excluded. He can at least, as do low-status and poorly educated patients everywhere, practice evasive techniques and act stupid in order to avoid some of what is expected of him. And while the patient can be involved in mutual participation by virtue of his similarity to the therapist, he is never wholly cooperative. Given the viewpoints of two worlds, lay and professional, in interaction, they can never be wholly synonymous. And they are always, if only latently, in conflict. Indeed, I wish to suggest that the most faithful perspective on interaction in treatment is one reflecting such conflict in standpoint, not on assuming an identity of purpose to be discovered by better education or a disposition to cooperate sometimes hidden by misunderstanding or by failure to cooperate.[19]

---

[19] For a more extended analysis of the conflict see Freidson, *Patients' Views, op. cit.*, pp. 171–191. And see the discussion in Carl Gersuny, "Coercion Theory and Medical Sociology," *Case Western Reserve Journal of Sociology*, II (1968), 14–20.

Hence, interaction in treatment should be seen as a kind of negotiation as well as a kind of conflict. This point is suggested in Balint's psychiatric sense that the patient is using his symptoms to establish a relationship with the physician[20] but more particularly in the sense of negotiation of separate conditions and of separate perspectives and understandings. The patient is likely to want more information than the doctor is willing to give him – more precise prognoses, for example, and more precise instructions. As Roth's study indicated, just as the doctor struggles to find ways of withholding some kinds of information, so will the patient be struggling to find ways of gaining access to, or inferring such information.[21] Similarly, just as the doctor has no alternative but to handle his cases conventionally (which is to say, soundly), so the patient will be struggling to determine whether or not he is the exception to conventional rules. And finally, professional healing being an organized practice, the therapist will be struggling to adjust or fit any single case to the convenience of practice (and other patients), while the patient will be struggling to gain a mode of management more specifically fitted to him as an individual irrespective of the demands of the system as a whole. These conflicts in perspective and interest are built into the interaction and are likely to be present to some degree in every situation. They are at the core of interaction, and they reflect the general structural characteristics of illness and its professional treatment as a function of the relations between two distinct worlds, ordered by professional norms. . . .

---

[20] See Michael Balint, *The Doctor, His Patient and the Illness* (New York: International Universities Press, 1957), *passim*.

[21] See Roth, *Timetables, Structuring the Passage of Time in Hospital Treatment and Other Careers* (Indianapolis: Bobbs-Merrill Co., 1963) and Julius A. Roth, "Information and the Control of Treatment in Tuberculosis Hospitals," in Eliot Freidson, ed., *The Hospital in Modern Society* (New York: The Free Press of Glencoe, 1963), pp. 293–318.

Chapter 14

Ellen Annandale

WORKING ON THE FRONT-LINE
Risk culture and nursing in the new NHS

From *Sociological Review,* 44, 1996: 416–51

Introduction

NURSES AND MIDWIVES increasingly talk of working in a climate of fear and uncertainty. The risks that they confront emanate not only from the long-standing concern with clinical uncertainty that has traditionally marked practice, but also from the great emphasis that health care organisations now place on nurses' and midwives' individual accountability. The reforms of the 1990s have sought to enhance quality and cost-effectiveness by breaking the traditional grip of the professions over clinical decision-making: competition has been injected into the system; sweeping reforms have taken place in the management of the health service; and responsibility (but not necessarily power) has been devolved to the point of contact with clients (Hunter, 1994; Harrison and Pollitt, 1994). This concern for individual accountability is heightened by the broader self-reflexive culture of late modern society. The shifting parameters of risk and uncertainty that thread through everyday life call for individuals to be constantly questioning, not only the conditions of their own lives, but also the authority of others (Lash, 1994). Thus, when expert individuals or expert-systems fall short of consumer expectations, they are increasingly called to account. The patient has been reborn as a 'consumer' who, in theory, is newly empowered to make health care choices and to hold providers to account through new citizens' rights embodied in the Patient's Charter (Walsh, 1994). These changes force risks to the surface that were previously veiled (such as errors of practice) evoking a new vigilance and heightened concern.

Developed responsibility and accountability to patients and colleagues need not in principle pose a problem for health care providers, but in a risk culture they can fuse to provoke stress and fear. The purpose of this paper is to explore the consequences that this has for practitioners as they engage in the everyday work of caring for patients. It will be argued that the increased surveillance of individual practice by self and others can have a backlash effect. Colleagues and patients are increasingly perceived as 'risk generators' who need to be watched at all times. While the self-protective strategies that emerge to cope with this pressure can enhance quality of patient care, they can also be counter-productive, generating defensive practices which are neither in the interest of health care providers nor patients. Moreover, it will be suggested that attempts to 'cover oneself' may be ineffective: since the practice decisions made *today* only become problems in the *future*, risks can never really be forestalled. The dilemma is that even though staff may come to appreciate this, they *still* feel compelled to do all that they can to colonise the future in order to protect themselves. Since protective strategies can themselves provoke problems a vicious circle is set in train. Herein lies the irony, for the panic culture that emerges, and the negative backlash that it effects, is itself a product of the consumerism and new managerialism that seeks, in fact, to achieve the opposite; that is, to enhance rather than undermine the quality of care that is provided.

The paper begins with a discussion of nurses' and midwives' perceptions of the risk climate in which they work and its associations with the culture of consumerism and the new NHS. This is followed by an analysis of the strategies that practitioners use to cope with the risk environment in which they work and the consequences that these coping strategies can have for the experience of staff and the quality of care that is provided for patients.

The data

The data come from a study of legal accountability in nursing and midwifery that was conducted in 1994. They are drawn from two sources: a questionnaire survey of all trained nurses and midwives who were employed in one hospital trust in late 1994, and in-depth interviews with nurses working for the neurology services of a different hospital trust.

The nursing workforce is made up of a number of categories of staff. As well as permanent full-and part-time workers, hospitals increasingly employ bank and agency nurses (Buchan, 1994). In addition, on any one day a significant number of staff are on annual leave, sick leave, maternity leave and so on. These factors, and the unavailability of centralised records listing staff by grade and area, meant that it was not possible to draw a stratified random sample for the survey. Consequently, questionnaires were handed out by and returned to the senior sister on each ward or area in the hospital over a one week period in November of 1994. The response rate is estimated to be approximately 60 per cent (n = 319).

The four page self-completion questionnaire, which had previously been piloted in the same hospital, was preceded by a brief summary of the research and an assurance of confidentiality. No names were recorded and only limited information was requested on the nurse or midwife's area of work, grade and whether s/he worked full or part-time. The questionnaires, which contained an equal balance of fixed-choice and open-ended questions, were very well completed.

The sample consists of 48 per cent full-time and 41 per cent part-time staff (information was missing for 11 percent). Their grades cluster at 'D' and 'E'. Thus, 27 per cent are 'D' grade and 36 per cent 'E' grade (i.e. staff nurses), with only 7 per cent at grades 'A' to 'C' and 26 per cent 'F' and above (information is missing for 4 per cent). They work in the wide range of clinical areas that is typical of a general hospital trust including outpatients, accident and emergency, orthopaedics, general medicine, intensive care, theatres, coronary care, care of the elderly, paediatrics, and maternity. For reasons of protecting confidentiality, as well as the relatively small number in each area, no attempt will be made to look at different perceptions and practices in response to risk by clinical area, although limited comparisons will be drawn between nursing (as a whole) and midwifery.

The interview sample consisted of 19 nurses who worked in the neurology services (consisting of neurological sciences, neuro-surgery, and an intensive therapy unit) of one the largest hospital trusts in the country. Neurology was not chosen by design, rather the senior nurse opted into the study when asked (along with others) if she would like her area to participate in the research. However, the area is a valuable site in which to consider nursing accountability and to explore the issue of risk since it covers both chronic and acute care. The sample is made up of 13 'D' and 'E' grade nurses, 1 auxiliary nurse, and 5 nursing sisters (4 'F' and 1 'H' grade). The interviews, which were semi-structured in style, took place privately in a room on the ward area. They lasted between forty-five minutes and an hour and covered a range of issues associated with nursing practice, nursing management, interaction with patients/relatives and colleagues, and concerns about legal accountability as they affect patient care. A total of thirteen interviews were taped and transcribed with the interviewees' consent. Since the remaining six preferred not to be tape-recorded, short-hand notes were taken during the interview and later transcribed.

The data extracts in the paper are presented verbatim except where the notation (. . .) is used. Where the staff designation is in parentheses (i.e. staff nurse) this indicates that the data come from the survey sample. Where interview data are used, the designation precedes the dialogue (i.e. staff nurse: . . .).

A climate of risk

> You can't really put your finger on it, what it is. And it's like at the moment you feel you've got to watch your back all the time. That's the sort of atmosphere it is. That you can't . . . if you're talking to somebody you've got to be careful. That's the feeling; the openness has gone. (sister)

> I think nursing *is* stressful, but as far as accountability is concerned . . . you see it's something you think about *all* the time. It's not here in front of your head, it's in the *background* and I think until something comes up, a mistake has been made, then you're made aware of it; that's when you start thinking about it. (staff nurse)

As these comments reveal, risk surrounds practice, it is in the *background*, there is an *atmosphere*: it is always there. As one staff nurse explained, it is 'always on your mind that you may be held responsible in a legal dispute for actions or words'. Or, as one sister more graphically, put it, 'litigation is the "bogey man" that stands behind my shoulder as I practise as a midwife'. This atmosphere engenders a feeling of vulnerability, a fear that you may do the 'wrong thing' or, more worryingly, that whatever you do may not be 'right'.

> You hear of others 'being held accountable' and begin to fear that what-
> ever you say or do may not be right. And you begin to feel more alone.
> (staff nurse)

Feeling vulnerable or under suspicion means working under

> a constant awareness that you may be subject to criticism, quite often in
> an unrealistic way. (sister)

The recognition that 'since we are all human, we can all make mistakes' only adds to this vulnerability, particularly when, as one nurse put it,

> I am constantly being made aware that every little thing that is done
> could in the future be used against me. (staff nurse)

Feelings of vulnerability, the sense that the future haunts actions in the present, can create a fair degree of stress. Indeed, only 23 per cent of the survey sample reported that concerns with legal accountability did not cause them 'any stress at all', while 60 percent said it caused them a 'little' and 17 per cent a 'great deal' of stress. . . .

Consumers as risk generators

The phrase 'patients are more aware of their rights' was a constant refrain in both the nurse interviews and survey data. This *awareness* seemed to be an omnipresent cloud hanging over daily practice. Although consumerism need not be viewed negatively, it was often taken to be a new and rather malevolent presence which was resented by staff,

> STAFF NURSE: The introduction of the Patient's Charter gets Joe Public to go
> to bat. It's quoted considerably in the hospital, people quote it
> to you. So there's an emphasis on 'my granny needs to see a
> surgeon', you get quite a bit of that. You got it even *before* the
> Patient's Charter came out, when it was a White Paper.
> INT: You mentioned talk about the White Paper around the hospital?
> STAFF NURSE: By patients and relatives. And in the community. People are
> more aware of what they're entitled to and expect standards to
> be higher than they used to be. Whether it's through the media,
> I don't know. But I've found that; they're very articulate.

INT: What about?
STAFF NURSE: Nursing care, waiting lists: 'My mother's not been seen.'

The notion of 'patient awareness', which is really a summary term for an assemblage of concerns, is perceived as something that is imported into the hospital from without. Thus, as illustrated in the preceding dialogue, it is seen as motivated by the Patient's Charter. Broader social changes are also seen as culpable.

> People are becoming more aware of their rights, and appear to be more concerned with mistakes and unreliability in all aspects of life unfortunately. (staff nurse)

They know more, want and expect more information,

> Before, I think people used to sit back and say oh, they're in hospital and, you know, 'let the doctors and nurses get on with it, they know what they're doing.' But with erm, there's so much hype, so much information from the media, they tend to question things because they're more aware of the things that *could* go wrong. (staff nurse)

The consumerist attitudes that are expressed in a desire for information can become particularly hard to take when they also involve a desire to blame someone for a 'bad outcome'. This is something that was particularly to the forefront of midwives' concerns.

> People generally have high, unrealistic expectations and think pregnancy, birth and newborns should be planned and perfect in line with their ideals. When it doesn't, they sue the pants off professionals. (sister)

The sense that patients and relatives are 'looking over the nurse's shoulder' undoubtedly generates personal vigilance over the nurse or midwife's actions and the actions of others,

> I think with the press, people are more aware of their rights and things like that . . . Whereas before people, if they weren't happy with some-thing, say they had a complaint to make, they perhaps wouldn't make it. Whereas now, I think they're more eager to because they're more aware of their rights from that point of view and you need to be *aware* of what you're doing more and more. I suppose you've always *been* accountable, *even more* so now because you need to document things more and be more aware of . . . it's always in the back of your head, you know, that you've got to be careful what you do because patients, you know patients are more likely to complain. (staff nurse)

But since patients' awareness is an awareness of nurses' and midwives' practice, it can also be experienced as a form of threat and a lack of trust,

> Although at the time you feel you have done the right thing, often people, mainly relatives, interfere and question if you have given the right treatment in an attempt to intimidate you by suggesting they will take further action. (staff midwife)

The concerns that we have seen expressed by nurses and midwives bear witness to the shift in relations of authority from producer to consumer that many commentators have deemed characteristic of late modern society (see Abercrombie, 1994). According to Giddens (1994), Beck (1992, 1994) and others, this shift is bound up with the inherently reflexive character of contemporary life. Reflexivity, which involves a process of self-monitoring as well as the monitoring of others, takes place against the backdrop of an implosion of information systems. In the context of health and illness individuals are effectively *forced* to confront the vast array of different 'knowledges' about 'health and lifestyle' and therapies which are displayed in the media. Health-related knowledge has become more visibly contested as the risks of applied science in the form of medical and nursing practice are paraded in newspapers, TV soaps, and documentaries. The reassuring face of medicine of yester-year has been replaced by visions of institutional risk. Financial cut-backs, bungled operations and incompetent practice are now at the heart of television medical dramas and news reports. This new knowledge can bear down heavily on the individual health care 'consumer' creating a sense of anxiety and the felt need to question and challenge. . . .

Coping with risk

The most general way that respondents cope is by engaging in a constant process of *checking*, and re-checking what they do and say. Checking and covering are defensive strategies that may have both positive and negative effects on the care that patients receive. They are also more or less successful as risk reduction strategies. As we have seen, nurses and midwives feel quite strongly that concern about legal accountability influences their practice in terms of how they document material in patients' records; and how they communicate with patients and their relatives, and with colleagues . . .

One of the most noticeable effects was a heightened concern with accuracy. This was highlighted by 49 per cent of the survey sample in reference to documentation. Comments like, 'everything must be written clearly leaving no room for misinterpretation' 'concern ensures accurate and thorough documentation' were made frequently. Patient records are an important resource for the different members of staff who are involved in caring for the patient over the course of the day. Their accuracy, therefore, should contribute significantly to information exchange and, through this, to quality of care. But, there is no doubt that the quest for accuracy is also bound up with covering oneself,

> You feel pressured to document minor irrelevant detail to 'cover yourself'. (sister)

> You are more personally responsible *now*. Everything needs to be documented, however trivial – at the end of the day it falls back on *you*. (enrolled nurse)

These respondents suggest that nurses and midwives might write too much, much of it trivial, in the process of covering themselves. Documenting 'everything' is a defence strategy: since they never know what may come back on them at a future date, they feel that they must write it all down 'just in case'. Thus there is a feeling that they must write things down to prove that they have done such diverse things as given a drug, noted and told others about a change in the patient's condition, discussed the patient's conditions with his or her relatives, noted a complaint or even just the possibility of a complaint,

> You find yourself documenting everything i.e. a conversation you had with relatives, for instance, if you get the slightest feeling that somebody is not happy. (staff nurse)

Respondents were well aware that medical and nursing records are legal documents that can be used in a court of law. Contemporaneous records offer a sense of security since they can be evoked as 'proof' of action at a future time when memories have faded. Thus records become simultaneously a crutch and a site of risk in their own right; as one staff nurse put it, they can be 'your saviour or your downfall'. Quite simply, respondents questioned how sure they could ever be that they had covered themselves adequately. The following interview extract illustrates the way in which documenting creates both security and insecurity for nurses and midwives precisely because they can never totally predict which actions or aspects of a patient's care may be defined as a problem at a future date,

SISTER:	We're very careful about documentation to ensure it's thorough and complete (. . .).
INT:	So is that a positive thing?
SISTER:	Yes, it's a good instrument for the nurses, to protect themselves.
INT:	Some people have said [in interview] that they feel anxious about documenting (. . .). Is that something that concerns you?
SISTER:	. . . I'm very *aware* about documentation. I'm very aware how much *time* it takes. Erm, it doesn't make me *anxious* particularly, I'm getting *fast* to the stage of thinking no matter *how* much you write, you never seem to write exactly what would be needed if, you know, there was a complaint. Erm, sometimes you just miss the one vital thing that you can't imagine that would come back at you. So I think all you can do is just be as precise and concise as you *can* be, *hope* you've covered what you need to cover (. . .).
INT:	(. . .) Are you aware of the legal side when you *are* documenting?
SISTER:	Oh definitely.

INT: Is it in the *back* of your mind?

SISTER: Yes, yes it's *constantly* there, and *especially* so if you've had a difficult patient or difficult relatives. You know, you can sit and write a thesis almost trying to cover every aspect that may come back at you. And, as I say, very often it's the *one* thing that you felt was *far* too trivial to document that *does* come back at you (. . .).

INT: Obviously you're documenting on any one day on a number of patients. You've just mentioned a *difficult* patient, how do you know you've got a difficult patient, is it intuitive?

SISTER: Yes, you already know your patients that are complaining, or your relatives that are complaining about things, and just discontented patients. You know the type of patient and you need to be as *absolutely* thorough as you can be with them. Obviously, people are encouraged to be thorough with *every* patient, but there are particular patients that you just *need* to ensure that absolutely *everything* is documented. Obviously you do get patients who complain who you *didn't* think would complain and *have*, but you know documentation should be thorough for *every* patient. But sometimes you just need to be that little bit more careful.

Even though documenting is a way for nurses and midwives to protect themselves against patients, the principle protection strategy of 'writing everything down' does not seem to be to the patient's detriment, except insofar as it takes time away from direct patient care. As several respondents implied, it is not really possible to separate out the extent to which the extra (in the minds of some, excessive) documentation that now takes place is for the purposes of good patient care and the extent to which it is done to cover oneself.

The same is broadly true when we consider the risks that nurses and midwives face when administering drugs. Undoubtedly, staff have *always been* concerned to make sure that patients receive the right drug, at the right dose, at the correct time. But this concern is heightened as a litigious climate has made trust management increasingly concerned about drug errors. The fact that many wards now have single nurse administration of drugs, means that the come-back is squarely on the individual who has signed for the drug,

> For oral drugs, it's one nurse administration, therefore, one nurse accountability. (sister)

But, of course, even though they *feel* individually accountable, nurses do not work independently. Health care work is inherently collective which means that any one individual's work is invested with the (correct and incorrect) actions of others. Hence an important source of vulnerability is the opening up of the nurse or midwife's work to scrutiny by others who are fearful that other people's actions will bounce back onto them. As one nurse put it,

> It's as if every move and decision is being watched and pulled to pieces making me less confident. (staff nurse)

Simultaneously, stress also occurs because respondents' own actions may be compromised by the actions of others who are less vigilant or aware. As with written documentation, the need to communicate verbally with colleagues is both a means of 'covering oneself' *and* of enhancing quality of care. In all, 43 per cent of the survey sample said that more effective communication occurred as a result of concern about legal accountability. For example,

> Unclear communication could potentially lead to errors in patient care. Each practitioner – doctor and nurse – has a responsibility to their patients to ensure communication is clear and unambiguous. (staff nurse)

At the same time better communication covers one's own actions,

> There is much more contact with doctors to ensure that anything is passed on that is needed straight away in order to cover oneself. (staff nurse)

. . .

Concluding discussion

The provision of health care is in considerable flux at the present time. In an environment of apparently constant change the boundaries of individual responsibility and accountability need to be attended to on a continuing basis. The nurses and midwives in the current study reported the need to be almost constantly vigilant; 'looking over their shoulders' 'watching their backs' and 'covering themselves' in light of the risks of practice today that could come back on them in the future. In many instances the defensive coping strategies that they developed appear to contribute simultaneously to good practice (in terms of quality of care to patients) and to their self-protection. For example, taking extra care to write detailed notes in patient records and to pass on information clearly, would seem to benefit both the nurse or midwife *and* the patient. Yet, these practices can also have a backlash effect. Thus respondents reported that excessive documentation took precious time away from direct patient care, and that 'patients' awareness of their rights' could generate caution and restraint in communication. More generally, the need to be wary and 'covering oneself' all the time could generate stress,

> Stress is caused because I feel on occasion that I'm not doing my job properly in caring for the patients as I am too busy documenting certain patients more than others in order to protect myself. (staff nurse)

> I find it very difficult to come to terms with the extra amount of documentation I feel needs to be done 'just in case, to cover myself'. And I often hesitate before acting a lot more, making me feel less certain and confident in my actions. I also feel that if any actions were challenged hospital authorities would not support me as once they would have done. (staff nurse)

Although the data suggest that these concerns are of recent origin, it would be mistaken to view them as totally new. In fact, although many of the issues that have been raised take on a new form in the context of the NHS of the 1990s, they are at the centre of long-standing debates about professionalisation, nursing knowledge and accountability for practice. The professionalising strategies of nursing and midwifery have historically placed great emphasis on individual accountability. Indeed, accountability is often presented as a *corollary* of professional status signalling a degree of autonomy that has traditionally been denied to nurses and midwives (Pyne, 1992). Legal accountability is, in fact, multi-faceted. Thus, the nurse or midwife is personally responsible under common law, accountable to her or his employer, and professionally accountable to the UKCC professional codes of practice (Owens and Glennerster, 1990). Recent debates within nursing and midwifery have highlighted the conflicts that can arise between professional accountability and accountability to the employing organisation. For example, staff may fear reprisals from employers if they fulfil their professional obligation to report circumstances when patient care is unsafe, or they may feel pressured to take on patient care tasks (such as giving intravenous drugs) that they do not feel competent to carry out. Here we can see an ironic sense of coherence between nursing and midwifery's *own* long-standing push for autonomy and individual accountability, and the strong emphasis that management now places on *individual* responsibility. As respondents themselves explained, now more than ever before, 'errors and inaccuracies come back on the individual'. Consequently, 'at the end of the day, it's your neck on the line'. In the eyes of many nurses and midwives, these problems are exacerbated by the loss of nursing line management in hospitals following the Griffiths reforms of the 1980s (Owens and Glennerster, 1990) and the introduction of a general management structure which is seen to be remote from the everyday concerns of staff working on the wards.

The risks that confront nurses and midwives in their day-to-day work are closely bound up with broader changes in the conceptualisation of citizenship. As Walsh (1994: 192) relates, a new model has emerged in which 'the market is the most effective means of enabling citizenship to be maintained, and the citizen is best seen as a customer'. In these terms, better and more cost efficient care is to be achieved through the individual acting in a simulated market. The environment in which nurses and midwives work is certainly marked by the individualistic ethos of the market and, ultimately, it is this ethos that fosters the sense of risk that surrounds practice. Although the patient as consumer is undoubtedly valued and cared for, he or she is also viewed as someone who *generates* risk. There is a strong ideology of 'partnership with patients', a sense of developing a unique knowledge where the 'nurse's role is seen partly as that of teacher or facilitator, enabling patients to marshal their own healing resources; involving patients as partners in care' and thereby increasing their knowledge and control of their health (Salvage, 1992: 13). But the likelihood of this approach being put into practice seems remote, when patients are simultaneously seen as risk generators. This generates a keen sense of ambivalence about patients on the part of nurses and midwives. In similar terms, team work and fostering a sense of collective identity as a basis for action (something which has always been illusive to nursing) are almost bound to be compromised when colleagues, who are generally viewed as supportive and good at their job, must always be watched as a potential source of risk.

Since risks tend to be future-oriented it can be difficult for nurses and mid-wives to actually *know* when actions taken to avert risk have been successful. Whatever they do, they may feel that they can never fully control the actions of others which may implicate them. Perhaps more worryingly, there is an accent on *self*-reflexivity where agency reflects on itself (Lash, 1994: 115). As we have seen, respondents were concerned that they personally could always miss something by chance, that they could never really predict which patient might complain. In large part, then, concern is generated because of the contingency that accompanies actions in the present. Lash (1994: 121) contends that 'life chances in reflexive modernity are a question of access not to productive capital or production struc-tures but instead of access to and place in the new information and communication structures'. The risk culture that marks the NHS of the 1990s signals the exclusion of the majority of nurses and midwives who work on the front lines of patient care from the knowledge/power complex of these information and communication structures. As well as being recast as reflexive actors (monitoring others and them-selves in a bid for security), they are caught up in public sector reforms that stress internal competition (between provider units) and individual accountability for action as hospital trusts increasingly operate in a climate of competition for con-tracts and for markers of quality. Fearful of lack of support from colleagues, in a climate of quite intense job insecurity, nurses and midwives may self-consciously turn to defensive practices that are not in the interest of good patient care in an attempt to create a tract of security and to close-off personal risk.

References

Abercrombie, N., (1994), 'Authority and consumer society', in *The Authority of the Consumer*, R. Keat, N. Whitley, and N. Abercrombie, (eds), London: Routledge, 43–57.

Beck, U., (1992), *The Risk Society*, London: Sage.

Beck, U., (1994), 'The reinvention of politics: towards a theory of reflexive moderniza-tion' in *Reflexive Modernization*, U. Beck, A. Giddens and S. Lash, Cambridge: Polity, 1–55.

Buchan, J., (1994), *Further Flexing. NHS Trusts and Changing Working Patterns in NHS Working*, London: Royal College of Nursing.

Giddens, A., (1994), 'Living in a post-traditional society' in *Reflexive Modernization*, U. Beck, A. Giddens and S. Lash, Cambridge: Polity, 56–109.

Harrison, S. and Pollitt, C., (1994), *Controlling Health Professionals*, Buckingham: Open University Press.

Hunter, D., (1994), 'From tribalism to corporatism: the managerial challenge to medical dominance' in *Challenging Medicine*, J. Gabe, D. Kelleher and G. Williams, (eds), London: Routledge, 1–22.

Lash, S., (1994), 'Reflexivity and its doubles: structure, aesthetics, community', in *Reflexive Modernization*, U. Beck, A. Giddens and S. Lash, Cambridge: Polity, 110–173.

Owens, P. and Glennerster, H., (1990), *Nursing in Conflict*, London: Macmillan.

Pyne, R., (1992), 'Changing the Code', *Nursing Times*, 88: 20–21.

Salvage, J., (1992), 'The new nursing: empowering patients or empowering nurses?' in *Policy Issues in Nursing*, J. Robinson, A. Gray, and E. Elkan (eds), Milton Keynes, Open University Press.

Walsh, K., (1994), 'Citizens, charters and contracts' in *The Authority of the Consumer*, R. Keat, N. Whitley and N. Abercrombie (eds), London: Routledge, 189–206.

Chapter 15

Deborah Lupton

CONSUMERISM, REFLEXIVITY AND THE MEDICAL ENCOUNTER

From *Social Science and Medicine,* 45 (3) 1997: 373–81

Introduction

WHEN THE HIGHLY PAID SPECIALIST said the decision to have a fancy medical test was up to me, I knew "empowerment" had gone too far. I was paying him to make the decisions. But he was acting like the junior partner in my health care. I might have yelled "Power to the People" in some demo 20 years ago when he was clawing his way into the Macquarie Street medical establishment, but I didn't actually mean power to me over every technical decision that would crop up in my life. I didn't seek to be "empowered" in matters that bored me, like tax, or that totally baffled me, like expensive tests. I long for the old doctor-as-God, for the expert who would tell me what to do rather than lay out the odds. (Horin, 1995)

Since the 1970s, the contention that lay people are moving towards a more "consumerist" approach when seeking health care has emerged in a range of forums. The discourse of consumerism has been adopted in a number of different sites with differing political objectives, including both the state and advocacy groups seeking to challenge the state (Grace, 1994). Community organizations such as the Consumers' Health Forum of Australia have adopted the principles of liberal humanism in their efforts to achieve equitable access to health and medical care and the best possible outcome for lay people when they seek such care. They tend to focus on patients' rights and capacity for autonomy. In contrast, participants in the development of public policy working from a rightwing approach have often made calls for increased Consumerist behaviour on the part of patients to accompany their suggestions that health care should be reformed by being subjected to a free market model. The conservative government in Britain has argued since the late 1980s for this approach to health care delivery, as have members of rightwing "think tanks" in Australia (see, for example, Logan et al., 1989) and the conservative New Zealand government in power in the early 1990s (Grace, 1994).

Proponents of the market economy approach believe that "medical services should be treated just like any other commodity that can be efficiently produced and consumed under competitive market conditions" (Logan et al., 1989, p. 163). Those who have adopted this model of doctor–patient relations view doctors simply as suppliers of services, competing amongst themselves and seeking to maximize their income by selling their professional expertise. It is assumed that consumers will benefit from a return to the free market because of increased competition, which will supposedly "weed out" inferior services and ensure optimal quality, consumer choice and price. For the community consumer advocates, health care is also represented as "just like any other commodity". Patients qua consumers are urged to refuse to accept paternalism or "medical dominance" on the part of the doctor, to "shop around", to actively evaluate doctors' services and to go elsewhere should the "commodity" be found unsatisfactory (see, for example, Commonwealth Department of Health, 1985; Australian Consumers Association, 1988).

Similarly, much previous research looking at the doctor–patient relationship has tended to be couched in terms of "measuring patient satisfaction" with medical care using quantitative scales, with a move towards the standardizing of such instruments (for example, the research reviewed in Buetow, 1995). Here again, the notion of the rational, autonomous subject is privileged. As Meredith notes,

> Patient satisfaction surveys implicitly rely on a conception of the patient as a "rational evaluator" who is willing, wishing and able to judge all aspects of hospital care relatively dispassionately and reasonably reliably. (Meredith, 1993, p. 599)

Indeed, the very concept of "satisfaction" is one that is largely imposed by the impetus towards evaluation from public policy. It assumes the patients will be ready and willing to adopt the "consumerist" approach to health care without first questioning what the concept of "satisfaction" means for them (Williams, 1994).

In all usages of the notion of the patient qua consumer, regardless of political orientation, the dominant and privileged representation is that of the dispassionate, thinking, calculating subject. This notion draws largely on psychological and neoclassical models of consumer behaviour. According to the classical economic theory of expected utility, consumers are rational economic decision-makers who have complete sovereignty over the choice of how to use their resources to their best advantage, or to their "maximum utility" (Fine, 1995). The archetype that is generally set up in opposition to this model of the idealized patient/consumer is that of the "passive" or "dependent" patient. This subject position is viewed as undesirable because of the implications of dependency and unquestioning compliance to an authoritative Other. Such compliance deviates from current dominant and privileged notions in Western societies about the importance of the autonomous self, the self who governs personal behaviour via reason rather than emotion. The philosopher Charles Taylor has characterized this ideal as the

> disengaged self, capable of objectifying not only the surrounding world but also his [sic] own emotions and inclinations, fears and compulsions, and achieving thereby a kind of distance and self-possession which allows him to act "rationally". (Taylor, 1989, p. 21)

As Taylor's language implies, this ideal also tends to privilege masculinity over femininity, because the former is associated with a greater degree of control over the emotions.

The "consumerist" subject also fits the sociological notion of the "reflexive project of the self". This draws upon the assumption that in late modern Western societies individuals constantly seek to reflect upon the practices constituting the self and the body and to maximize, in an entrepreneurial fashion, the benefits for the self (see, for example, Giddens, 1992, 1994). Life, in this formulation, is carried out as an enterprise, demanding a continual search for knowledge to engage in self-improvement. Instead of simply accepting the "way things are", individuals must continually make decisions from a variety of options as part of everyday life. It is argued, therefore, that individuals experience self, the body and the social and physical worlds with a high degree of reflection, questioning, evaluation and uncertainty. Consonant with this concept of contemporary subjectivity is the contention that expert knowledges, such as medicine and science, are no longer simply accepted on face value. Rather, it is asserted that these knowledges are now open to scepticism and to challenge on the part of lay people due to an increasing public awareness of their uncertainties (Beck, 1994).

There is, therefore, a congruence between the notions of the "consumerist" patient and the "reflexive" actor. Both are understood as actively calculating, assessing and, if necessary, countering expert knowledge and autonomy with the objective of maximizing the value of services such as health care. Both tend to portray a type of subject that is non-differentiated; for example, there is little discussion of how gender, sexual identity, age, ethnicity, social class and personal biography or life experiences affect the taking up of "consumerist" or "reflexive" positions. Further, neither approach tends to take into account the role played by cultural, psychodynamic and affective processes in individuals' everyday life choices, decisions and actions. That is, there is little understanding of the consumption of health care *qua* commodity as a dynamic and intersubjective sociocultural process rather than as an outcome of an individualized calculation.

As a counter to some of the more quantitative assessments of patient "satisfaction", sociological studies using qualitative methods to explore the ways that people experience and approach the medical encounter have attempted to go beyond description to interpreting the meaning of the encounter (recent examples include Wiles and Higgins, 1996; Broom and Woodward, 1996; May *et al.*, 1996; Williams and Calnan, 1996). This research, while varying in the extent to which the data were theorized using contemporary sociocultural theory, has pointed to the importance of acknowledging the complexity of the medical encounter on the interpersonal level and the tensions, ambivalences and contradictions that both patients and doctors may experience. The majority of this research, however, has focused on the British context. The study presented here was an attempt to explore these issues with Australians; more specifically, using in-depth individual interviews with 60 lay people living in Sydney, eliciting their responses to general issues around the role played by medical practitioners in their lives and their opinions of medicine and the medical profession.

The study

The genesis of this research was in a previous predominantly quantitative study of consumerism among a sample of Australians. In early 1990 I was involved as a co-researcher in a study that surveyed over 300 people attending general practices in Sydney, seeking to explore their attitudes to selecting and evaluating their doctors. The study used a self-administered questionnaire with both "tick the box" and open-ended questions to elicit data. The general findings were that the sample in general did not display a high level of consumerist approaches to the selection and evaluation of their medical care. Indeed, the majority of respondents did not tend to position themselves as "consumers" or doctors as the purveyors of a "commodity". Rather, we concluded, they still expressed a desire to conform to the "patient" role and an unwillingness to approach the medical encounter from a position where they distrusted the doctor. In the openended questions, words such as "trust" and "faith" were frequently used by the respondents when describing their own doctor. We did find significant differences, however, related to age and social class. Older people were far less likely than younger people to demonstrate consumerist behaviour (such as seeking recommendations from others or deciding to change their doctor), as were people living in socioeconomically disadvantaged areas of Sydney compared with those from more advantaged areas (Donaldson et al., 1991; Lupton et al., 1991; Lloyd et al., 1991). . . . .

The subsequent study was funded by a grant that provided the resources to interview in depth 60 lay people living in Sydney. (A group of 20 medical practitioners also participated in interviews, but these data will not be discussed here.) In the interviews, carried out between late 1994 and mid 1995, the participants were asked to talk about their own experiences with medical practitioners over their lifetime, their strongest memories of doctors, the ways in which doctors are portrayed in the mass media, their notions of "good" and "bad" doctors and their opinions on whether the medical profession had lost some of its status in recent times. Efforts were made to recruit the lay people from a wide range of occupations, education level and ethnic backgrounds. As a result, the final group ranged from socioeconomically privileged people with high levels of formal education and professional occupations to blue-collar workers, retired people living on pensions, the unemployed and those who had left school early. Equal numbers of women and men were interviewed. The ages of the lay participants ranged from 16 to 81 years: 23 per cent of the participants were aged 30 or younger, 40 per cent were in the 31–49 years age group and 37 per cent were 50 years or older. Sixty-two per cent were Australian-born of Anglo–Celtic ethnicity, 22 per cent were of non-English-speaking European ethnicity (either born in continental Europe or first-generation Australian-born with European parents), 7 per cent were of Chinese ethnicity and 5 per cent were British-born of Anglo–Celtic parents. Two participants had mixed Anglo–Celtic and European parentage and one participant was of half-Aboriginal and half-Scottish descent.

As one would expect of the "rich" data that are collected in one-to-one interviews of an average of 45 minutes to one hour in length, there were many areas that could have been taken up and analysed in detail. Issues to do with trust relations and the emotional dimensions of the medical encounter have been discussed in detail elsewhere (Lupton, 1996). In the present article, issues pertinent to consumerism in the medical encounter as they were articulated by lay people are explored. The interview data were treated as texts, in which narratives were recounted by the participants. Such data are treated not as "*the truth*" of people's thoughts and experiences but as "a situated truth" that inevitably is shaped through the particular context in which it is elicited. That is, it was assumed that as in any account of behaviour, experiences, thoughts and opinions, the nature of the interview context itself influences the data in ways that are impossible to eliminate from the research process. Influential factors include the types of questions asked, the gender, social class, ethnicity and age of the interviewer (in this case, the project's research assistant, a middle class, Anglo–Celtic Australian woman in her late 30s), her manner, the mood of the interviewee and so on. The accounts of the participants, therefore, are a joint construction with the interviewer as well as with the person interpreting the data for analysis.

The interviews were transcribed and the transcripts were then analysed for recurring discourses, or patterned ways of articulating points of view and conveying meaning. The present analysis first focuses on two of the major topics upon which the participants were asked to expound their views and experiences: the changing role and status of doctors and biomedicine vs alternative therapies. The differences emerging among the participants in terms of age and social class are then discussed.

The changing role and status of doctors

When the participants were asked whether they thought the social status of medical practitioners in Australian society had changed over time, nearly everyone agreed that it had. A common observation put forward by the participants was that while doctors may still be generally respected in Australia, they are now subject to more criticism. In doing so, regardless of their age, the participants routinely drew comparisons between the medical practitioners they remembered from their childhood, and those they had dealings with today. An almost mythological account was given of a kindly (almost invariably middle-aged, white male) doctor, the traditional archetype of the "family doctor" who had visited the house and given close and caring attention to them as children:

> [The family doctor] would come to the bed of the child who was ill with my mother. He would take blood pressure, temperature, generally, you know, a gentle hands on approach, and he was actually very comforting. His nature was a very comforting nature. I suppose we all revered him in a way because it was the general feeling in that period that the family doctor was someone you really listened to and respected. (Carol, part-time counsellor and postgraduate student, age 41)[1]

These days, it was often contended, this ideal figure of the "family doctor" had been challenged by increasing publicity around medical negligence or mistakes, sexual harassment or assault of patients by doctors, medical fraud and so on. There was no general agreement, however, about the extent to which doctors' status had fallen in recent years. The participants were extremely variable in their negative comments about the medical profession. In the interviews they tended to oscillate back and forth between expounding their support of medicine and doctors and criticizing them. Some participants were vehement in their opinion that the image of medical practitioners had been severely damaged:

> I think [doctors] are perceived as money hungry, as incompetent, often not being able to diagnose properly. And you often hear conversations about or participate in conversations about things that have gone wrong with you, and the doctor has given completely the wrong thing or they have prescribed something for the sake of prescribing something without really knowing what they are doing. And I think the community perception of doctors is a poor one. (Graham, pensioner on sickness benefits, 41).

Others, however, were less adamant about the change in doctors' social position and authority, arguing that doctors are still highly respected by members of the general public and that people tend not to challenge them. Even those people who expressed a strong dislike of doctors, contending that they avoided going to see them if at all possible, would often then go on to mention times when doctors had helped themselves or a family member, and the gratitude they felt for this help.

The major emphasis of the criticism of the medical profession articulated in the interviews was not the extent to which medicine had gained power, but rather the proficiency with which individual doctors used their medical knowledge and dealt on a personal level with their patients. The participants tended to be highly aware of the way doctors interacted with them and to judge them harshly if they felt they had been badly treated. This was particularly the case if the doctor had responded to them in what they considered to be an "uncaring" or abrupt manner, appearing to be insensitive to their feelings or not wanting to take the time to listen. Such doctors, it was contended, could not be trusted with one's health. Such "atrocity stories"

---

[1] All names are pseudonyms. Unless otherwise stated, individual participants referred to in this article are of Anglo–Celtic ethnicity.

relating to the doctor's personal manner have been identified in other qualitative research studies with lay people (for example, Meredith, 1993). . . .

Biomedicine vs alternative therapies

There is evidence that people in Western societies, including Australia, are seeking the help of alternative therapists in greater numbers (Lloyd et al., 1993; Saks, 1994). Some commentators have suggested that this represents a greater cynicism on the part of lay people towards the claims and expertise of biomedicine. The findings of the present study, however, suggest that faith in biomedicine remains strong. Most participants, when asked if they believed in medical science as a good remedy for illness and disease, agreed that they did. Several participants expressed the opinion that medical science itself, while not necessarily possessing the cure for every ill, is continually progressing and will eventually discover a solution. Indeed, for many people, the developments in medical knowledge could only be described as beneficial for society, by dealing with illnesses and diseases that previously were not easily treatable. As Jason, a 16-year-old school student, commented:

> Well, I mean you look at the transplants, heart transplants, livers, kidneys, lungs, cancer – the latest cure for cancer is slowly getting better and improving with new methods and treatments. And so I think the medical system, whether it be the research teams, the development teams, whatever, they deserve some respect for the job that they're doing, the work they're accomplishing.

Other participants acknowledged that perhaps medical expertise was taken for granted, and that patients need to acknowledge that doctors are not saint-like figures, but are just as susceptible to human foibles as anyone else:

> I think it's a very difficult profession. Look, I am an accountant and I did make a few mistakes in my life, in my work. But it always can be rectified. Ah, well, a doctor is a doctor making a mistake. He is only a human being. So I think it's a very difficult profession and maybe we expect too much. (Peter, Hungarian, accountant, age 81)

> I suppose very simply I see doctors as very clay-footed. They are, of course, very able in all sorts of ways but they are human like the rest of us too. (Sheila, arts administrator and postgraduate student, age 52)

Despite this general expression of faith in medical science, several of the participants had sought alternative therapies for illnesses or conditions they thought had not been adequately treated by biomedicine. This did not mean that they had avoided medical treatment, however. Typically they had sought alternative therapy after orthodox medicine had first been tried. In some cases, alternative therapies were combined simultaneously with biomedical treatment. For example, Julia, who was receiving treatment for breast cancer at the time of her interview, as a nurse is herself trained in orthodox medicine. Despite her background, she has tried herbalism and naturopathy for her condition. Nonetheless, she commented that orthodox medicine:

> . . . will be my first line of defence. Like when I went and saw the herbalist a couple of weeks back, he said, "Oh, if you really want to take my advice, don't have the chemotherapy and we will go from there." And I just said, "No, I have just got to have"—what is the word I am looking for—"conventional treatment and then I will back it up with all the herbs and things."

For some people, alternative therapies offer the empathetic interaction with a health provider they feel many doctors lack the time or inclination to provide. Rochelle, 23 years old and unemployed, who had had chemotherapy treatment for a brain tumour, said she found the experience extremely alienating:

> At times you just felt like you were just another like animal coming in for the check-in station and getting, you know, they'd measure the size of it, they'd put your skull on that, get out like the callipers and like, a couple of words said here and there but just like a job more than anything. They were going through the motions.

By contrast, Rochelle commented, the naturopath she now sees twice a year for more minor health problems is far more interested in her as an individual. She thinks that compared to naturopaths, many doctors are not as interested in people's emotional states and personal relationships and how they affect health:

> . . . when you go and see a naturopath, sure you might pay a bit extra, but I would rather pay the 50 dollars to see my naturopath at the holistic medical centre where I get to see her for an hour or an hour and a half. She goes through everything, from what I've eaten in the last month that I can remember, to mood swings, to the effect that the weather plays on people, to everything—pollution, I mean, you know, being in the city . . . Doctors don't think of it like that. They're just willing to hand out the drugs without actually thinking that there could be another problem.

These comments underline the importance that most people tend to place upon the affective aspects of health care. If patients think that doctors cannot provide the emotional support and personal interest they feel they need, then they may seek treatment from other kinds of practitioners. Nevertheless, the authority and expertise that attend biomedicine and those who are medically trained still carry much weight, and no participants had completely rejected biomedicine in favour of alternative therapies.

Differences among participants: the influence of age and social class

Previous research (Blaxter and Paterson, 1982; Calnan, 1988; Donaldson *et al.*, 1991) has suggested that older people are more deferential than are younger people towards the medical profession, and that people who are university educated and in professional occupations themselves are more likely to challenge the authority of doctors and seek detailed information on their medical condition. These differences were also evident in the present study. The participants who were aged in their 70s or 80s were more likely to express extremely positive and grateful attitudes about doctors and to state that they had never had a bad experience with a doctor compared with younger participants, who tended to express somewhat more cynical views. Some of the older people had been seeing the same doctor for 30 or more years, growing old with her or him. The older participants were also much less likely than the younger participants to say that they had sought treatment from alternative therapists. Ray, for example, a retired accountant who was 79 years old at the time of the interview, said that he had been very satisfied with the medical care he had received over his life. When asked what he considered the qualities of a "bad doctor" were, he said:

> Well, I don't know—I have experienced such good relations with doctors that I can't imagine what a bad doctor would be like. A bad doctor would be one that was slap happy and would not care for you as much as he should for your health. That is what I imagine a bad doctor to be. I haven't had an experience of bad doctors in my opinion, so I can't help you there.

Similarly, 78-year-old Dolly expressed the opinion that doctors are still highly respected today for their capacity to heal and save lives: "Well, I think they should be—they save lives, don't they?"

People with lower levels of education were also somewhat more reverent when discussing doctors, often because of their respect for the years of university education and arcane knowledge that doctors had acquired to become medical professionals. One example is Joe, aged 66, who left school at the age of 15 and has worked in a number of manual occupations, including transport driver and fisherman. Joe said that he accepts what doctors say without question as "the umpire's decision", because "probably I don't know any better. To argue with them and say, 'I haven't got bronchitis', but they say 'You have'—okay, I have." So too, Paul, a 28-year-old storeman, argued that he thought people generally respected doctors because "they've done all their studies. Like if you've studied for so many years you're going to know a lot more than I'd know if I went to a doctor. Yes, I respect them."

In contrast to these participants were people such as Helen, a 56-year-old teacher and writer with a Master's degree. She is perhaps typical of the archetypal middle class consumer who highly values self-autonomy and choice. At the time of the interview, Helen had recently developed leukaemia, and recounted in her interview how she was told by her medical specialists that she should have chemotherapy and bone marrow transplants. According to Helen, four of the specialists she had consulted insisted that she should have this treatment. She refused their advice, however, because she was feeling well at the time. Helen also did not have a partner or children to look after her, and knew that she would be ill for a long time after the suggested treatment. She presented herself in the interview as someone who was actively resisting medicalization in the attempt to retain her sense of self as an autonomous, independent woman:

> I couldn't explain to [the specialists] that there was a point beyond which I could not go. I didn't want to become hospitalized, I didn't want to become medicalized. I still wanted my dignity. They became fixated on the fact that I kept saying that I didn't want to lose my hair. But the hair just was a symbol of what I would be losing. It was—I didn't want to turn into a poor thing. I didn't want to be dependent, I didn't want to be bleating to friends, "Please help me." Because as you can see from what I have said, my entire attitude to illness has been you are stoic, you must bear it, you manage yourself, you don't go under. And that is simply so intrinsic to the way I think that I won't have it [treatment].

. . .

11096

Discussion

The interview data, while revealing some points of general agreement about medicine and the medical profession, also demonstrate conflicting opinions. There seems little argument among the participants that the status of the medical profession has diminished in recent years and that doctors as a group are no longer necessarily viewed or unproblematically accepted as "heroes in white coats". The data here presented suggest that for many people the discourse of consumerism and the reflexive subject position are important parts of the contemporary medical encounter. All participants expressed strong opinions about how they would characterize and distinguish between a "good" and a "bad" doctor, and some told "atrocity stories" involving cases of medical negligence. Factors such as social class and age or generation group appear to continue to shape the ways that lay people approach the medical encounter, while other factors such as gender and ethnicity seem not to be as influential.

Despite a general agreement that the medical profession is subject to more criticism than in previous times, most people still articulated respect for doctors and faith in medical science. Even those people who had appeared to support and adopt the discourse of consumerism suggested that at least on some occasions they would be willing to invest their trust and faith in a particular doctor, should that doctor earn this trust. This suggests the importance of acknowledging the personal experiences of individuals, including the embodied and affective dimension of illness, and how their interaction with experts is part of their ceaseless construction and reconstruction of subjectivity. As Wynne has noted, people informally but incessantly problematise their own relationship with expertise of all kinds, as part of their negotiation of their own identities. They are aware of their dependency, and of their lack of agency even if the boundaries of this are uncertain. (Wynne, 1996, p. 50)

If we are to position health care as a commodity, we need to acknowledge that while the selection of many commodities and services may be undertaken from purely rationalist motivations in response to the perception of a need, many other forms of consumption take place at the subconscious or unconscious levels, involving a high level of emotional investment. As recent literature on the socio-cultural aspects of consumption has contended, the commodity not only has "use value" or need-fulfilling value for the consumer but also has an "abstract value", consisting of the cultural, symbolic and emotional meanings around the good (see Bocock, 1993; Richards, 1994). There are resonances in this literature for under-standing health care. Health care, of course, incorporates the use of several kinds of tangible and quite prosaic consumables: drugs, vaccines, lotions, bandages, ointments and so on. The major component of health care, however, is more intangible, involving body work and affective exchanges and outcomes. Thus, for example, the physical examination involves the doctor looking at and touching the patient, using her or his knowledge to search for signs of illness to make a diagnosis. The touch of the doctor and the way she or he interacts with the patient, the doctor's tone of voice, the manner, the words chosen, are all central to the "consumption" experience, as is how the patient "feels" during and after the encounter.

It has often been pointed out by critics of the consumerist approach to health care that lay people simply lack the specialized knowledge that medical professionals possess, and this is regarded as a major barrier to consumerism. Over and above this "asymmetry of knowledge", however, is the almost unique nature of the medical encounter in relation to embodiment and emotional features. Dependency is a central feature of the illness experience and the medical encounter and serves to work against the full taking up of a consumer approach. Illness, disease, pain, disability and impending death are all highly emotional states, and they all tend to encourage a need on the part of the suffering person for dependency upon another (Stein, 1985; de Swaan, 1990; Cassell, 1991). As noted earlier, the late modern notion of reflexivity presented by writers such as Giddens and Beck tends to privilege, above all, a conscious and rational state, involving continual monitor-ing and criticism based on a challenging approach that is itself reliant on know-ledge. The privileged representation of the patient as the reflexive, autonomous consumer simply fails to recognize the often unconscious, unarticulated depend-ence that patients may have on doctors. This representation also tends to take up the mind/body separation in its valorizing of rational thought over affec-tive and embodied response. It is as if "the consumer" lacks the physically vulnerable, desiring, all-too-human body which is the primary object of medical care . . .

A more nuanced interpretation of reflexivity may be to acknowledge the ways that knowledges are constructed via embodied and affective experiences which are both accumulative and dynamic over a person's lifetime . . .

To conclude, there seems little reason to attempt to position one particular kind of response to bodily or psychic distress or pain as more appropriate than the other, for example, by urging people to adopt the "active consumer" rather than the "dependent patient" approach. Calls for the increased and continual undermining of professional claims to medical expertise and authority, as advocated by the proponents of consumerism and as supported by the sociological concept of reflexivity, threaten to undermine the beneficial aspects of the doctor–patient relationship, particularly in a context in which uncertainty is inevitable (Katz, 1984). If we cannot invest our trust and faith in the expertise of at least some of the medical practitioners to whom we have access, relying on embodied and affective experience and judgement as guides, the alternative may be paralysis and distress in the face of conflicting options.

References

Australian Consumers Association (1988) *Your Health Rights.* Australasian Publishing, Sydney.

Beck, U. (1994) The reinvention of politics: towards a theory of reflexive modernization. In *Reflexive Modernization: Politics, Tradition and Aesthetics in the Modern Social Order*, eds U. Beck, A. Giddens and S. Lash, pp. 1–55. Polity, Cambridge.

Blaxter, M. and Paterson, E. (1982) *Mothers and Daughters: A Three Generational Study of Health Attitudes and Behaviour.* Heinemann, London.

Bocock, R. (1993) *Consumption.* Routledge, London.

Broom, D. and Woodward, R. (1996) Medicalisation reconsidered: toward a collaborative approach to care. *Sociology of Health and Illness* **18**(3), 357–378.

Buetow, S. (1995) What do general practitioners and their patients want from general practice and are they receiving it? A framework. *Social Science & Medicine* **40**(2), 213–221.

Calnan, M. (1988) Lay evaluation of medicine and medical practice: report of a pilot study. *International Journal of Health Services* **18**(2), 311–322.

Cassell, E. (1991) *The Nature of Suffering and the Goals of Medicine.* Oxford University Press, New York.

Commonwealth Department of Health (1985) *Health Care and the Consumer.* Australian Government, Canberra.

Donaldson, C., Lloyd, P. and Lupton, D. (1991) Primary health care amongst elderly Sydneysiders. *Age and Ageing* **20**, 280–286.

Fine B. (1995) From political economy to consumption. In *Acknowledging Consumption: A Review of New Studies*, ed. D. Miller, pp. 127–164. Routledge, London.

Giddens, A. (1992) *The Transformation of Intimacy: Sexuality. Love and Eroticism in Modern Societies.* Polity, Cambridge.

Giddens, A. (1994) Living in a post-traditional society. In *Reflexive Modernization: Politics, Tradition and Aesthetics in the Modern Social Order*, eds U. Beck, A. Giddens and S. Lash, pp. 56–109. Polity, Cambridge.

Grace, V. (1994) What is a health consumer? In *Just Health: Inequality in Illness, Care and Prevention*, eds C. Waddell and A. Petersen, pp. 271–283. Churchill Livingstone, Melbourne.

Horin, A. (1995) It's the price we pay for empowerment. *Sydney Morning Herald*, 7 October, p. 21.

Katz, J. (1984) Why doctors don't disclose uncertainty. *The Hastings Center Report* February, 35–44.

Lloyd, P., Lupton, D. and Donaldson, C. (1991) Consumerism in the health care setting: an exploratory study of factors underlying the selection and evaluation of primary medical services. *Australian Journal of Public Health* **15**(3), 194–201.

Lloyd, P., Lupton, D., Wiesner, D. and Hasleton, S. (1993) Socio-demographic character-istics and reasons for choosing natural therapy: an exploratory study of patients resident in Sydney. *Australian Journal of Public Health* **17**(2), 135–144.

Logan, J., Green, D. and Woodfield, A. (1989) *Healthy Competition*. Centre for Independ-ent Studies, Sydney.

Lupton, D. (1996) "Your life in their hands": trust in the medical encounter. In *Health and the Sociology of Emotion*, Sociology of Health and Illness Monograph Series, eds J. Gabe and V. James, pp. 158–172. Blackwell, Oxford.

Lupton, D., Donaldson, C. and Lloyd, P. (1991) Caveat emptor or blissful ignorance? Patients and the consumerist ethos. *Social Science & Medicine* **33**(5), 559–568.

May, C., Dowrick, C. and Richardson, M. (1996) The confidential patient: the social construction of therapeutic relationships in general medical practice. *Sociological Review* **44**(2), 187–203.

Meredith, P. (1993) Patient satisfaction with communication in general surgery: problems of measurement and improvement. *Social Science & Medicine* **37**(5), 591–602.

Richards, B. (1994) *Disciplines of Delight: The Psychoanalysis of Popular Culture*. Free Association Books, London.

Saks, M. (1994) The alternatives to medicine. In *Challenging Medicine*, eds J. Gabe, D. Kelleher and G. Williams, pp. 84–103. Routledge, London.

Stein, H. (1985) *The Psychodynamics of Medical Practice: Unconscious Factors in Patient Care*. University of California Press, Berkeley.

de Swaan, A. (1990) *The Management of Normality: Critical Essays in Health and Welfare*. Routledge, London.

Taylor, C. (1989) *Sources of the Self: The Making of the Modern Identity*. Cambridge University Press, Cambridge.

Wiles, R. and Higgins, J. (1996) Doctor–patient relationships in the private sector: patients' perceptions. *Sociology of Health and Illness* **18**(3), 341–356.

Williams, B. (1994) Patient satisfaction: a valid concept? *Social Science & Medicine* **38**(4), 509–516.

Williams, S. and Calnan, M. (eds) (1996) *Modern Medicine: Lay Perspectives and Experiences*. UCL Press, London.

Wynne, B. (1996) May the sheep safely graze? A reflexive view of the expert–lay knowledge divide. In *Risk. Environment and Modernity: Towards a New Ecology*, eds S. Lash, B. Szerszynski and B. Wynne, pp. 44–83. Sage, London.

Chapter 16

David Silverman

GOING PRIVATE
Ceremonial forms in a medical oncology clinic

From *Communication and Medical Practice: Social Relations in the Clinic,* London and New York: Sage (1987)

. . .

Variability in the doctor–patient relation

TO ASK ABOUT THE IMPACT of method of payment on the form of the doctor–patient relationship means controlling for the impact of such variables as doctors' consulting styles and patients' social class. Leaving out such traditional psychological and sociological factors, Strong (1977, 1982) notes that, by the mid-nineteenth century, the professionalization of medicine had meant that, within the consultation, clinical judgment reigned supreme. Doctors had many clients and used routinized practices based on their technical authority to assert their professional dominance.

The authority of doctors within the consultation was, however, matched by their inability to enforce their decisions. With certain limited exceptions, like mental illness, the state did not give any power of compulsion to the medical profession. Patients were thus free to decide when to visit the doctor and whether to comply with his (sic) advice.

Within what Strong calls this 'classical form' of the relation, competition between doctors had two interactional consequences. First, doctors tried to sell themselves. By being attentive to the personal wishes of their clientele, they offered a differentiated, personalized product. Second, doctors employed tacit idealizations of the character of their clientele. This 'politeness ethic' served two functions: it minimized 'upsetting' valuable clients and it fitted neatly with the medical predisposition to treat illness as a natural, rather than a social, phenomenon.

Strong's central argument is found in the title of his paper, 'Private Practice for the Masses'. According to him, the NHS simply transferred these interactional patterns from a private to a public setting. With one exception, 'the classical form survived and is now applied universally' (1977:7). The exception was the pattern of product differentiation. This is illustrated in Table 16.1.

The absence of private competition has meant that the NHS consultation typically offers 'a standard, somewhat impersonal product with a minimum of choice' (Strong, 1977). This impersonality is based on an appeal to 'collegial' authority – the authority of the institution rather than of any individual practitioner. Doctors tend to be anonymous and to avoid differentiating between themselves, their colleagues or, indeed, doctors in other NHS institutions. Conversely, the individualization of service in private medicine means that doctors are more likely to seek to personalize their communication methods and, in return, to expect patients to act more like the clients of any fee-paid service, i.e. to question the competence of the practitioner, to evaluate services and to shop around.

Sample and methods

A small-scale study of a private London oncology clinic carried out in 1982–3 provides the possibility of evaluating some of Strong's hypotheses. The study developed as an off-shoot of a comparative study of two oncology clinics at a London teaching hospital within the NHS (Silverman, 1982). One clinic dealt with patients with leukaemia, the other mainly with patients suffering from Hodgkin's Disease – a cancer of the lymph system which, of all the cancers, seems to respond best to treatment and to offer the most favourable prognosis.

The consultant physician running the Hodgkin's clinic offered access to his private practice. This allowed comparison of consultations, many of which involved the same doctor and the same condition, but with the distinguishing variable being the location and the method of payment. The number of consultations observed is noted in Table 16.2.

The sample of private patients had broadly the same age and gender distribution as the NHS sample. Predictably, however, only one manual worker was a private patient (an Asian working in the garment industry). Two out of five of the NHS

Table 16.1 Classical and NHS interactional forms – Strong's argument

	'Classical' medicine	*NHS*
Professional dominance	yes	yes
No state enforcement	yes	yes
Politeness ethic	yes	yes
Product differentiation	yes	no

Table 16.2 Consultations sample

	Consultations	*Clinic sessions*	*Doctors*
Leukaemia clinic (NHS)	55	6	4
Hodgkin's clinic (NHS)	49	10	5
Oncology clinic (Private)	42	9	1
Total	146	25	9*

* Doctor in private oncology clinic was also observed in the Hodgkin's clinic.

Table 16.3 Accompanying family

	Private clinic (n = 42)	*NHS clinic (n = 104)*
Family present	20	29
No family	22	75

Difference not significant at 0.10.

patients whose occupation was recorded were manual workers. Again, as expected, nine out of the forty-two private patients were foreign nationals. Although the mean length of their consultations was one minute longer than those involving British subjects, they tended to participate far less. This may have been due to language problems. Finally, private patients were rather more likely to be accompanied by family, friends, or in the case of foreign nationals, interpreters. This is shown in Table 16.3.

Data from the NHS clinics had shown a statistically significant relation between the presence of family and patient participation in the consultation (Silverman, 1983). Here, however, although patients who are accompanied do participate slightly more than patients on their own, the difference is not significant ($\chi^2 = 2.1$, 1d.f; not significant at 0.10).

The study was preceded by two weeks spent observing ward-rounds, case-conferences and day wards and informal interviews with in-patients. It was not possible to secure agreement to tape-record out-patient consultations. Normal methods of note-taking were therefore used but efforts were made to record 'routine' as well as deviant patterns and to establish any special forms that might arise in particular situations e.g. 'new' or medically qualified patients.

The researcher identified himself in the NHS clinics by a name badge that was commonly worn by doctors there. No such identification was used at the private clinic. In the NHS clinics, doctors varied as to whether they informed patients and asked consent for my presence. In the private clinic, the doctor usually asked for consent. Patient response to my presence is discussed below.

A simple coding form was developed and pre-tested in fourteen consultations drawn from a Hodgkin's and a non-Hodgkin's Lymphoma clinic, observed prior to the collection of the main sample. This allowed the generation of comparative, quantitative data across a number of variables (e.g. the length of the consultation, the number of questions asked or unsolicited statements made by the patient or patient's family, the extent of small talk between doctor and patient). In all, ten independent variables and fourteen dependent variables were counted and then related through chi-square tests. The comparison of the two NHS clinics is discussed in Silverman, 1982.

Observational methods necessarily concentrate on particulars deemed 'interesting' according to certain theoretical or practical frames of references. This study followed Strong in focusing on what he calls the 'ceremonial order of the clinic'. Closely tied to Goffman's model of the encounter (Goffman, 1961), this attends to the display of identities within rules of etiquette. It is particularly concerned with 'who is to be what . . . and what sorts of rights and duties they may expect, exert and suffer' (Strong, 1982: 3).

These interactionist concerns understandably are not representative of the majority of work concerned with the social and psychological aspects of health and illness. For instance, a review of the literature on social aspects of cancer care, carried out by the author, reveals a huge concentration of work on accounts offered by patients outside medical settings (e.g. in home interviews), an attention to dramatic medicine (e.g. childhood leukaemia, breast cancer) and a concern with medically defined issues (e.g. how to improve information-flow from doctor to patient).

Interactionism is used here as a means of gathering basic data on social processes in an unexplored area. Although it offers its own 'blinkers', it nonetheless frees the researcher from the varying forms of reductionism offered by purely structural sociologies or by adopting medically defined problematics. When wedded, as here, to simple methods of quantification, it seeks to combine theoretical insight with methodological rigour, while being sensitive to policy issues see Silverman (1989).

Similar forms

Some of the quantitative data discussed elsewhere (Silverman, 1982) has revealed that the private clinic offers important instances of continuity with the NHS clinic. This should not be so surprising if we remember Strong's argument that the NHS provides 'private practice for the masses'. Each of the three features of 'classical medicine' which he claims are reproduced today can be found in equal measure in both the private and NHS clinics.

1 Professional dominance

Private patients, like NHS patients, generally take the role of laypersons confronted by an expert. In a clinic which treats life-threatening diseases, the relief and satisfaction that greets the doctor's judgment that all is well at the moment is universal. However, even where the medical verdict is unfavourable and out of line with the patient's own feelings of wellness, it is generally accepted stoically. Take the case of Mrs A, a lady in her sixties, with a diagnosis of hypoblastic anaemia —

potentially an early stage of leukaemia. The doctor has just suggested that further extensive treatment is necessary and Mrs A (A) questions him closely about the outlook:

(P:7)
1 A: Don't you think this rights itself
2 D: It's going to continue to be a nuisance
3 A: So what's the point of feeling well if you're going to feel bad again?
4 D: (explains that the blood count will go very low unless Mrs A is transfused and takes a cytotoxic drug)[1]
5 A: I thought I wouldn't need more treatment. I've been feeling so much better . . . Oh well, there's always miracles. I'm a great believer in miracles.

The professional's judgment reigns supreme here as elsewhere in the private clinic. Despite the lack of fit between the patient's perceptions of feeling 'well' and 'better' and the proposed treatment, the doctor's version of the situation takes precedence. Notice, moreover, that the doctor dwells in the discursive space of clinical definitions at Utterance 4. Despite Mrs A's attempt at 3 to raise broader practical or everyday issues, the doctor stays firmly in the clinical realm, leaving homespun philosophy to the patient (as at 5).

It must be borne in mind that this is an example of specialist private medicine. Although they can always seek 'another opinion', these patients are much closer to 'the end of the line' than those receiving primary care. Specialist medicine, dealing with life-threatening, complex processes, may encourage simpler patterns of professional dominance in both NHS and private settings.

In specialist medicine, private as well as NHS, the patient may even come to doubt his own experience of 'wellness'. This possibility is raised in another male patient's (A) response to the elicitation question:

(P:8)
1 D: How are you?
2 A: Pretty well I think.

While too much weight should not be attached to the patient's 'I think', it is rarely found in answer to elicitation questions. After all, we can all be presumed to know how we feel and to know with reasonable certainty. Yet Mr A, with leukaemia, seems to have learned, like Mrs A, that his own experience of wellness gives no certain guide to his state of health. Like many patients with his diagnosis, the blood count rather than how he feels has become his own basis for assessing his wellness.

This form of specialist private medicine, then, is not salient in relation to many of the features of the 'normal' lay–professional encounter. This is well illustrated by a comparison with an NHS consultation involving a patient with some medical

---

[1] Brackets are used in these transcripts to summarize what was said where the words were not noted at the time or for reasons of space.

background – she works as a pharmacist. This generated this grossly atypical elicitation question:

(H:5)
> D: Clinically, how are you?

The use of the term 'clinically' underlines how the medically qualified patient is granted the ability to judge the significance of her own symptoms. Such a right even extends to medically qualified spouses of patients. As Strong (1979) has noted, nurses are treated as good informants. Thus, at the private clinic, the doctor breaks into the elicitation sequence to turn to the patient's wife – a nurse:

(P:4)
> D: How breathless did he seem to you? Did he go blue?

For most patients, NHS or private, subjective perceptions of 'wellness' are recognized to be merely one fact among many that only the doctor is in a position to weigh and assess.

However, we should not assume that this technical dominance of the doctor always carries over into all the forms of *social* control of the consultation that are usually associated with professional dominance. As we shall see later, although these private patients do not challenge the clinical judgments of the doctor, many claim the kind of extensive rights over the agenda of the consultation which are rarely claimed or granted in the NHS clinics observed in this study.

2 No enforcement of decisions

In none of the clinics do the doctors seek to enforce their decisions. They present their conclusions as 'advice' which patients are free to reject, at their own risk. However, this does not mean that doctors are constrained from expressing their displeasure when patients seem like taking a contrary line. When, for instance, the pharmacist (B) shows concern at the possible effect of cytotoxic drugs on her ovaries (and hence her fertility), she is firmly put in her place:

(H:7)
> 1   B: Will it affect my ovary?
> 2   D: I think that's neither here nor there. We're dealing with a question of life and death. It actually doesn't affect the ovaries but the important thing is that (you should be in the right shape for looking after children).

While the issue of cancer treatment and fertility questions is discussed elsewhere (Silverman, 1982), we are here concerned with the aggressive response generated by patient questioning of medical advice over matters of 'life and death'.

In this case, the patient accepts the treatment. At the private clinic, where another patient (Mrs B) had rejected treatment for her cancer of the colon and had now developed lung secondaries, the doctor once again made his displeasure clear. The patient makes extensive displays of deference to professional dominance:

(P:8)

1   B: You're the doctor . . . (further discussion of the blood transfusions she is to have as a palliative measure)

2   B: Forgive me . . . to my lay mind . . . can I have it (the blood) over separate days?

Despite these statements acknowledging her lay status, Mrs B will not budge from her refusal to accept active treatment of her cancer. The doctor makes his displeasure clear, avoiding eye contact throughout and sternly remaining in his professional role.

3 Politeness ethic

At all clinics, patient's moral worth is never directly questioned. As Strong found, in a paediatric clinic, even potentially disturbing social information elicited from a parent rarely led to further questioning (Strong, 1979). An indirect example of this is to be found in the private clinic. Following a form of social elicitation much more commonly found here than in the NHS, as we shall show later, disquieting news is allowed to drop:

(P:4)

1   D: Wife well?

2   B: No. She's got a problem at the moment.

Despite Mr B's statement, the doctor changes the topic. It seems that, in the clinic, the doctor's question is to be seen as a polite enquiry, which is not intended to maintain its topical status whatever reply is elicited.

The only departure from the normal avoidance of 'personal' issues arises in the discussion of diet and alcohol. Nevertheless, the doctor's advice in both clinics is always presented in a light-hearted, bantering manner. The first two extracts below are taken from the private clinic.

(P:4)

[After discussion of patient's alcohol intake]

1   D: I'm not giving you any moral homilies but I think it's a message you're getting.

2   C: Sounds like a dry Christmas, doesn't it?

3   D: No, the last thing I'm trying to say is to change your life. Don't ruin your Christmas.

    D: You've lost a stone you say; you could do with losing another.

(H:6)

    D: You'll have to lose some weight won't you?

We may add to these similarities between the clinics certain other forms, some of which seem specific to oncology clinics. As so much popular and academic attention has focused on how much to tell the cancer patient, we should not be surprised that this is a common thread at both NHS and private clinics. Sometimes this is taken up by the family:

(P:3)

[*Patient is in the examination room getting dressed*]

DAUGHTER: [*to doctor*] He doesn't know it's a malignant tumor, he thinks it's benign.

Sometimes the patient wants to avoid letting the family know, Mrs B, for instance, asks the doctor not to 'let on' to her children while she is an in-patient; because 'they can't do anything' she does not want them troubled.

In all cases, doctors are very sensitive about informing the newly presenting cancer patient. Invariably the first question that is asked, prior to any diagnosis statement, is some form of: 'What have they told you so far?' In the light of that information, the news is broken to the patient: the term 'cancer' appearing rapidly or slowly according to the patient's present state of awareness. At subsequent consultations, the usual preferred term is 'the disease', while, in the course of the elicitation sequence, all doctors have a preferred form of euphemism about the spread of the condition:

(P:8)

D: Any lumps or bumps?

I have heard this phrase used by nearly all the nine doctors I have observed. . . .

Conclusions

1 A distinctive product?

The debate about private medicine often centres upon the issue of resources. On one side, there is the argument that (like private education) the more money is ploughed into private medicine, the more resources are freed for the public sector. This is countered by the claim that the growth of private medicine will establish a two-tier standard of treatment and that private medicine has high administrative costs and high rates of (possibly unnecessary) clinical tests and surgery.

For instance, the *New Statesman* (19 September 1986) reported an *Economist* estimate in April 1984 that, although the USA spends around $1,500 a year per head on health care, nearly four times what Britain spends, its people are no healthier. Indeed, the health care in countries like the USA seems increasingly polarized between extensive services offered to those who can pay and very limited services for the poor.

The Guardian (5 August 1985) headed a report from Washington 'Hospitals offload poorer patients'. It went on:

> A growing number of poor patients are being dumped – often in need of emergency care – on to public hospitals because they cannot afford

treatment at private hospitals. In the hospital jargon their 'wallet biopsies show a low green count'. Dollar bills are green.

Conversely, GP care, for those who can pay, is being redefined as a medical industrial complex. In Australia, we read that:

> the traditional suburban surgery is being metamorphosed into the 'boutique practice' in which perhaps two GPs offer an intensive service to patients who are prepared to pay high fees. The personalized doctor–patient relationship remains and there is an emphasis on preventive care with a wider range of strictly non-medical services such as counselling. (*Sydney Morning Herald*, 5 November 1986)

The evidence gathered from this London oncology private clinic cannot arbitrate between these arguments about inequalities of health care. The NHS clinic, where the doctor works, has no waiting list and the resource impact of his private practice is unclear. We can be a little clearer about what is, rather than what ought to be: about individual gains and losses, rather than social utility. The market principle is sometimes used in support of private medicine. People will only pay for a product that they regard as distinctive and worthwhile. The data give us an opportunity, on an objective basis, to answer the question: precisely what are these patients buying?

In brief, we have shown how these private patients buy a setting which is territorially and socially organized to provide for a personalized service, based on an individualized, non-bureaucratic authority and personally orchestrated care. In social terms, these patients seem to obtain the best kind of individualized, GP service in the context of highly qualified, specialist treatment for life-threatening conditions.

These gains are balanced by potential and real losses. Socially, isolation can be the other side of the coin to this kind of individual care. Because these patients do not attend large clinics, they cannot call upon the kind of peer-group support that I have observed in the NHS leukaemia clinic. They simply do not see other patients on a regular basis and so cannot share their burdens or appeal to a comparative reference group.

The argument is problematic in the same way as the choice between public wards and private rooms: what is support to one patient may be intrusion to another. All we can objectively say that these patients are losing is the opportunity to observe the peer-group relations that arise in the NHS clinics and to become involved if it should suit them.

Even on the medical side, there are three problematic aspects of private care: (1) Unlike the NHS clinic, other appropriate specialists, like radiologists and pathologists, are not at hand. Much of the orchestration of care that develops here is necessitated by the isolated form of consultation. As the doctor concerned has told me, at this clinic it is much harder to sort out the patient's treatment programme very rapidly. (2) The doctor also feels that, ironically, he is 'not on such a tight schedule' in his NHS clinic and so can give more time to patients there. At the private clinic, the perceived need to avoid keeping patients waiting produces a much more uniform consultation length, perhaps less responsive to the special needs of new patients who, as we have seen, actually get slightly shorter consultations than NHS patients. (3) The patients at the private clinic have a broader range of cancers, as well as other conditions, than those seen at either of the NHS clinics. There might be an issue of losses and gains in less specialized, more diffuse medicine versus highly specialized medicine.

2 A continuum of ceremonial forms

It would be completely mistaken to assume that the ceremonial forms observed here are unique to private medicine. Nearly every one has a parallel in the NHS clinics. Four factors, in particular, seemed to push the NHS consultations observed here in this direction:

The type of setting The leukaemia clinic discussed in another paper (Silverman, 1982) was composed entirely of patients who had survived their first treatment. It was an informal clinic where the patients, who all knew the ropes, took on the role of 'old lags'. There was extensive social elicitation and patients were seen to evaluate medical work, to influence the agenda and, like the private patients, were expected to orchestrate some of their own care.

The patient's occupation As is commonly suggested, doctors who are patients are given a position of much greater interactive equality than others and this can lead to the kind of personalized encounter found in the private clinic (for instance, the definition of medical history by citing doctors' surnames). Again, certain other professionals may have skills that are relevant in obtaining personalized treatment. A senior social worker, for instance, just 'popped in' to the leukaemia clinic and set up a 'joint chat' with two doctors and himself and his wife to discuss his 'future'.

The patient's condition Where the patient is approaching a terminal condition, all the normal rules may be waived. Such a patient, observed at the leukaemia clinic, broadly defined his own preferred consultation disposal, was more or less in control of the agenda, and was promised a home phonecall that day in response to his requests.

The patient's social background Here the evidence is patchy. Nonetheless at the NHS clinic, one clearly upper-class lady (Mrs J) (who I was told would have been a private patient if the consultant concerned had taken them) got personalized treatment to a degree not seen in other patients. For instance.

(L:2)
1   D: We've got an audience. I hope that's OK.

        . . .

2   D: John (the consultant) is in America.
3   J: Lucky him.

Finally, where a patient at another NHS clinic was married to the son of a surgeon, the husband speedily raised the question of private care and an immediate scan was set up at the BUPA Centre because the NHS hospital had a two-week delay in the pre-Christmas period. Like many private consultations, the encounter ended with X-rays being passed into the keeping of the patient.

3 Further research

This chapter began by citing Strong's work which hypothesized that 'product differentiation' based on individual, non-collegial, authority would be the distinguishing mark of private consultations. This small-scale study has largely borne out this hypothesis, although I have added a note of caution about the continuum of forms to be found within NHS medicine. Further research should broaden the database to include a range of private practitioners and private practice. A study of private general practice would usefully complement these data on a specialist private clinic. If the former can generate situations, as observed here, in two cases, where the GP accompanies his patient to the specialist, it is likely to offer a data-rich area for comparative study.

References

Goffman, E. (1961) *Encounters*, Indianapolis: Bobbs-Merrill.

Silverman, D. (1982) ' "Is It Cancer Doctor?" Interpersonal Relations in Two NHS Oncology Clinics', mimeo, London: Goldsmiths' College.

Silverman, D. (1983) 'The Clinical Subject: Adolescents in a Cleft-Palate Clinic', *Sociology of Health and Illness* 5(3): 253–74.

Silverman, D. (1989) 'Telling Convincing Stories', in B. Glassner and J. Moreno (eds), *The Qualitative–Quantitative Distinction in the Social Sciences*. Dordrecht: Kluwer.

Strong, P. (1977) 'Private Practice for the Masses: Medical Consultations in the NHS', mimeo. Aberdeen: MRC Medical Sociology Unit.

Strong, P. (1979) *The Ceremonial Order of the Clinic*. London: Routledge.

Strong, P. (1982) 'Power, Etiquette and Identity in Medical Consultations', mimeo, Open University.

Chapter 17

Sarah Cant and Ursula Sharma

A NEW MEDICAL PLURALISM?

From *A New Medical Pluralism: Alternative Medicine, Doctors, Patients and the State*, London: UCL Press (1999)

. . .

Motivations to consume

THERE ARE A NUMBER of possible individual motivations for turning to alternative medicine. However, we need to examine these reasons more carefully to assess whether they offer general explanations for the increased popularity and the rise of the new medical pluralism. At the most simplistic level the examination of the dissatisfactions with biomedicine and the attractions of alternative medicine offer some insight into this question, but as we shall see the picture is rather more complicated and is not a case of individual consumers weighing up costs and benefits in a calculated manner. The decision making process is a complex one and incorporates perceptions of the body, desire for inclusion and power in the healing process.

Let us first take the more straightforward explanations as given by the consumers. Sharma's study offers ample evidence of the costs and benefits of using alternative and orthodox medical services. We can link the use of alternative medicine to wider concerns about modern science. Specifically, it appears that many consumers are genuinely concerned about the side effects of drugs and are anxious about taking medication that seems to them to be made of artificial substances and chemicals. In contrast, the apparent harmlessness of alternative medicine and its concentration on natural products is an attraction:

> Jason had a very bad skin rash which would not clear up, and I thought it
> might be eczema. The doctor prescribed cortisone creams and steroids

> which I thought was rather drastic. We went to a homoeopath who dealt
> with the problem more or less. It was a relief not to have put cortisone
> cream and stuff like that all over his hands . . . I was always worried
> about having medicine in the house and I was relieved that homoeopathic
> medicines are non-poisonous. If you take a whole bottle full you are not
> going to die even though it may be labelled "belladonna" or something
> like that. (Sharma 1996:236)

Or

> I tried all the tablets the GP gave me for my migraine. I have had all
> kinds, Migraleve, Migril etc. which I don't believe in because they have
> got ergotamines and I feel the side effects are too great and I am not
> prepared to risk it. I think it is too much. (Sharma 1996:237)

Of course, consumers may be under some misapprehension if they automatically equate alternative medicine with safety and the BMA has gone to great lengths to point out the potential harm that can come from consultations with alternative practitioners (BMA 1986, 1987). These include the failure of alternative practitioners to identify serious medical conditions and the side effects associated with alternative medical products (this was the basis of the campaign to ban comfrey, although in this case, as Whitelegg (1996) shows, the evidence against the herb was far from convincing).

It is also the case, as we have already seen, that consumers of alternative medicine are concerned about the effectiveness of biomedicine and its ability to provide answers to chronic health problems (Donnelly et al. 1985, Moore et al. 1985, Furnham and Smith 1988). MacGregor and Peay (1996) showed that while users of alternative medicine were not necessarily dissatisfied with their recent visits to their biomedical practitioners, they expressed lower levels of confidence in bio-medicine in general. Perhaps the most obvious reason for continuing to use alterna-tive medicine is the experience that it is efficacious, and a number of respondents in Cant's (1996) study suggested that they had been won over to homoeopathy because they had experienced positive results: "I really had bad ovulating pain, he gave me a remedy and it worked. That was what converted me. Homoeopathy worked in five minutes, no more pain. It was so miraculous."

Another interviewee recognized that she could not prove that it was homoeopathy that had made her feel better: "The remedy worked in a very gradual way, I mean you could be getting better yourself. That's the airy fairy nature of homoeopathy."

Indeed, surveys of users have found widespread satisfaction with alternative medicine. For example, in a *Guardian* (1996) survey all except four of the 386 respondents claimed to have experienced some improvement in their condition. Maybe the continued motivation to use this sector is a pragmatic one? It is important to try and locate the foundations upon which feelings of satisfaction are based, as it is unlikely that alternative medicine is judged purely on clinical efficacy but also the extent to which consumers feel that their experiences are taken seriously and given due attention and time.

This leads us to another area of concern to consumers – the amount of time that is spent with the practitioner. All studies have revealed that consumers are drawn to consultations where they have more opportunity to discuss their problem in depth.

> They [complementary practitioners] give you more time. Obviously most of them charge you, so they would do. But most of them treat the individual symptoms as the individual's problem not just some Latinised name (Sharma 1996:242).

Or as a respondent in Cant's study also explained,

> I tend to get depressed and then I get fat because I eat more. The general practitioner said to go out more and use Prozac. You just get a prescription but you don't get to the bottom of why you are depressed because they haven't got the time to get to the root cause and because they have not been trained to treat you totally and wholly.

Most first consultations with alternative practitioners tend to last well over an hour (Sharma 1992, Cant and Calnan 1991) although again we must be cautious about making generalizations. Some therapists do not need to spend as long with the patient, for example the average consultation with a chiropractor lasts between 15 and 20 minutes (Cant and Sharma 1994). Perhaps in the case of chiropractic it is the pragmatic and physical relief that is important rather than the detailed discussion of a person's emotional, and spiritual well-being, as might be the case in a two-hour session with a homoeopath? Certainly, the attraction of time is not peculiar to alternative medicine and studies of the private biomedical sector have revealed this to be an important reason for choosing to pay (Calnan et al. 1993). The issue of time, however, is also a contentious one; discussions within therapy groups about the advantages and disadvantages of incorporating their practice into the National Health Service always reveal concerns that such a move would necessarily curtail the amount of time the practitioner could spend with their patients.

If we move beyond the straightforward costs and benefits to patients of biomedicine versus alternative medicine another range of explanations become available, in particular motivations that resonate with wider cultural changes. The increased availability of information and the knowledge of risks may have provided for a more reflexive and questioning consumer – an explanation that of course precedes those of costs and benefits. In Sharma's study there was evidence of interviewees who had developed greater confidence in their capacity to choose between therapies: "I make up my own mind about these things now . . . Now I feel I am in control of my life" (Sharma 1995:51).

It appears that patients also desire more control in the consultation. In longer consultations patients have the opportunity to provide more information about their complaint and take on board information provided by the practitioners (Johannessen 1996). Qualitative studies have revealed that patients respond to being treated as an equal and desire a more participative relationship with their practitioner. Such a possibility derives from the fact that most alternative medicine proposes a form of holism, which rejects the treatment of symptoms in isolation but seeks to understand them in the context of a person's total health profile (their spiritual and emotional responses as well as their experience of their social situation). Such an approach requires both an individualistic approach to treatment and the need to extract detailed information from the patient about the circumstances of their illness and their feelings about it. Consequently, the patient is given the position of "expert", having valuable knowledge about themselves and this is clearly enjoyed. As one respondent in Sharma's study revealed: "When I saw her I thought she is of my intelligence, she treats me as an equal" (Sharma 1995:51).

Similarly in Cant's study, the positive aspects of mutuality again were expressed: "He takes my opinion more seriously, I have more time and it is more two way definitely, but obviously he makes the decision about the remedy." Or, "I really connect with him, I have a relationship with him, I feel comfortable and trust the person. He's not just your clinician, he's caring."

Many of the respondents in this study spoke about their practitioner as being a friend or confidante as much as a practitioner. As one woman said: "He's the third most important man in my life after my husband and son."

In many of the cases this made the relationship a rather ambiguous one, for after all the practitioner is not usually a friend, although the patient may feel that they have connected with him/her in the consultation room and experience feelings of closeness. The following extract from Cant's study is revealing,

> I unburden myself and he listens . . . I still go now that I am well and talk
> to him about any old thing. But he has suggested that I do not see him for
> a while. I feel really quite sorry, my husband is away a lot and I enjoyed
> unburdening myself.

Indeed one respondent talked of how she had expected the homoeopath to check up on her on an occasion when she had been admitted to hospital and "I felt really upset when he did not ring – I felt let down really."

Thus, a more mutual and sharing relationship also brings ambiguities, ones that have to be dealt with carefully. One homoeopath told how she had two phones in her home, one number for her personal friends and one for her patients, that she could leave on the answer machine and monitor if patients were becoming too intrusive (Cant 1996). The professional associations that represent practitioners have also had to reflect upon this problem and have drawn up clear codes of conduct so that any claims of harassment or misunderstanding made by patients can be dealt with in a clear manner.

Although all the respondents that were questioned in Cant's study felt that they had a role to play in the consultation, the majority were not at all informed about the medication that they had been prescribed or indeed about homoeopathy in general; indeed only one respondent said that they had read up about the remedy that they had been given: "I never know which remedy I have been given. I never know what the remedy is – I did read and go to lectures, I got hooked really, but he (the homoeopath) discouraged me and told me to think that it is all magic."

Such a description of the consultation suggests a number of possible interpretations. Perhaps there is a level where patients do not wish to exercise knowledgeability and consumerism, just as in the private biomedical sector where the patients do not make the choice of consultant (Calnan *et al.* 1993). It may also be the case that practitioners only want to encourage a degree of participation, partly no doubt to maintain their own distance and boundaries of expertise. Or perhaps there is a concern to protect the patient; for example, in homoeopathy there is often a reluctance to tell patients about the chosen remedy, which is linked to a whole range of social and emotional traits (e.g. tearful, greedy, etc.) because the practitioners are concerned that the patient may read the descriptions and make assumptions about how the practitioner viewed their personality. Overall, however, patients talked of feeling that they were participating in the medical encounter. According to Taylor (1984) this shift links more to changes in the political rather than medical culture and demands for the democratization of decision-making. Certainly, this view would link in with Giddens's (1990) discussion of the growing disillusionment with the expert, and processes of re-skilling by the lay populace.

This idea also resonates with an explanation offered by medical anthropologists that suggests alternative medicine offers more meaning to the patients and allows them to link their illness to wider cultural, personal and social frameworks. We know that the lay public have a wide range of frameworks that they use to make sense of illness episodes and that they use illness episodes to re-interpret their own biographies. These frameworks – such as a previous experience or the health of other family members – are not generally drawn upon by the biomedical doctor. In contrast, alternative medical practitioners usually spend a long time questioning the patients about their family, their lifestyle and environment (indeed questions can be so probing and seemingly irrelevant that new patients can feel perturbed about their relevance). Helman puts great emphasis on the sense making potential of alternative medicine, especially that which it gives to suffering:

> Many patients have an unfulfilled sense of wanting to be connected once again, to some wider context, to locate their suffering in a wider framework – even to somehow contain themselves within the many cycles of nature . . . Complementary practitioners often help people make sense of their situation in a more meaningful way than does medicine, often utilising more traditional modes of dealing with misfortune . . . many of them utilise traditional cultural beliefs in order to explain to the patient why they have been affected by that particular illness at that particular time. (Helman 1992:12)

Certainly there seems to be some evidence that patients feel that alternative medicine does help them make sense of their situation even if it is by simply linking their health problems to those of their family. As one respondent in Sharma's study outlined,

> I had to do a massive questionnaire about my family background. No-one had ever asked me to do this before. I had to ring my mother and go back to bronchial asthma in my family before the turn of the century . . . all this seems to come together and it was *my* body and *my* temperament. (Sharma 1996:243)

Thus, alternative medicine may offer new ways of looking at health and illness that move beyond reductionist accounts and allow for more varied and plural understandings that converge with those held by the patient. Johannessen (1996) argues that the individualized treatment bestows meaning to the patient and allows them to create order in a situation of personal chaos, created by the illness episode. The explanations offered by the alternative practitioner purport to be and are experienced by the patient as "tailor made" to their own biography and experiences and can in turn engender changes to the person's perception of their health and social situation. Such a stance clearly also allows the patients the opportunity to develop and extend their pluralistic understandings of their bodies and bodily suffering and to construct multiple possibilities for comprehending the relationship between their body, self and social context (Busby 1996).

It is also possible that the motivations to use alternative medicine may stem from changes to attitudes held about the body, although it is difficult to establish whether it is ideas about the body that motivate use or whether consumers alter their perception of their body as a consequence of visiting an alternative therapist. Certainly, at a time when the body has come to be seen as a "project" (Giddens 1991, Shilling 1993), it is not hard to see the attraction of therapeutic practice that places great emphasis on a holistic approach to health care and which makes links between physical complaints and the emotional and spiritual levels of a person and indeed offers hope that good health can be achieved and maintained. According to Coward, alternative medicine is premised on very different ideas about the body and assumes that perfect health is an achievable aim. "The body has a whole new centrality as a place of work and transformation" (Coward 1989:194).

The long term users of homoeopathy in Cant's study had found that they were more aware of their bodies and tended to monitor physical changes more closely, especially recognizing that these may be a sign that they were emotionally unwell. Such body monitoring is often encouraged by the therapists who sometimes ask their patients to keep a diary of how they are feeling and to chart any bodily changes they experience. Respondents felt they had altered in their perceptions of themselves:

> It has done something to me – what am I trying to say, my body tells me what is happening all the time. My body leads me now . . . if the psoriasis starts I know now that I am emotionally stressed . . . I make the connection between emotional and physical signs. I don't check my body all the time but I do monitor it.

Another interviewee said:

> Maybe you become a bit of a hypochondriac. I think everything is now relevant. I think about my whole body and how it might be connected. The body constantly surprises you when you monitor it.

Others talked about how they had become more obsessed with their good health and made sure that they did all possible to ensure that a state of such "good health" was maintained: "I am more aware of my body, its strengths and weaknesses. I go to the homoeopath because I am worried about the winter and I go for a boost . . . my health rules my life really."

These extracts concur with Lloyd *et al.*'s (1993) findings that users were concerned about having a healthy lifestyle but this also places responsibility upon the individual to ensure they monitor and judge all physical, mental and spiritual changes that they experience. There was evidence in many of the interviews (Cant 1996) that using homoeopathy had provided the interviewees with a broader understanding of their bodies, their health and a recognition of their obligations if they wished to achieve perfect wellbeing: "I've learnt to exercise more and to eat differently and I am aware that everything is connected." Or, "Homoeopathy touches your whole life and you understand yourself, I do not know how I lived without it."

Such commentary can explain the continued use of alternative therapies and also illustrates the connection between alternative medical practice and "healthism" (Crawford 1980) – the desire to retain and maintain perfectibility in health and put much of the emphasis upon the individual. This emphasis can of course be interpreted as empowering, offering individuals the opportunity to know themselves (Busby 1996) or as disciplining, deflecting the responsibility away from society and operating as a surveillance function (Braathen 1996). Crawford (1980) would use the latter interpretation, arguing that alternative medicine does not empower the individual as this would require effective social and political analysis of the causes of ill health. Certainly alternative medicine seems to demedicalize personal health by encouraging the individual to be less dependent on biomedicine but paradoxically it remedicalizes life, bringing all areas of a person's emotional and spiritual life under scrutiny (Lowenberg and Davis 1994). . . .

References

Braathen, E. 1996. Communicating the individual body and the body politic. The discourse on disease prevention and health promotion in alternative therapies. In *Complementary and alternative medicines. Knowledge in practice*, S. Cant and U. Sharma (eds), 151–62. London: Free Association Books.

British Medical Association 1986. *Alternative therapy report of the board of science and education*. London: BMA.

British Medical Association 1987. *The BMA guide to living with risk*. London: Penguin.

Busby, H. 1996. Alternative medicines/alternative knowledges: putting flesh on the bones using traditional Chinese approaches to healing. *Complementary and alternative medicines. Knowledge in practice*, S. Cant and U. Sharma (eds), 135–51. London: Free Association Books.

Calnan, M., S. Cant, J. Gabe 1993. *Going private. Why people pay for their health care*. Buckingham: Open University Press.

Cant, S. 1996. From charismatic teaching to professional training. In *Complementary and alternative medicines. Knowledge in practice*, S. Cant and U. Sharma (eds) 44–66. London: Free Association Books.

Cant, S. and M. Calnan 1991. On the margins of the medical marketplace? An exploratory study of alternative practitioners' perceptions. *Sociology of Health and Illness* **13**, 34–51.

Cant, S. and U. Sharma 1994. *The professionalisation of complementary medicine*. Project report to ESRC.

Coward, R. 1989. *The whole truth*. London: Faber & Faber.

Crawford, R. 1980. Healthism and the medicalization of everyday life. *International Journal of Health Services* **10**(3), 365–88.

Donnelly, W.J., J.E. Spykerboer, Y.H. Thong 1985. Are patients who use alternative medicine dissatisfied with orthodox medicine? *Medical Journal Australia* **142**, 539.

Furnham, A. and C. Smith 1988. Choosing alternative medicine: a comparison of the patients visiting a GP and a homoeopath. *Social Science and Medicine* **26**, 685–7.

Giddens, A. 1990. *The consequences of modernity*. Cambridge: Polity Press.

Giddens, A. 1991. *Modernity and self-identity*. Cambridge: Polity Press.

Guardian 1996. Back to our roots. *Guardian*, 9 January.

Helman, C. 1992. Complementary medicine in context. *Medical World* **9**, 11–12.

Johannessen, H. 1996. Individualised knowledge: reflexologists, biopaths and kinesiologists in Denmark. In *Complementary and alternative medicines. Knowledge in practice*, S. Cant and U. Sharma (eds) 114–32. London: Free Association Books.

Lloyd, P., D. Lupton, D. Wiesner, S. Hasleton 1993. Choosing alternative therapy: an exploratory study of socio-demographic characteristics and motives of patients resident in Sydney. *Australian Journal of Public Health* **17**(2), 135–41.

Lowenberg, J. and F. Davis 1994. Beyond medicalisation-demedicalisation: the case of holistic health. *Sociology of Health and Illness* **16**(5), 579–99.

MacGregor, K. and E. Peay 1996. The choice of alternative therapy for health care. Testing some propositions. *Social Science and Medicine* **43**(9), 1317–27.

Moore, J., K. Phipps, D. Marcer 1985. Why do people seek treatment by alternative medicine? *British Medical Journal* **290**, 28–9.

Sharma, U. 1992. *Complementary medicine today. Practitioners and patients*. London: Routledge.

Sharma, U. 1995. *Complementary medicine today. Practitioners and patients*. (revd edn). London: Routledge.

Sharma, U. 1996. Using complementary therapies: a challenge to modern medicine. In *Modern medicine: lay perspectives and experiences*, S. J. Williams and M. Calnan (eds) London: UCL Press.

Shilling, C. 1993. *The body and social theory*. London: Sage.

Taylor, C. R. 1984. Alternative medicine and the medical encounter in Britain and the United States. In *Alternative medicines. Popular and policy perspectives*, Warren Salmon, J (ed.), 191–228. London: Tavistock.

Whitelegg, M. 1996. The Comfrey controversy. In *Complementary and alternative medicines. Knowledge in practice*, S. Cant and U. Sharma (eds), 66–87. London: Free Association Press.

Chapter 18

Cathy Charles, Amiram Gafni and Tim Whelan

DECISION-MAKING IN THE PHYSICIAN–PATIENT ENCOUNTER

Revisiting the shared treatment decision-making model

From *Social Science and Medicine*, 49, 1999: 651–61

Introduction

ALTHOUGH SHARED TREATMENT decision-making is a concept that has gained widespread appeal to both physicians and patients in recent years, there is still confusion about what the concept means. To help clarify this issue, we published a paper which tried to define shared treatment decision-making and its key characteristics and to show how this interactional model differs from other commonly cited approaches to treatment decision-making such as the paternalistic and the informed models (Charles *et al.*, 1997a). The paternalistic model is by now well known and articulated (Emanuel and Emanuel, 1992: Levine *et al.*, 1992: Beisecker and Beisecker, 1993; Deber, 1994; Coulter, 1997). Hence, we concentrated on exploring the differences between the informed and the shared models because these two labels have often been used interchangeably to describe quite different types of interaction between physician and patient in treatment decision-making.

The context for our discussion was a life threatening disease where several treatment options were available with different possible outcomes (benefits and risks or side effects), outcomes could vary in their impact on the patient's physical and psychological well-being and outcomes in the individual case were uncertain. In this context, we argued that a shared treatment decision-making model could be identified as such by reference to four necessary characteristics (Charles *et al.*, 1997a) as follows:

1   At a minimum, both the physician and patient are involved in the treatment decision-making process.

2   Both the physician and patient share information with each other.
3   Both the physician and the patient take steps to participate in the decision-making process by expressing treatment preferences.
4   A treatment decision is made and both the physician and patient agree on the treatment to implement.

In this paper we revisit and add elements to our conceptual framework based on further analytic thinking and our current research on the meaning of shared decision-making to women with early stage breast cancer and to physicians who specialize in this area (Charles *et al.*, 1998). Our revised framework (1) identifies different analytic stages in the treatment decision-making process: (2) provides a dynamic view of treatment decision-making by recognizing that the approach adopted at the outset of any given physician–patient encounter may change during the course of that encounter; and (3) identifies different approaches that lie in between the three predominant treatment decision-making models. Before exploring these issues, we briefly review factors that have led to the development of new treatment decision-making models as alternatives to the traditional paternalistic approach.

The rise and fall of paternalism

Prior to the 1980s, the most prevalent approach to treatment decision-making in North America was paternalistic with physicians assuming the dominant role. Underlying this deference to professional authority were a number of assumptions. First, that for most illnesses, a single best treatment existed and that physicians generally would be well versed in the most current and valid clinical thinking. Second, physicians would not only know the best treatments available, they would consistently apply this information when selecting treatments for their own patients. Third, because of their expertise and experience, physicians were in the best position to evaluate tradeoffs between different treatments and to make the treatment decision. Fourth, because of their professional concern for the welfare of their patients, physicians had a legitimate investment in each treatment decision. This legitimation of physician control was further buttressed by professional codes of ethics which bound physicians to act in the best interests of their patients (Lomas and Contandriopoulous, 1994; Charles *et al.*, 1997b). All of these assumptions led both physicians and patients to expect a dominant role for physicians in treatment decision-making. Status differences between physicians and patients in terms of education, income and gender also contributed to power differentials in the medical encounter.
    During the 1980s and beyond, the credibility of the above assumptions began to be questioned. For an increasing number of illnesses, for example, there was no one best treatment and a more murky and complex decisional context evolved where different treatments had different types of tradeoffs between benefits and risks. Since the patient rather than the physician would have to live with the consequences of these tradeoffs, the assumption that physicians were in the best position to evaluate and weigh these was increasingly challenged (Eddy, 1990; Levine *et al.*,

1992; Lomas and Lavis, 1996). At the same time, research into the quality of medical care began to focus on the effectiveness and appropriateness of a wide range of services delivered by physicians (Roos, 1984; Chassin et al., 1986, 1987b: Roos et al., 1988: Berwick, 1989; Lomas, 1990; Wennberg, 1990). The research on small area variations, for example, found consistent evidence that physician procedures for the same disease often varied considerably across small geographic areas and that these variations did not seem to be related to differences in the health status of the respective populations (Roos, 1984: Chassin et al., 1986, 1987a; Wennberg et al., 1987; Roos et al., 1988: Leape et al., 1993: Iscoe et al., 1994). Variations in treatment patterns were also found for diseases for which clinical guidelines had been developed on best practices (Lomas et al., 1989). Patient preferences may have accounted for some of this variation, but the data also suggested that either some physicians were unaware of recommended best practices for the treatment of particular diseases or that they were aware, but were not implementing the recommended guidelines.

Concern with rising health care costs in both Canada and the United States was another health policy issue focusing attention on the medical profession (Katz et al., 1997). The joining together of cost and quality concerns resulted in recommendations to make physicians more explicitly accountable to patients, the public, and in the case of the United States, to third party payers. In addition, the twin principles of caveat emptor (let the buyer beware) and consumer sovereignty gained popularity (Haug and Lavin, 1981, 1983: Charles and DeMaio, 1993), as manifested in new legislation precluding treatment implementation without informed consent and in legislation safeguarding the rights of patients to be informed about all available treatment options (Nayfield et al., 1994: Ontario Ministry of Health, 1994). These two principles were also evident in the emergent interest among both patients and physicians in developing and advocating new approaches to treatment decision-making which would incorporate a larger role for patients in the decision-making process (Brody, 1980; Quill, 1983; Thomasma, 1983; Eddy, 1990; Hughes and Larson, 1991; Emanuel and Emanuel, 1992; Ryan, 1992; Deber, 1994; Llewelyn-Thomas, 1995; Cahill, 1996; Quill and Brody, 1996; Charles et al., 1997a; Coulter, 1997; Gafni et al., 1998).

Models of treatment decision-making

Both the informed and the shared models of treatment decision-making were developed largely in reaction to the paternalistic model and to compensate for alleged flaws in the latter approach. These three models are the most prominent and widely discussed in the treatment decision-making literature. Key characteristics of each model and how they differ from one another are summarized in Table 18.1. In Table 18.1 treatment decision-making is subdivided into three analytically distinct stages, even though, in reality, these may occur together or in an interative process. The steps are: information exchange, deliberation about treatment options and deciding on the treatment to implement. The latter is the outcome of the deliberation process.

Table 18.1 Models of treatment decision-making[a]

Analytical stages	Models	Paternalistic (in between approaches)	Shared (in between approaches)	Informed
Information exchange	Flow			
	Direction	One way (largely) Physician → patient	Two way Physician ⇆ patient	One way (largely) Physician → patient
	Type	Medical	Medical and personal	Medical
	Amount[b]	Minimum legally required	All relevant for decision-making	All relevant for decision-making
Deliberation		Physician alone or with other physicians	Physician and patient (plus potential others)	Patient (plus potential others)
Deciding on treatment to implement		Physicians	Physician and patient	Patient

[a] Illustration for an encounter focusing on the case of a (treating) physician–patient dyad. For more complex cases see text.
[b] Minimum required.

Information exchange

Information exchange refers to the type and amount of information exchanged between physician and patient and whether information flow is one or two way. Types of information that the physician might communicate to the patient include: the natural history of the disease, the benefits and risks (side effects) of various treatment alternatives, a description of the treatment procedure(s) to be used and community resources and information that the patient could access about her disease. These are primarily technical types of knowledge which most patients will not have. Information that the patient might reveal to the physician include: aspects of the patient's health history, her lifestyle, her social context (e.g. work and family responsibilities and relationships). her beliefs and fears about her disease and her knowledge of various treatment options obtained from lay networks and/or other information sources. Except for the latter, these are primarily types of self-knowledge that the patient brings to the encounter and that the physician typically has no way of knowing except through direct communication with the patient in this or in prior consultations. In addition, at the outset of the encounter, either the physician, the patient, or both may exchange preferences regarding their own and each other's role in the decision-making process. The goal of this exchange is to make explicit how each expects the decision-making process to proceed.

The flow of information exchange may be one way or two way. In the paternalistic model, the exchange is largely one way and the direction is from physician to patient. At a minimum, the physician must provide the patient with legally required information on treatment options and obtain informed consent to the treatment recommended. Beyond this, the patient as depicted in this model is a passive recipient of whatever amount and type of information the physician chooses to reveal. In some cases, the physician may ask the patient about specific issues such as pain tolerance or allergies that could affect the latter's reaction to the treatment selected by the physician. In general, this model assumes that the physician knows best and will make the best treatment decision for the patient. In addition, information exchange from patient to physician is not seen as a major prerequisite to completing this task.

In a shared decision-making model, the information exchange is two way (Charles et al., 1997a). At a minimum, the physician must inform the patient of all information that is relevant to making the decision, i.e. information about available treatment options, the benefits and risks of each and potential effects on the patient's psychological and social well being. The patient needs to provide information to the physician on issues raised above, e.g. her values, preferences, lifestyle, beliefs and knowledge about her illness and its treatment. The first type of information exchange ensures that all relevant treatment options are on the table; the second ensures that both the physician and patient evaluate these within the context of the patient's specific situation and needs rather than as a standard menu of options whose impact and outcomes are assumed to be similar for clinically similar patients.

In the informed model, information exchange is one way, from physician to patient. This exchange is the very crux of the model, defining the boundaries of the physician's clinical role in decision-making. The physician in this model is assumed to be the primary source of information to the patient on medical/scientific issues about the patient's disease and treatment options. To fulfil this role, the physician, at a minimum, needs to give the patient all relevant information from the highest quality research evidence on the benefits and risks of various treatments so that she will be enabled to make an informed decision. Beyond information transfer, the physician has no further role in the decision-making process. The remaining tasks of deliberation and decision-making are the patient's alone. Eddy (1990, p. 442) describes the rationale for restricting physician involvement in these latter two steps as follows:

> the people whose preferences count are the patients, because they are the ones who will have to live (or die) with the outcomes . . . Ideally, you and I are not even in the picture. What matters is what Mrs. Smith thinks . . . It is also quite possible that Mrs. Smith's preferences will differ from Mrs. Brown's preferences. If so, both are correct, because 'correct' is defined separately for each woman. Assuming that both women are accurately informed regarding the outcomes, neither should be persuaded to change her mind.

Not only the direction of information exchange but also the amount of information exchanged can vary across decision-making models. So far, we have focused on minimum amounts for each model but have not specified outer boundaries. The amount of information that the physician could convey to the patient, for example, is, theoretically, infinite. The physician could provide detailed information on issues like the biology of the disease or detailed aspects of the molecular basis for the disease. However, in practice, the amount of information exchanged will be influenced by time and money constraints, both of which raise issues of equity and costs. Time spent by physicians with a given patient, for example, depletes the time available to them for other needy patients in their practice. This issue seems particularly salient to a shared decision-making approach. Because the information exchange is two way rather than one way, as are processes of deliberation and decision-making, this approach is likely to take more time than either the paternalistic or informed approaches, each of which requires less interaction and consensus building. . . .

Decision aids which present scientific information to patients about treatment benefits and risks are developed to create more informed patients and to encourage 'evidence-based decision-making'. This approach assumes that if only physicians knew how to transfer scientific information to patients in an accurate and unbiased way, the latter could be filled up (like an empty glass) with new knowledge and thereby transformed into informed and willing decision-makers. However, patients are not empty vessels. They come to the medical encounter with their own beliefs, values, fears, illness experiences and, increasingly, information about various treatment options. Moreover, patients are not so much interested in average outcomes for aggregate groups of patients as they are in knowing what this information means for themselves specifically. Patients interpret information on average treatment outcomes in order to make them personally meaningful within the decision-making context they face (Adelsärd and Sachs, 1996; Turney, 1996; Charles et al., 1998). In so doing, their own values and beliefs act as filters in processing what information is allowed in and how it is understood (Williams and Calnan, 1996). In this interpretive process, the intended message to the patient may be lost, altered or transformed (Parsons and Atkinson, 1992; Whelan *et al.*, 1995; Charles *et al.*, 1998). Research into decision aids and other communication mechanisms that focus only on defining the specific message to be conveyed and the most appropriate means of doing so, fail to consider patient factors that might also affect how information is processed and understood. This latter type of data would be useful to clinicians who want to be part of the deliberation process, to better understand their patients and to recognize potential differences between lay and medical world views (Mishler, 1984).

Deliberation

The deliberation stage of decision-making refers to the process of expressing and discussing treatment preferences. The minimum requirement for who is involved in this process varies across decision-making models. In the paternalistic approach, the treating physician weighs the benefits and risks of each option alone or in consultation with other physicians. The treating physician dominates the deliberation process while the patient passively listens. Physician dominance is justified by clinical judgement and experience. The label paternalistic is an apt term for this model because it evokes the image of a parent–child relationship where the authority figure (physician) has the right to decide what is best for the child (patient), even if the child disagrees (Parsons, 1951).

The treating physician may verbally communicate to the patient only the ultimate treatment decision, failing to reveal knowledge and values considered in the selection process and how these were weighted. Decision-making in this context can be completed fairly quickly if the physician feels well informed to make the decision and unrestrained by the need to have patient input into this process. Of course, the lack of patient input is precisely the reason why this model is viewed by many as undesirable.

The defining characteristic of deliberation in the shared decision-making model is its interactional nature (Charles *et al.*, 1997a). This is both its major strength and weakness. The emphasis on interaction ensures patient input into the process; but it also makes the process more cumbersome and time consuming. Both physician and patient are assumed to have a legitimate investment in the treatment decision, the patient because her health is at stake and the physician out of concern for the patient's welfare.

For a shared model to work, both physicians and patients have to perceive that there are treatment choices. Otherwise, there is nothing to decide (Charles *et al.*, 1998). Patients typically face one of two alternative treatment decisional contexts. The first is a choice between two different treatments: the second is a choice between doing nothing (e.g. watchful waiting) and doing something (e.g. implementing a specific intervention such as radiation). In an earlier study, we found that women with early stage breast cancer attending a regional cancer centre for consultation re: adjuvant therapy did not perceive the latter situation as one of choice. Many women felt they had no choice but to accept the treatment offered so that they could reassure themselves that they had done everything possible to fight the disease and to alleviate the possibility of post-decision regret should the disease return. As one woman said: 'Doing nothing is no choice' (Charles *et al.*, 1998).

In a shared approach, each person needs to be willing to engage in the decision-making process by expressing treatment preferences, in addition to whatever information they exchange. Some have argued that if information is exchanged, this is sufficient to view the interaction as shared. We view information as only the first step in the overall treatment decision-making process. It is the basic building block to enable a shared process to occur but it does not, in and of itself, constitute that process.

In a shared model, the interaction process to be used to reach an agreement may be explicitly discussed at the outset of the encounter or may evolve implicitly as the interaction unfolds. The process is likely to be consensual if both parties start out fairly close together in their thinking about the preferred treatment. If they are wider apart in their views, a process of negotiation is likely to occur. Negotiating as equal partners, however, is not easy for the patient because of the inherent information and power imbalance in the relationship. Physicians, in the usual case, will have superior knowledge of the technical issues involved in treatment decision-making and perhaps years of clinical experience with similar types of patients. The physician bears the officially legitimized title of 'expert' while the patient may feel particularly vulnerable and frightened during the medical encounter. When education, income, culture and/or gender differences also exist between the physician and patient, the patient may feel too intimidated to freely and openly express her preferences, let alone negotiate for them with the physician. Creating a safe environment for the patient so that she feels comfortable in exploring information and expressing opinions is probably the highest challenge for physicians who want to practise a shared approach (Guadagnoli and Ward, 1998). At the other end of the patient spectrum are those who are well informed about their illness and various treatment options and who have no difficulty expressing preferences. Some of these patients may have already made the treatment decision before entering the physician's office. If the patient's preference is different from the physician's and the physician is not able to change the patient's view, then the process will become conflictual. . . .

Each of the above examples assumes that only two parties are involved in the decision-making process. This is the most simple case but probably not the usual case. The patient may decide to share any or all of the decision-making steps with persons other than or in addition to the physician. For example, some women with early stage breast cancer in our study of shared treatment decision-making shared the information exchange component of the process with their oncologist but consulted with family, friends or their family physician in selecting the most appropriate treatment for themselves. These latter individuals knew the patient personally and were sought out during the deliberation and decision-making stages precisely for this reason. Including others in the decision-making process introduces additional complexity since it expands both the nature and the number of decisions to be made as well as increasing the need for co-ordination so that consultations with all persons involved can occur. In addition, some decisions require third party agreement as a necessary pre-condition for implementation. For example, a physician and patient may decide that the latter would do better being cared for at home, even though a high level of constant and close supervision is required. If there is no care-giver willing to step in and either organize or undertake this task, the decision cannot be implemented.

These examples illustrate that, in many instances, a given physician–patient interaction is only one slice of a larger decision-making process that involves others in key roles and that takes place outside the context of the medical encounter. To the extent that our conceptualizations of treatment decision-making fail to incorporate these others or to recognize their influence, they fail to capture important slices of the reality of this process. Concepts, particularly sensitizing concepts, serve as analytic guides, defining, at least initially, the boundaries of what to look for empirically to better understand a phenomenon or process of interest (Blumer, 1969; Charmaz, 1990; van den Hoonaard, 1997). If conceptualizations of treatment decision-making fail to incorporate a potential role for significant others outside the physician–patient dyad, empirical research will focus solely on this micro-system, excluding important external influences. Focusing on the physician–patient dyad may yield a lot of information about this particular slice of reality, but relatively little about the importance of this slice in the overall treatment decision-making process.

In the informed model, as noted earlier, the patient proceeds through the deliberation and decision-making process on her own. The physician's role is limited to providing medical/scientific information that will enable her to make an informed decision. Underlying this model are two assumptions. The first is that as long as patients possess current scientific information on treatment benefits and risks, they will be able to make the best decision for themselves. The second is that physicians should not have an investment in the decision-making process or in the decision made (Eddy, 1990). To do so, would go beyond the boundaries of an appropriate clinical role because the physician might harm the patient by inadvertently steering her in a certain direction which reflects the physician's own bias. Underlying this concern is the assumption that the interests and motivations of the physician and patient may not be the same. This consumer oriented model emphasizes patient sovereignty and patients' rights to make independent, autonomous choices (Quill and Brody, 1996). . . .

The use of evidence-based clinical guidelines in treatment decision-making provides a useful context within which to consider this issue. Increasingly, clinical guidelines are being developed, based on the highest quality research evidence available, to inform treatment decision-making. Underlying the evidence-based approach is an assumption that whatever treatment is shown by the evidence to be the most effective is the best treatment and the 'rational' choice to implement. Some physicians go further to argue that if an informed patient with an expressed desire to 'get well' chooses a different treatment, this choice must be the result of 'irrational' thinking and it is the physician's duty to try to change the patient's mind (Brock and Wartman, 1990). In such situations, evidence may be used by the physician to prescribe the 'right' treatment. Consumer sovereignty takes second place to the physician's own belief system about what ought to determine the treatment decision. This role for evidence is not compatible with either a shared or an informed model of treatment decision-making. A role that is compatible lies in using scientific information to help create more informed patients and to enhance patient choice.

When physicians and patients have different ideas about which decision-making model should be used to structure the decision-making interaction, they are headed for conflict. Decision-making using any of the above models will be prone to set-backs if the physician and patient are not in step with each other. In our earlier paper (Charles et al., 1997a), we made the analogy that shared decision-making takes 'two to tango'. For the two parties to dance together, the physician needs to know what kind of dance the patient prefers and the steps that this involves. Otherwise, the dance will be punctuated with false starts and missteps, creating tension between the partners and impeding their ability to work together. This analogy can be extended. For a certain type of dance, it seems appropriate that the physician take the lead (for example, in transferring technical information to patients). However, when the music changes to another type of dance, the patient may well take the lead, being more of an expert in the new steps required to fit with this particular beat (for example, patient preferences for different health states). In a shared treatment decision-making model both the physician and patient can take turns 'leading' specific discussions depending on which person has more expertise and experience to contribute on a given issue.

Decision on the treatment to implement

The final task in the decision-making process is choosing a treatment to implement. In the paternalistic and informed models, the decision-maker is one person; in the first case, the physician and in the second, the patient. However, in both cases the decision-maker is not totally autonomous because each faces constraints in actually implementing the decision. The physician must have the patient's informed consent before proceeding and the patient needs the physician's agreement to implement her preferred treatment (unless no treatment or an alternative therapy is preferred). In the shared model, both parties, through the deliberation process, work towards reaching an agreement and both parties have an investment in the ultimate decision made. The extent to which patient involvement in decision-making is associated with a greater commitment to the agreed upon treatment is an important area for study. . . .

Conclusion

In this paper we have revisited and expanded our earlier conceptual framework of different treatment decision-making models. We think this framework is more flexible than its predecessor and recognizes more clearly the dynamic nature of treatment decision-making. Practical applications of the framework have also been discussed. Over the course of our research we have learned that treatment decision-making is a complex process that takes place over time and can involve many individuals rather than an event that takes place at a fixed point in time and is restricted to the physician–patient dyad. Our thinking on treatment decision-making will continue to evolve as we move in an iterative process, empirically studying different aspects of this process and using the information to clarify our conceptual thinking.

References

Adelswärd, V., Sachs, L., 1996. The meaning of 6.8: numeracy and normality in health information talks. *Social Science & Medicine* 43, 1179–1187.

Beisecker, A., Beisecker, T., 1993. Using metaphors to characterize doctor–patient relationships: paternalism versus consumerism. *Health Communication* 5, 41–58.

Berwick, D.M., 1989. Health services research and quality of care: assignments for the 1990s. *Medical Care* 27, 763–771.

Blumer, H., 1969. *Symbolic Interactionism: Perspective and Method*. Prentice Hall. Englewood Cliffs. NJ.

Brock, D.W., Wartman, S.A., 1990. When competent patients make irrational choices. *New England Journal of Medicine* 322, 1595–1599.

Brody, D.S., 1980. The patient's role in clinical decision-making. *Annals of Internal Medicine* 93, 718–722.

Cahill, J., 1996. Patient participation: a concept analysis. *Journal of Advanced Nursing* 24, 561–571.

Charles, C., DeMaio, S., 1993. Lay participation in health care decision-making: a conceptual framework. *Journal of Health Politics. Policy and Law* 18, 881–904.

Charles, C., Gafni, A., Whelan, T., 1997a. Shared decision-making in the medical encounter: what does it mean? (Or, it takes at least two to tango). *Social Science & Medicine* 44, 681–692.

Charles, C., Lomas, J., Giacomini, M., et al., 1997b. The role of medical necessity in Canadian health policy. Four meanings . . . and a funeral? *The Milbank Quarterly* 75, 365–394.

Charles, C., Redko, C., Whelan, T., Gafni, A., Reyno, L., 1998. Doing nothing is no choice: lay constructions of treatment decision-making among women with early-stage breast cancer. *Sociology of Health and Illness* 20, 71–95.

Charmaz, K. 1990. 'Discovering' chronic illness: using grounded theory. *Social Science & Medicine* 30, 1161–1172.

Chassin, M.R., Brook, R.H., Park, R.E., 1986. Variation in the use of medical and surgical services by the medicare population. *New England Journal of Medicine* 314, 285–290.

Chassin, M.R., Kosecoff, J., Park, R.E., et al., 1987a. Does inappropriate use explain geographic variations in the use of health care services? *Journal of the American Medical Association* 258, 2533–2537.

Chassin, M.R., Kosecoff, J., Solomon, D.H., et al., 1987b. How coronary angiography is used. Clinical determinants of appropriateness. *Journal of the American Medical Association* 258, 2543–2547.

Coulter, A., 1997. Partnerships with patients: the pros and cons of shared clinical decision-making. *Journal of Health Services Research and Policy* 2, 112–121.

Deber, R., 1994. Physicians in health care management. 7. The patient–physician partnership: changing roles and the desire for information. *Canadian Medical Association Journal* 151, 171–177.

Eddy, D.M., 1990. Anatomy of a decision. *Journal of the American Medical Association* 263, 441–443.

Emanuel, E.J., Emanuel, L.L., 1992. Four models of the physician–patient relationship. *Journal of the American Medical Association* 267, 2221–2226.

Gafni, A., Charles, C., Whelan, T., 1998. The physician as a perfect agent for the patient versus the informed treatment decision-making model. *Social Science & Medicine* 47, 347–354.

Guadagnoli, E., Ward, P., 1998. Patient participation in decision-making. *Social Science & Medicine* 47, 329–339.

Haug, M.R., Lavin, B., 1981. Practitioner or patient: who's in charge? *Journal of Health and Social Behavior* 22, 212–229.

Haug, M., Lavin, B., 1983. *Consumerism in Medicine*. Sage, Beverly Hills.

Hughes, T.E., Larson, L.N., 1991. Patient involvement in health care: a procedural justice viewpoint. *Medical Care* 29, 297–303.

Iscoe, N.A., Goel, V., Wu, K., *et al.*, 1994. Variation in breast cancer surgery in Ontario. *Canadian Medical Association Journal* 150, 345–352.

Katz, S.J., Charels, C., Lomas, J., Welch, H.G., 1997. Shooting inward as the circle closes. *Journal of Health Politics, Policy and Law* 22(6), 1413–1431.

Leape, L.L., Hilborn, L.H., Park, R.E., *et al.*, 1993. The appropriateness of use of coronary artery bypass graft surgery in New York State. *Journal of the American Medical Association* 269, 753–760.

Levine, M.N., Gafni, A., Markham, B., *et al.*, 1992. A bed-side decision instrument to elicit a patient's preference concerning adjuvant chemotherapy for breast cancer. *Annals of Internal Medicine* 117, 53–58.

Llewellyn-Thomas, H.A., 1995. Patients' health-care decision making: a framework for descriptive and experimental investigations. *Medical Decision Making* 15, 101–106.

Lomas, J., 1990. Quality assurance and effectiveness in health care: an overview (editorial). *Quality Assurance in Health Care* 2, 5–12.

Lomas, J., Contandriopoulous, A.P., 1994. Regulating limits to medicine: towards harmony in public- and self-regulation. In: Evans, R.G., Barer, M.L., Marmor, T.R. (Eds). *Why are Some People Healthy and Others Not? The Determinants of the Health of Populations*. Adline De Gruyter. New York, pp. 253–283.

Lomas, J., Lavis, J., 1996. *Guidelines in the mist*. CHEPA Working Paper #96-231996. Centre for Health Economics and Policy Analysis. McMaster University, Hamilton. Ontario.

Lomas, J., Anderson, G.M., Karin, D.P., *et al.*, 1989. Do practice guidelines guide practice? The effect of a consensus statement on the practice of physicians. *New England Journal of Medicine* 321, 1306–1311.

Mishler, E.G., 1984. *The Discourse of Medicine*. Ablex Publishing Corporation. New Jersey.

Nayfield, S.G., Bongiovanni, G.C., Alciatti, M.H., *et al.*, 1994. Statutory requirements for disclosure of breast cancer treatment alternatives. *Journal of the National Cancer Institute* 86, 1202 1208.

Ontario Ministry of Health, 1994. *Consent to Treatment: A Guide to the Act*. Ontario Queen's Printer for Canada. Ontario.

Parsons, E., Atkinson, P., 1992. Lay constructions of genetic risk. *Sociology of Health and Illness* 14, 437–455.

Parsons, T., 1951. *The Social System*. The Free Press. New York, Chapter 10.

Quill, T.E., 1983. Partnership in patient care: a contractual approach. *Annals of Internal Medicine* 98, 228–234.

Quill, T.E., Brody, H., 1996. Physician recommendations and patient autonomy: finding a balance between physician power and patient choice. *Annals of Internal Medicine* 125, 763–769.

Roos, N.L., 1984. Hysterectomy: variations in rates across small areas and across physicians' practices. *American Journal of Public Health* 74, 327–335.

Roos, N.L., Wennberg, J.E., McPherson, K., 1988. Using diagnosis-related groups for studying variations in hospital admissions. *Health Care Financing Review* 9, 53–62.

Ryan, M., 1992. *The Economic Theory of Agency in Health Care: Lessons from Non-economists for Economists* Health Economics Research Unit Discussion Paper, 03 921992. University of Aberdeen, Scotland.

Thomasma, D.C., 1983. Beyond medical paternalism and patient autonomy: a model of physician conscience for the physician–patient relationship. *Annals of Internal Medicine* 98, 243–248.

Turney, J., 1996. Public understanding of science. *Lancet* 347, 1087–1090.

van den Hoonaard, W.C., 1997. Working with Sensitizing Concepts: Analytical Field Research. In: *Qualitative Research Methods Series*, 41. Sage. Thousand Oaks, CA.

Wennberg, J.E., 1990. Better policy to promote the evaluative clinical sciences. *Quality Assurance in Health Care* 2, 21–29.

Wennberg, J.E., Freeman, J.L., Culp, W.J., 1987. Are hospital services rationed in New Haven or over-utilized in Boston? *Lancet* 1, 1185–1188.

Whelan, T.J., Levine, M.N., Gafni, A., Lukka, H., Mohide, E.A., Patel, M., Streiner, D.L., 1995. Breast irradiation post-lumpectomy: development and evaluation of a decision instrument. *Journal of Clinical Oncology* 13, 847–853.

Williams, S., Calnan, M., 1996. The 'limits' of medicalization? Modern medicine and the lay populace in 'late' modernity. *Social Science & Medicine* 52, 1609–1620.

PART FOUR

Chronic illness and disability

IN CONJUNCTION WITH ISSUES OUTLINED in the first three Parts of the Reader, the study of illness experience has been one of the most productive areas of research in medical sociology, especially the study of chronic illness. There are many reasons for this interest, including, of course, the widespread nature of chronic conditions and difficulties in medical treatment. As with mental illness, if medicine were able to offer cures, the social as well as personal significance of these disorders would be reduced. Their often intractable character leads to problems of everyday living and to difficulties in lay and medical management. Alongside living with pain and discomfort, making sense of seriously disruptive symptoms frequently initiates a 'search for meaning' on the part of the patient, in an attempt to construct or reconstruct a sense of biographical continuity. In the first article in this part, Gareth Williams offers an analysis of the 'narrative reconstructions' people develop in coming to terms with their altered bodies and altered situations. Though some of the accounts collected by Williams in his research referred to possible external causes of the illness (arthritis), including those that might have come from hazardous working conditions, the general tenor of the narratives was to sustain a claim to moral worth. Williams argues that together with other elements, such as religious sentiments, patient narratives challenge the assumption that medical expertise has a dominant hold on people's understandings. While medical knowledge may be of great importance, resistance to it can come from other competing sources of meaning.

In the next extract, by Kelly and Field, Williams' argument about disrupted bodies and disrupted social relationships in chronic illness is taken a step further. Drawing on the sociology of the body, Kelly and Field show how disabling illness threatens to compromise people's display of cultural competence. Their argument is that with the onset of symptoms that alter bodily functioning, self-identity and relationships with others must also change. In this way, biological and social realities are closely related

– an issue which sociologists have sometimes found it difficult to appreciate. Kelly and Field's argument in essence is that recognition and acceptance of being socially competent depends in no small measure on the control and presentation of the body. By extension, poor 'performance' resulting from the onset of illness compromises the ability to meet the demands of social roles. A focus on body management and body display helps bring together not only biological and social processes, but also helps to unite two traditions of social enquiry in the study of illness, one that emphasises illness as a form of 'crisis', and one that emphasises its negotiated character.

It is still a moot point, of course, as to where the difficulties in self-presentation and thus identity originate. An interactionist view of social life would emphasise the interplay between self and society. A more radical view would focus on social structural and material sources of personal difficulties. In the field of chronic illness and disability considerable debate has grown up around such issues, especially with the growth of the disability movement. Exchanges between medical sociologists and members of this movement have sharpened some of the lines of agreement and disagreement. In the first of two pieces from this debate, Bury takes on the main thrust of the radical case, namely that disability should be seen as wholly social in character (hence the 'social model' of disability) and separate from matters to do with illness and the body. Bury points out, however, that such separation is easier to state than to demonstrate. The charge that the sociology of chronic illness is too much concerned with interactional difficulties, and not enough with sources of social oppression and exclusion, has to be set against the empirical evidence that sociologists of chronic illness have gathered. This, as we have noted above, speaks to an *interaction* between impairments and the social context in which they unfold. Bury also notes that official definitions of disability, sometimes derided by activists, have revealed both the material disadvantage of disabling illness and its crucial relationship to later life.

In the article that follows, Oliver attempts to defend the 'social model' of disability, and deal with the difficulties it presents – some of which have been identified from within the disability movement as well as by medical sociologists. Oliver argues that it is not the intention of the 'social model' to deny the reality of illness or impairment. The point is, however, that the social model aims to highlight the inadequacies of current social arrangements in meeting the needs of disabled people. In particular, 'oppressive' practices that exclude or bar people from social participation should be identified and tackled. For Oliver, the differences between medical sociologists and disability activists could be avoided if illness and impairment were separated off, and regarded as have nothing to do with disablement. From this viewpoint, attention could then be focused on those matters that are medical in character on the one hand, and those that are social on the other. Once this is achieved, Oliver argues, the essentially *political* character of disablement can then come to the fore. Though, to repeat, medical sociologists have found this kind of separation difficult to recognise in everyday settings, Oliver tries to meet the point by arguing that the 'social model' is not designed to cover all eventualities. Its main aim is to draw attention to those aspects of experience that relate to social barriers and are subject to political action.

One of the issues raised by this debate is how far research should document the problems created by chronic illness and disability, whether interactional or social structural. An emphasis on the relentlessly negative nature of disability, and on disruption and disadvantage, may miss the point that individuals and groups are active agents in dealing with their problems. The final two contributions in this Part of the Reader tackle this issue head on. The first, by Carricaburu and Pierret, reports on a study comparing the responses of HIV/AIDS and haemophiliac men in Paris. In fact, the relationship between resources and interaction were the key to understanding the differences between the two groups studied. For haemophiliac men the advent of HIV/AIDS threatened to overwhelm an already difficult situation, leading to a withdrawal from interaction. Gay men, on the other hand were able to be more active in their responses, mobilising friendship networks and using a variety of resources, including health services. For these men, Carricaburu and Pierret argue, a form of 'biographical reinforcement' occurred, giving a sense of continuity to an otherwise threatening and disruptive experience. In this study, therefore, features of social context, biography and interaction were all seen to be of importance.

The last extract in this Part takes a wider view of the culture surrounding chronic and disabling illness. In North American culture an emphasis on positive responses to adversity is now widely observable, giving credence to the saying that if one is given lemons the best thing is to make lemonade. In Arthur Frank's work this cultural motif is particularly prominent. Frank argues that such is the prevalence of chronic illness and different forms of disability, as well as the many situations where people have recovered or are recovering from impairments or illness, that we can now speak of living in a 'remission society'. As noted in the general introduction to the Reader, self-reported health problems seem to have grown massively in recent years. For Frank, the response of many lay people to such a situation is to emphasise a form of 'growth through adversity', in which narratives express a desire to 're-colonise' illness from the medical profession. In a postmodern culture, Frank argues, medical dominance loses its grip over matters medical. Indeed, one can see the disability movement in developed societies as one example of this. But Frank also has in mind the myriad forms of advocacy and 'narration' that give shape to experience and help people 'move on'. The ambiguities of treating chronic illness and disability almost as positive experiences need to be recognised, but the title of Frank's book, from which the extract included here is taken – *The Wounded Storyteller* – has a resonance which goes far beyond traditional views of health and illness.

Chapter 19

Gareth Williams

THE GENESIS OF CHRONIC ILLNESS
Narrative reconstruction

From *Sociology of Health and Illness*, 6, 1984: 174–200

Introduction

WE ARE SEATED IN THE LIVING-ROOM of a modern, urban council house somewhere in the north-west of England. Bill, the fifty-eight year-old man with whom I have been talking for almost an hour, leans forward. Then, in a strained voice and with a look of exasperated incomprehension on his face, he says: 'and your mind's going all the time, you're reflecting . . . "how the *hell* have I come to be like this?" . . . because it isn't me' (B13.6).

Bill has rheumatoid arthritis (RA), which was first diagnosed eight years ago following two years of intermittent pain and swelling in his joints; a serious heart attack has added to his difficulties. We have never met before. His words indicate the way in which a chronic illness such as RA may assault an individual's sense of identity, and they testify to the limitations of medical science in delivering a satis-factory explanation for the physical and social breakdown to which such an illness can lead.

In the *Collected Reports* on the rheumatic diseases published by the Arthritis and Rheumatism Council, and with a beguiling acknowledgement of the popular image of the scientist as Great Detective, the experts admit their limitations and pro-nounce RA to be 'one of the major medical mysteries of our time'.[1] What is striking about Bill's interrogative, however, is that it points to a concern with something more than the cause of his arthritis, and what I would like to do in this paper is to examine the nature of his question, and those of one other, and to consider the significance of the answers they provide. That is to say, I want to elucidate the styles of thought and modes of 'cognitive organization'[2] employed by two people suffering from RA in making sense of the arrival of chronic illness in their lives. I will not be claiming that these two cases are 'representative' in any statistical sense, but I *do* suggest that they symbolise, portray, and represent something important about the experience of illness. They are powerful, if idiosyncratic, illustrations of typical processes found in more or less elaborate form throughout my study group.

The fieldwork on which this study is based consisted of semi-structured, tape-recorded interviews with thirty people who had been first diagnosed as suffering from RA at least five years ago prior to my contact with them. The rationale guiding selection of people at this point in their illness was that in pursuing a general interest in what might be called the structured self-image of the chronically sick person it seemed sensible to talk to those who were 'seasoned professionals' rather than novices in the difficult business of living with a chronic illness. Four members of my study-group were in-patients on rheumatology wards and the rest were out-patient attenders at rheumatology clinics at two hospitals in north-west England. The in-patients were interviewed in a relatively tranquil side-room off the busy ward while the out-patients were first approached in the clinic and subsequently interviewed in their own homes. Of the 30 respondents, 19 were women and 11 were men, so my group had proportionately more men than one would expect to find in the general population.[3] Their ages ranged from 26 to 68 years at time of interview; thirteen being between 26 and 49, eleven between 50 and 64, and six were 65 years of age or over. Twenty-two were married, the rest being a mixture of single, widowed, and divorced or separated.

The interview covered a variety of themes relating to the experience of living with arthritis, and the data were elicited according to a simple checklist of topics. The duration of the interview as a whole and the sequencing of particular topics were influenced more by contingent features of the interview process than by any well-considered plans of my own. Where I had to compete with an obstreperous budgerigar or a boisterous young child, the interviews would likely be short and fragmented. On better days, with a minimum of interruption and an eager and lucid respondent, the interview could last for three or even four hours.

Although my central concepts – *narrative reconstruction* and *genesis* – are, I believe, novel,[4] the issues they are designed to address – how and why people come to see their illness as originating in a certain way, and how people account for the disruption disablement has wrought in their lives – have been the subject of innumerable investigations. Sociological and anthropological research into illness behaviour and health beliefs and psychological research into processes of attribution have all, in one way or another, attended to related issues; but there is so much of it! I cannot possibly indicate all my debts, but perhaps the body of work which has had most influence on this paper is that which examines lay beliefs or folk theories about the causes of specific diseases or illness in general.[5] Although much interesting material has been collected in this line, it has tended to rest content with treating people's casual beliefs as simply that: beliefs about the aetiology of illness. However, it seems to me that if, in some fundamental way, an individual is a social and historical agent with a biographical identity (in the fullest sense) and if the prime sociological importance of chronic illness is the 'biographical disruption'[6] to which it gives rise, then an individual's account of the origin of that illness in terms of putative causes can perhaps most profitably be read as an attempt to establish points of reference between body, self, and society and to reconstruct a sense of order from the fragmentation produced by chronic illness. . . .

Theoretical prologue

The concept of 'narrative' does not hold an established theoretical place in any sociological school or tradition. In general speech it is often used, in noun form, as a synonym for 'story', 'account', or 'chronicle'. When used as an adjective, as in 'narrative history', it typically refers to the process of relating a continuous account of some set of events or processes. When A.J.P. Taylor, for example, refers to himself as a 'narrative historian', as he often does, he implies both a concern with telling a good story and also a preference for a common-sense, empirical reading of historical events, unencumbered by any theoretical baggage be it marxist, structuralist, or psychoanalytic.

As I see it the term has two aspects: the routine and the reconstructed. In its routine form, it refers to the observations, comments, and asides, the practical consciousness which provides essential accompaniment to the happenings of our daily lives and helps to render them intelligible. In this sense narrative is a process of continuous accounting whereby the mundane incidents and events of daily life are given some kind of plausible order. If 'biography' connotes the indeterminate, reciprocal relationships between individuals and their settings or milieux and between those milieux and the history and society of which they are a part[7] then narrative may be seen as the cognitive correlate of this, commenting upon and affirming the multiform reality of biographical experience as it relates to both self and society. . . .

Bill: narrative reconstruction as political criticism

A significant portion of Bill's working life had been disrupted. In fact, he had had a tough time. He had worked as a skilled machine operator in a paperworks and, shortly before the first appearance of symptoms, was promoted to the position of 'charge hand' which entailed his supervising three floors in the factory. It was shortly after assuming his expanded responsibilities as a 'working gaffer' that things began to go wrong:

> I was a working gaffer . . . but, you know, they were mostly long hours and the end result, in 1972, was every time I had a session like, my feet began to swell and my hands began to swell. I couldn't hold a pen, I had difficulty getting between machines and difficulty getting hold of small things.

At this time he also had a massive heart attack and was off work for five months. A series of blood tests were done by his heart specialist who then referred him to a rheumatologist, and within the space of a couple of weeks he was hospitalized. At the time this unpleasant sequence of events was ambiguous and confusing, but over ten years Bill had become clearer about it:

> I didn't associate it with anything to do with the works at the time, but I think it was chemically induced. I worked with a lot of chemicals, acetone and what have you. We washed our hands in it, we had cuts, and we absorbed it. Now, I'll tell you this because it seems to be related. The men that I worked with who are all much older than me – there was a crew of sixteen and two survived, myself and the gaffer that was then – and they all complained of the same thing, you know, their hands started to puff up. It seems very odd.

Yes, very odd indeed. If I were simply interested in identifying his central aetiological motif no more need be said because the rest of the discussion was essentially a reiteration of this connexion. However, in order to understand the strength of his attachment to this belief, in the face of highly plausible alternatives, it is necessary to examine how his view of life has called forth this essential connextion between work and illness.

An important point about narratives, whether they be routine or reconstructed, is that they are necessarily co-authored.[8] The interview, of course, is itself a particularly clear case of co-authorship, but, more generally, narratives are bounded by and constructed in relationship with various individual people and organizations. With regard to illness, any narrative built around it needs to take account of the medical world within which the official definition of that illness has been specified. Bill described how, following the diagnosis of 'rheumatoid arthritis' resulting from clinical and laboratory investigations, the doctors disclaimed any interest in his hypothesis about workplace toxicity and pursued alternative hunches:

> I was assured by them (the doctors) that this is what it was, it was arthritis. Now, it just got worse, a steady deterioration, and I put it down that it was from the works. But with different people questioning me at the hospital, delving into the background, my mother had arthritis, and my little sister, Ruth, she died long before the war, 1936/7, and she had not arthritis, just rheumatism and that naturally did for her.

From a clinical perspective and, indeed, from a common-sense appreciation of 'inheritance', there appeared to be a strong case for accepting an explanation in terms of genetic transmission. Certainly, in rheumatological circles, genetic and viral hypotheses are those receiving most serious and sustained attention. Why was he not content with this? . . .

Bill recognized the pressure to accept the doctors' analysis as legitimate, but in the light of his practical knowledge he felt that their analysis was inadequate:

> But putting it out of my mind, and having spoken to the specialists, they say: 'No way.' So you take their word for it. But it seems a bit . . . thinking in my mind when I go to bed . . . I can't go to sleep straight

away, I have to wait until I get settled and your mind's going all the time, you're reflecting 'How the *hell* have I come to be like this?', you know, because it isn't me.

Bill has gone some way towards answering the question. He has identified a causal agent which seemed to explain his arthritis as well as symptoms in others, and he has described the milieu in which the causal nexus was situated. He has also portrayed a critical consciousness and a feeling of revolt amongst the workers which helps to explain his own unswerving attachment to his explanation when faced with a plausible clinical alternative. But is this observation of work experiences also part of a far more pervasive image of the world? . . .

Following the excursions into the subjects of his wife's accident and an incident with the police, we returned to his own illness and disablement, and Bill related more scenes from his working life:

> 'cause there you had extremes of heat, in the tapes section, we were doing computer tapes. There was a special section, and that was quite hot up there. Your entry and exit was through the fire door, and there was no air intake, no fresh air from the outside because it had to be at a particular temperature. And even the chemist down there realised that they're like ovens. It's totally enclosed, it's double thick glass, and they always had the damn things shut till we opened them. We said: 'Get us a vent in here or we're not running.' And he got one in – that's the chairman who is now dead – he got us an intake. But it was too late for them lads. They had been in it all the time and they were much older than me, and I think their age was against them. They had minimum resistance.

Not only, then, was there a sense of revolt amongst individual workers but a collective refusal by a number of workers to continue what they were doing until certain health and safety measures were instigated. It was not clear how long it was from the workers' recognition of detrimental effects to management compliance, but it was certainly too long for some of them. In this way, Bill's particular arthritic symptoms and their origin became absorbed into a public issue, the issue of health and safety at work, and the original question about the causes of his arthritis was transformed into an examination of the power struggle between workers and management. . . .

Betty: the transcendence of causality and narrative reconstruction

. . . Betty was in her early sixties, married, and had worked full-time and then part-time in a shop until developing disablement made continuation impossible. She had had arthritis for about seven years. Her life was not a comfortable one, and she had worked, as she put it, 'out of necessity', in order to supplement her husband's low wage, to pay off the mortgage, and to maintain a base equilibrium in the home economy. The loss of her wage rendered the future profoundly insecure. I asked her why she thought she got arthritis:

> The Lord's so near, and, you know, people say 'why you?' I mean this man next door, he's German, and of course he doesn't believe in God or anything (sic) and he says to me, 'you, my dear, why he chose you?' And I said, 'Look, I don't question the Lord, I don't ask (. . .), He knows why and that's good enough for me.' So he says, 'He's supposed to look after . . .' [and] I said, 'He is looking after his own (. . .) and he does look after me,' I said, I could be somewhere where I could be sadly neglected (. . .), well, I'm not. I'm getting all the best treatment that can be got, and I do thank the Lord that I'm born in this country, I'll tell you that.

Instead of simply affirming that her arthritis originated in the mysterious workings of God's will, Betty tells a story that locates her attitude to her illness within a framework of justification that has been called forth on other occasions by non-believers. She suggests that her personal misfortune can only be approached within an understanding of the good fortune in other aspects of her life. The goddess Fortuna faces both ways. The secular search for cause and meaning or what Alasdair MacIntyre calls the 'narrative quest'[9] is redundant because the cause, meaning, and purpose of all things is pre-ordained by God:

> I've got the wonderful thing of having the Lord in my life. I've got such richness, shall I say, such meaning. I've found the meaning of life, that's the way I look at it. My meaning is that I've found the joy in this life, and therefore for me to go through anything, it doesn't matter really, in one way, because I reckon that they are testing times . . . You see, He never says that you won't have these things, He doesn't promise us that we won't have them, He doesn't say that. But He comes with us through these things and helps us to bear them and that's the most marvellous thing of all.

So, for Betty, biographical robustness, narrative order, and the personal *telos* were not actually contingent upon what happened to her in the profane world. In fact the idea of a separate and vulnerable 'personal' *telos* would make little sense in the context of her essential relationship with God's purpose. MacIntyre argues that teleology and unpredictability coexist in human lives and that the intelligibility of an individual life depends upon the relationship between plans and purposes on the one hand, and constraints and frustrations on the other. The anxiety to which this might give rise did not exist for Betty because the unpredictability of say, pain and illness, are part of an ulterior teleology.

This kind of interpretation of life and its difficulties is hard to appreciate in the context of a secular society with its mechanical notions of cause and effect. In talking of 'God's purpose' as a component in people's understanding of the genesis of illness, it is important to think carefully about what exactly is entailed in the use of such expressions. When Betty talked about God and personal suffering, she did not imply that God's will was an efficient or proximate cause in the development of her arthritis, rather He is the cause of everything and, as such, makes narrative quests unnecessary. Nonetheless, from a sociological viewpoint, Betty's concept of 'God' had similarities to Bill's notion of 'work' in that it transcended linear frameworks of cause and effect so as to define a symbolic and practical relationship between the individual, personal misfortune, social milieu, and the life-world. However, although Bill went beyond a linear explanation of disease by placing his experience of illness within a political narrative reconstruction of his relationship to the social world, Betty's 'God' implied a principle of meaning that transcends the social world as such. Betty did not have to reconstruct order through narrative because God, existing 'outside' both the individual and society, encompasses within his plans what appear to us as biological caprice and senseless biographical disruption. Physical suffering was only important insofar as it signified a feature of her essential relationship to God and so her sense of identity was not unduly threatened by the body's afflictions. The body itself is nothing as was made clear when, elsewhere in the interview, Betty aired her thoughts on donating her body to medical science:

> Your body is dust and that is what it goes to. I mean the spirit goes to the Lord, the part of me that's telling you all that I am and what goes to the Lord.

Although much that Betty said of her material life would suggest profound disruptions in socio-economic circumstances, there was no sense of disruption because her life was part of God's unfolding purpose. Moreover, 'God's will' does not imply self-blame where the individual is bad and illness is retribution; at least, there is no direct relationship:

> You see, it's got nothing to do with Man's goodness. It's all to do with Christ, all to do with Him being born to save me, to suffer my sins and everything I've ever done. I'm made righteous and sanctified by the wonder of that cross and that to me is marvellous, that to me is the jewel of life (. . .). You see, there's a beauty about everything and you can sort of go through it in this way, you know, talking to the Lord and entering into it. He knows all about it. So people say, 'why you?' Well, why not me? Better me who knows the Lord.

Because she did not see herself as the author of her own narrative there was nothing for her to reconstruct or explain. For Betty the course and end of her life were defined outside herself and history:

> And I think that, yes, it's helped me to understand, and even to the [point where] it can have a mental depressive [effect] on some people, because if they haven't got the Lord in their lives, of course, it must do. You know, 'why am I here? why this, that and the other?' To me there's an end to it, something the Lord has for it, and He knows best what to do. I reckon, you know, that with faith I'll go through with this to an extent and that'll be it, and God will say, 'well, that's it'.

The interview with Betty was a particularly difficult one to conduct because my sociological questions appeared insignificant and redundant in the face of the teleo-logical certainty of her beliefs. When interviewing someone with such a profound sense of meaning, it seemed almost meaningless to ask whether the illness had damaged her sense of self-worth or whatever. For Betty, most people live their lives in the immediacy of personal and material interests. Their lives follow a narrative thread defined by everyday events and happenings and routines, and when major problems occur in their social world their identity is bound to be threatened and it is not surprising that they should become lost and depressed. But for her 'there is an end in it' and all analytic puzzlement and personal doubt evaporate in the glare of God's purpose.

Conclusion

. . . The body is not only an object amongst other objects in the world, it is also that through which our consciousness reaches out towards and acts upon the world. This is the dual nature of the body referred to by Sartre,[10] and within this duality chronic illness is a rupture in our relationship with that world. However, consciousness is itself biographically framed, so that consciousness of the body and the inter-pretations of its states and responses will lead us to call upon images of the private and public lives we lead. Narrative reconstruction is an attempt to reconstitute and repair ruptures between body, self, and world by linking-up and interpreting different aspects of biography in order to realign present and past and self with society. In this context, the identification of 'causes' creates important reference points in the interface between self and society. My respondents were, perhaps, not so different from the *baladi* women in Evelyn Early's study for whom 'The dialectic between the diagnosis and the life situation is crystallized in the illness narrative, where somatic progression and social developments are both documented.'[11]

For Bill, illness developed out of a working life but where the significance of work could only be understood by elaborating an image of the kind of society in which that work was situated. His attachment to workplace toxicity as a causal factor could be understood only in terms of his image of society as a place of exploitative relationships and power inequality. . . . For Betty, the genesis of illness was seen to reside in the transcendental realm of God's purpose. This is not to say that God was seen as an efficient cause of her illness, but rather that her illness was necessitated and justified by reference to her intrinsic relationship to a suffering God.

These accounts all speak of illness experience at one moment in time. Their pasts were the pasts of those presents in which they were interviewed, and I have no evidence for or against the proposition that their image of the past would have been substantially different in other presents. To test that would require an altogether more sophisticated piece of research. Within the constraints, what I have attempted to demonstrate is that causality needs to be understood in terms of narrative reconstruction and that both causal analysis and narrative reconstruction may be rendered redundant in the presence of an embracing theodicy. For medical sociologists such an approach suggests caution in attributing particular belief models to individuals out of relation to other aspects of their narrative, and for doctors it could alert them to reasons for the apparent resistance of some patients to clinical explanations.

Notes

1   The Arthritis and Rheumatism Council for Research, *Reports on Rheumatic Diseases. Collected Reports 1959–1977*, London: ARC, 1978, p. 6.

2   D. Locker, *Symptoms and Illness: The Cognitive Organization of Disorder*, London: Tavistock, 1981.

3   P. H. N. Wood (ed.), *The Challenge of Arthritis and Rheumatism: A Report on Problems and Progress in Health Care for Rheumatic Disorders*, London: British League Against Rheumatism/Arthritis and Rheumatism Council, 1977.

4   The term 'genesis' is used by Claudine Herzlich in her monograph: *Health and Illness: A Socio-Psychological Approach*, London: Academic Press, 1979. Although I employ a somewhat different definition, I have been much influenced by both the style and substance of that excellent book.

5   For example, J. H. Mabry, 'Lay concepts of aetiology', *J. Chron. Dis.*, vol. 17, 1964, pp. 371–86; R. G. Elder, 'Social class and lay explanations for the aetiology of arthritis', *J. Hlth. Soc. Behav.*, vol. 14, 1973, pp. 28–38; M. Linn, B. Linn, and S. Stein, 'Beliefs about causes of cancer in cancer patients', *Soc. Sci. Med.*, vol. 16, 1982, pp. 835–9; R. Pill and N. Stott, 'Concepts of illness causation and responsibility: some preliminary data from a sample of working class mothers', *Soc. Sci. Med.*, vol. 16, 1982, pp. 43–52; M. Blaxter, 'The causes of disease: women talking', *Soc. Sci. Med.*, vol. 17, 1983, pp. 59–69.

6   M. Bury, 'Chronic illness as biographical disruption', *Sociology of Health and Illness*, vol. 4, no. 2, 1982, pp. 167–82.

7   See P. Berger and B. Berger, *Sociology: A Biographical Approach*, Harmondsworth: Penguin, 1976; C. W. Mills, *The Sociological Imagination*, Harmondsworth: Penguin, 1970; D. Bertaux (ed.), *Biography and Society: The Life History Approach in the Social Sciences*, New York: Sage, 1981.

8   A. MacIntyre, *After Virtue: A Study in Moral Theory*, London: Duckworth, 1981.

9   A. MacIntyre, op.cit.

10 J-P. Sartre, *Sketch for a Theory of the Emotions*, London: Methuen, 1971.

11 E. A. Early, 'The logic of well-being: therapeutic narratives in Cairo, Egypt', *Soc. Sci. Med.*, vol. 16, 1982, p. 1496.

Chapter 20

Michael P. Kelly and David Field

MEDICAL SOCIOLOGY, CHRONIC ILLNESS AND THE BODY

From *Sociology of Health and Illness*, 18, 1996: 241–57

Introduction

THE PURPOSE OF THIS PAPER is to raise questions and develop the debate about how the body might be integrated into sociological accounts of the experience of chronic illness in a way that acknowledges both biological and social facts. Illness, like life itself, is a multi-phenomenal experience and therefore a multi-layered object of analysis. From the perspective of the person who has the illness and in whose body the physical or psychological pathology exists, or is defined as existing, the illness will be felt in a variety of ways. There may be intrusive symptoms such as pain or nausea. There may be interruptions to usual physical and social routines. There may be cognitive disorientation and confusion and the behaviour patterns of self and others may take on new and particular forms. If the pathology is asymptomatic, the phenomena may not have a subjective or experiential dimension at all, and in the case of functional psychiatric disorders there may be no lesion as such, but discomfort, distress and disruption may be very real indeed. From the point of view of the sufferer and of significant others – family or carers – the experience may be described and labelled using various expert or lay languages. These provide professionals, families and carers, as well as the sufferer, with various bench-marks against which the experience may be evaluated. These languages also provide explanations – scientific and lay – of what is happening.

These points are commonplace in medical sociology. Over several decades sociologists have provided numerous accounts of these social and biological processes. Thus the importance of the social construction and definition of illness experiences (Freidson 1970, Scheff 1966), the kinds of social structures which constrain human behaviour in the face of discomforts and disruptions (Locker 1983, Navarro 1978), the means and the mechanisms whereby the bearers of expert languages are able to define the situation in various and sometimes self-serving ways (Hollingshead and Redlich 1958, Mercer 1972, Scheff 1966, Scott 1969), the divergence between expert and lay languages (Freidson 1970), the nature of the power relationships between patients and professionals (Freidson 1970, Kelly and May 1982, Jeffery 1979, Lorber 1975), and the contingent nature of diagnosis (Dingwall 1976) have all been described sociologically. Some authorities have written their sociology in ways which eloquently express physical limitations and bodily difficulties (Strauss *et al.* 1984) or directly address the interactions between physical and social aspects of human life and their consequences for illness (Freund, 1982; Freund and McGuire 1991, Lawler 1991). However, in most types of socio-logical narrative about chronic illness, the body remains theoretically elusive. Its existence is seldom explicitly denied, but its presence has a kind of ethereal quality forever gliding out of analytic view.

The understatement of the body in medical sociology has been noted by others (Turner 1992). Nevertheless, the point needs to be emphasised that in chronic illness the obdurate nature of the physical reality of 'bad' bodies is such an all-embracing aspect of the experience that an adequate sociology of the physical experience would appear to be the *sine qua non* for analysis (Moos and Tsu 1977, Anderson and Bury 1988, Radley 1993). Perhaps the omission is not very surprising. Sociological discourse, with its foci on agency and structure, and its rejection of methodological individualism, drives attention away from the body. Thus the physical reality of illness tends mostly to be treated by sociologists in two broad ways. First, as an *a priori* category which legitimately belongs to other realms of discourse – medicine or biology (Friedson 1970). Second, as something socially constructed and/or socially mediated, possibly of doubtful ontological status, and therefore of little sociological interest other than in terms of the forms of narrative and accounting which provide for the means of 'doing' the social construction and mediation (Armstrong 1983, Foucault 1973, Shilling 1993, Turner 1992).

It is probably the case that these tendencies have been reinforced in medical sociology from Parsons onwards (Parsons 1951a, 1951b) by the influence of accounts of psychological illness. Parsons' insistence on treating illness as a form of deviance took the sick role into a moral realm. Indeed in his discussion of the sick role in *The Social System* (1951a) he was strongly influenced by his interests in psychoanalysis. During the 1960s and 1970s many other writers were also fascinated by psychiatric problems as an arena in which to do medical sociology (Goffman 1970, Lemert 1962, Rose 1962, Scheff 1966). More recently, as medical sociology has expanded its range of interests, the disorders which have attracted particular attention have not infrequently been the more exotic ones (Conrad 1976, Conrad and Schneider 1980). Epilepsy has received a great deal of attention for example (Jacoby 1994, Scambler and Hopkins 1986, Scambler 1989, West 1986). Intractable illnesses about which medicine can do little by way of alleviation have also been prominent in medical sociology. In this latter respect terminal illness (Field 1989, Hockey 1990) and especially cancer (Glaser and Strauss 1965, McIntosh 1977, Schou 1993), rheumatoid arthritis (Locker 1983, Wiener 1975, Williams 1984), multiple sclerosis (Robinson, 1988) and Parkinson's disease (Pinder, 1990) spring to mind. Conversely, common illnesses which in terms of incidence, prevalence and caseload are those which preoccupy most general medical practitioners are less well represented in the sociological cannon. For example, in recent years disorders like gall bladder disease, ulcers, back pain, stroke and bronchitis pale into significance sociologically, compared to studies of AIDS/HIV (Field and Woodman 1990, Barbour and Van Teijlingen 1994). Even where writers have focused on the apparently physical, as in the case of pain, it is the cognitive mediation and interpretation of pain (Bendelow 1993, Kotarba 1983) or the ways in which professionals make sense of it (Baszanger 1992) which is of sociological interest, rather than the bodily experience of pain itself. That is, the meanings of pain are given precedence over its physical restrictions and discomforts – even though it is precisely these which have greatest weight in shaping interpretations and the attribution of meaning by sufferers. . . .

The body and illness

There are few accounts of chronic illness which do not acknowledge that basic to the experience of that illness is the disruption of the normal and usually desired routines of everyday life. Some early accounts attended only to the disruption (Lawrence 1958), while subsequently others explored the ways in which the experience is reconstructed and rendered meaningful by sufferers, family, friends and carers (Davis 1972, Davis and Horobin 1977, Darling 1979, Finlayson and McEwen 1977, Voysey 1975, Anderson and Bury 1988, Radley 1993). What is usually central to both types of approach is a concern with the coping behaviours which people use in the face of illness (Moos and Tsu 1977). We suggest that central to the coping task is dealing with the physical manifestations of illness, and that coping with the physical body has to precede coping with relationships, with disruptions and indeed with any social reconstruction of events (Kelly 1991). At the very epicentre of the coping experience and from which other social coping processes flow, is the management of the physical problems which the chronic illness generates. The physical aspects of living such as eating, bathing, or going to the toilet are the prime focus of the experience of chronic illness, because above all else coping with chronic illness involves coping with bodies – not just for people who are chronically ill themselves but also for their families and familiars (Anderson and Bury, 1988). As Parker (1993) has shown, the intimate physical care which is often required is overlaid with symbolic meanings which may transform relationships between husbands and wives. In part, attacks on medical sociology from the politics of disability movement (Morris 1993, Oliver 1990, 1994) arise precisely because medical sociology has understated the central facts of bodily difficulties which are entailed in illness and disability.

One of the virtues attached to using the concepts of self and identity as a means of describing the physical and social reality of illness lies in their usefulness in describing change. Bodies change in chronic illness. Chronic illness also involves changes in self-conceptions which are reciprocal to bodily experiences, feelings and actions. The person as known to themself (i.e. their self-conceptions) undergoes considerable transformation. Illness may also involve changes in the ways in which others perceive and define (i.e. construct the identity of) the sufferer as the illness takes hold. However, feelings about self-conceptions and the feelings about identities applied by others fluctuate and vary. They do not change in a coterminous, simultaneous or deterministic way (Kelly, 1986). The problem of meaning, which so many sociological accounts of chronic illness focus on, is another way of looking at the tension which is generated between self and identity in illness. This tension is well described by Goffman (1963) in his analysis of the discrepancy between the 'virtual identities' imputed by others on the basis of appearance (e.g. crippled, sad and dependent) and the individual's self-conceptions based on the 'actual identities' of what they are able to do (e.g. wife, librarian, music buff).

Self and identity not only change in chronic illness but they also have an enduring quality (Kelly 1992). As an individual moves from situation to situation, as their body changes and as their illness develops, there is still an important sense in which they are the same person they were before their body began to alter, albeit in a different social situation. They are also known, at least to significant others, as the person they were before they became ill and although some identities may change other core identities will remain unaltered. Just as the body which is diseased is the same body as it was pre-morbidly, so too are self and identity. Yet with the onset of illness the body changes and self-conception changes too as the individual objectifies themself as someone in pain and discomfort and with a restricted range of activities. The body, which in many social situations is a taken for granted aspect of the person, ceases to be taken for granted once it malfunctions and becomes more prominent in the consciousness of self and others. It has to be acknowledged as limiting or interfering with other physical and social activities, especially in the early phases of an illness. The important tension between continuity and change – which is the central problematic in many sociological accounts of chronic illness – is therefore also embraced by the concepts of self and identity.

Illness is a negotiated state which results in a change of identity when others define the person as sick, typically after consulting a physician who legitimates their sickness, thereby constructing or confirming a new identity. In an acute episode, like a bout of influenza or appendicitis, the label of sickness has an existential and ontological reality for the sufferer, and the feelings of being unwell are highly salient to self. However, this state of affairs is recognised both by the person and by others as temporary and neither self nor identity are fundamentally changed. The sick person is expected to, and usually will, get better (Parsons 1951a, 1951b). In a chronic illness however, and in disability more generally, the alterations to self and identity are more substantial and permanent than acute illness, although this fact may neither be recognised nor acknowledged at first. The sick role in a Parsonian sense will not be completely relinquished but will become transformed (Parsons 1951a, Gallagher 1976, Gerhardt 1989, Kassebaum and Baumann 1965) and periods of being sick and living with the problems of impaired functioning will become permanent features of self and of publicly defined identity. Thus, the nature of the chronic illness and its bodily consequences have to be incorporated permanently into conceptions of self and are likely to become a basis for the imputation of identity by others. The body is central because the biological bases of experience as perceived by self and others have very important effects on the construction of self and identity. The relation between self and identity in chronic illness is a social process which alters through time, as the bodily contingencies change. These bodily contingencies may be cyclical, intermittent and unpredictable, or they may be ever downward as in a terminal illness. Living biological systems are not static. Neither are their manifestations nor the sensations and experiences of these manifestations. These experiences are not merely socially constructed, they are contingencies exercising varying degrees of salience for self and others through time and place (Strauss *et al.* 1984).

At one extreme for example, an illness like well-controlled diabetes demonstrates our point (Kelleher 1988). To all intents and purposes this disease is invisible to all but intimate others. Hence identity may remain unchanged. However, the individual's sense of self will be intricately tied into the routines attached to managing the illness with respect to physical activities like insulin regimes, urine testing and dietary control. So long as the self-management practices remain private or concealed in ordinary interactions, the identity of a well person can be maintained. In contrast, at the other extreme, someone whose condition is visible and cannot be hidden, for example if they are in a wheelchair, will be in social situations where, whatever the salience of their impairment for self at any given moment, their public identity is always constrained by the wheelchair. The wheelchair gives a physical salience and presence for identity construction. Between these extremes lie a large number of diseases and conditions in which the progress may be unpredictable, the intrusiveness of symptoms may fluctuate, and the prognosis may be uncertain. The consequences for self and identity are therefore highly variable. Someone with psoriasis may be involved in permanent self-care routines at the level of self which makes the illness highly salient, while their public identity may change in terms of the obviousness of the disease to others (Jobling 1977). Someone in the early stages of cancer may have had their sense of self completely shattered as they ruminate on their own mortality but to their neighbour, their workmates, to their fellow travellers on the morning commuter train, their identity remains unaltered, until either they show external signs of deterioration, or other cues are given off intentionally or unintentionally which signal the need for a revision in identity. In other illnesses the transformations in identity may not only be highly salient but also highly stigmatising. External signals deriving from the disease may be of such symbolic significance, say in uncontrolled epilepsy or frank schizophrenia, that the identity is overlain by all kinds of other negative and stigmatising labels (Albrecht *et al.* 1982, Goffman 1963, Jones *et al.* 1984).

Discussion

In a theoretical review of medical sociology Gerhardt (1989) has made a distinction between two ways in which sociologists have been influenced by the interactionist tradition from which the ideas of self and identity used in this paper derive. She calls these the crisis model and the negotiation model. The crisis model is typified by the work of Becker (1963), Scott (1969) and Lemert (1962). In the crisis approach, becoming ill is about identity change. The sociological interest is in irreversible status passage and changes in the person's placement in the social structure. The negotiation model, in contrast, characterises chronic illness as a process of loss of self as the individual struggles or works to be as normal as possible. The negotiation model is exemplified by the work of Strauss *et al.* (1984), Charmaz (1983, 1987), Bury (1982) and Williams (1984).

Bringing the body into analytical focus helps to show that these are not really two separate traditions but rather different ways of dealing with the salience of the body. In the crisis approach symptoms of body alterations lead to societal reactions (identity change) which in turn lead to internalisation and alterations in the self. The logic of the explanation runs from body to self to identity. The degree to which interaction is self-driven or driven by the social reactions of others depends on the salience of body to either self or others. An obvious point perhaps, but made the more obvious when one considers that the crisis model happens to be derived from studies of blindness (Scott 1969) and paranoia (Lemert 1962) neither of which condition can be easily bracketed out of social interactions by others. In the negotiation model the illnesses dealt with – rheumatoid arthritis, colitis, emphysema – do not *necessarily* make people look especially unusual. The physical symptoms of this latter group of illnesses do not always and invariably impinge directly on interactions and will not inevitably be taken account of by others in interactions. They do, however, have continuous salience for the sufferer. Differently diseased bodies therefore affect interaction differentially.

It is also helpful to consider the role of language in these processes. In a paper considering some of the methodological issues associated with the validity of accounts of illness produced and analysed qualitatively, West (1990), following Cornwell (1984), draws a distinction between private and public accounts and the apparent inconsistency between the two. Public accounts are those produced by subjects which affirm and reproduce the moral order. These tend to be 'ought' types of expressions of an approved or an acceptable kind: 'Oh I'm doing fine', 'I can't complain', or 'Mustn't grumble' are public accounts of this type. Private accounts, in contrast, refer to meanings derived from the experiential world – a world of body experience and pain – often at odds with the public account of things. They arise out of bodily experience, including all those difficult and socially unacceptable aspects of body experience and outpourings like blood, vomit and faeces. In public accounts social order is maintained, and to echo both Mary Douglas (1966) and Norbert Elias (1994), dirt is kept in its place and civilisation upheld. In other words, the very nature of the accounting process, the way people talk about, or are permitted to talk about illness, reflects the salience and the immediacy of the bodily experience of self.

Most public accounting practices help direct attention away from the potentially stigmatising nature of illness, and much social interaction is geared to repairing or overlooking *faux pas*, to covering up mis-understanding and generally making inter-action work (Goffman 1961, Schutz 1970, Garfinkel 1967). That the interaction between someone who is sick and others is like this is not, in sociological terms, very surprising. However, when the body of the sick person intrudes into interaction in ways which others cannot overlook or ignore this kind of public accounting may be sorely tested, demonstrating the importance of the body to social interaction. There are also the private accounts *about* the sufferer produced by others, which may sometimes involve negative stereotyping. This is the type of accounting process in which 'normal people' reaffirm their normality with reference to the deviance of the sufferer. The fear of this kind of negative stigmatisation – the private accounts of others – can have a far more pervasive effect on the sufferer than outright discrimination as has been demonstrated in the case of epilepsy (Scambler and Hopkins 1986, Jacoby 1994). Once again, these private accounts flow from the cues of the bodily differences of the negatively labelled individual. Once this type of private account goes public, the individual has to organise their life around their public and 'deviant' identity. No amount of euphemism or politically correct discourse can detract from the centrality of the public and physical difference. It cannot be socially constructed out of existence. The body is central both to the experience and feelings associated with illness (self) and in the social processes involved in its management (identity).

We can summarise the body's role in chronic illness as threefold. First, it is the point at which self is in touch with itself; it is the point of immediate salience for self. Second, the body is an obvious, though sometimes ambiguous, point of reference for external labels. It is an important and easily available cue to the nature of the appropriate public identities which may be bestowed. Third, labelling and identification feed back directly to self-conception as the chronically ill person constructs and reconstructs the meaning of their bodily malfunctioning and the responses of others to this.

The interplay between self and identity provides a theoretical bridge to manage sociologically the relation between biological and social facts. The biological and physical facts are significant sociologically because (a) they impinge directly on self, (b) they provide the signals for identity construction, and (c) they act as limiting factors on social action for the sufferer. The physical facts have a physical reality *sui generis* and hence may be described in the language of bio-physical science. That language may lead to significant physical interventions which have both physical and social consequences for the illness career. They also have a social reality *sui generis* which can be articulated through the analytic constructs of self and identity. Biological facts become social facts because others respond to the person in terms of their physicality. They are also social facts for the individual because the individual sufferer is aware of, and has to take steps to cope with, that physical reality. At the same time the sufferer and his or her significant others have to balance the demands of social life with the compelling demands of the subjective feelings and the physical demands and restrictions on the body.

Over the years, a great many sociological accounts of chronic illness have made these points, if only by implication. However, the impact of this kind of sociology has not been as marked as it should have been because of the elusive characterisation of the body and its physical manifestations. The human suffering and misery occasioned by diminished bodily capacity must be captured in the sociological analysis of illness. Our argument is that by reintegrating a substantive conceptualisation of the body into the analysis of chronic illness linked to the concepts of self and identity, it is possible to produce a language that enables us to reconcile levels of analysis which while they may be treated quite separately and independently, provide a more satisfactory form of understanding when related to each other.

References

Albrecht, G., Walker, V. and Levy, J. (1982) Social distance from the stigmatised: a test of two theories *Social Science and Medicine*, 16, 1319–27.

Anderson, R. and Bury, M. (eds) (1988) *Living with Chronic Illness: The Experience of Patients and their Families*. London: Unwin Hyman.

Armstrong, D. (1983) *Political Anatomy of the Body: Medical Knowledge in Britain in the 20th Century*. Cambridge: Cambridge University Press.

Barbour, R. and Teijlingen, E. (eds) (1994) *Medical Sociology in Britain: A Register of Research and Teaching* (7th Edition). British Sociological Association Medical Sociology Group.

Baszanger, I. (1992) Deciphering chronic pain, *Sociology of Health and Illness* 14, 181–215.

Becker, E. (1963) *The Birth and Death of Meaning*. Glencoe, Ill: Free Press.

Bendelow, G. (1993) Pain perceptions, emotions and gender, *Sociology of Health and Illness*, 15, 273–294.

Bury, M. (1982) Chronic illness as biographical disruption, *Sociology of Health and Illness*, 5, 168–95.

Charmaz, K. (1983) Loss of self: a fundamental form of suffering of the chronically ill, *Sociology of Health and Illness*, 5, 168–95.

Charmaz, K. (1987) Struggling for a self: identity levels of the chronically ill. In Roth, J.A. and Conrad, P. (eds) *The Experience and Management of Illness*. Greenwich, Conn and London: JAI Press.

Conrad, P. (1976) *Identifying Hyperactive Children: The Medicalization of Deviant Behaviour*. Lexington, Mass: D C Heath.

Conrad, P. and Schneider, J.W. (1980) *Deviance and Medicalization: From Badness to Sickness*. St Louis: Mosby.

Cornwell, J. (1984) *Hard Earned Lives: Accounts of Health and Illness from East London*. London: Tavistock Publications.

Darling, R. (1979) *Families Against Society: A Study of Reactions to Children with Birth Defects*. New York and London: Sage.

Davis, A. and Horobin, G. (1977) *Medical Encounters: The Experience of Illness and Treatment*. London: Croom Helm.

Davis, F. (1972) *Illness, Interaction, and the Self*. Belmont, California: Wadsworth.

Dingwall, R. (1976) *Aspects of Illness*. London: Martin Robertson.

Douglas, M. (1966) *Purity and Danger: An Analysis of Concepts of Pollution and Taboo*. London: Routledge and Kegan Paul.

Elias, N. (1994) *The Civilising Process: The History of Manners and State Formation and Civilisation* (Trans E. Jephcott) Oxford: Blackwell.

Field, D. (1989) *Nursing the Dying*. London: Tavistock/Routledge.

Field, D. and Woodman, D. (eds) (1990) *Medical Sociology in Britain: A Register of Research and Teaching* (6th Edition). British Sociological Association Medical Sociology Group: Leicester.

Finlayson, A. and McEwen, J. (1977) *Coronary Heart Disease and Patterns of Living*. London: Croom Helm.

Foucault, M. (1973) *The Birth of the Clinic: An Archaeology of Medical Perception*. London: Tavistock.

Freidson, E. (1970) *Profession of Medicine: A Study of the Sociology of Applied Knowledge*. New York: Dodd Mead.

Freund, P. (1982) *The Civilised Body*. Philadelphia: Temple University Press.

Freund, P. and McGuire, M.B. (1991) *Health Illness and the Body: A Critical Sociology*. Engelwood Cliffs, NJ: Prentice Hall.

Gallagher, E.B. (1976) Lines of reconstruction and extension in the Parsonian sociology of illness, *Social Science and Medicine*, 10, 207–18.

Garfinkel, H. (1967) *Studies in Ethnomethodology*. Engelwood Cliffs, New Jersey: Prentice Hall.

Gerhardt, U. (1989) *Ideas about Illness: An Intellectual and Political History of Medical Sociology*. London: Macmillan.

Glaser, B.G. and Strauss, A.L. (1965) *Awareness of Dying*. Chicago: Aldine.

Goffman, E. (1961) *Encounters*. New York: Bobbs-Merrill.

Goffman, E. (1963) *Stigma: Notes on the Management of Spoiled Identity*. Englewood Cliffs, NJ: Prentice Hall.

Goffman, E. (1970) *Asylums: Essays on the Social Situation of Mental Patients and Other Inmates*. London: Penguin.

Hockey, J. (1990) *Experiences of Death*. Edinburgh: Edinburgh University Press.

Hollingshead, A.B. and Redlich, R.C. (1958) *Social Class and Mental Illness*. New York: Wiley.

Jacoby, A. (1994) Felt versus enacted stigma: a concept revisited: evidence from a study of people with epilepsy in remission, *Social Science and Medicine*, 38, 269–74.

Jeffery, R. (1979) Normal rubbish: deviant patients in casualty departments, *Sociology of Health and Illness*, 1, 90–108.

Jobling, R. (1977) Learning to live with it: an account of a career of chronic dermatological illness and patienthood. In Davis, A. and Horobin, G. (eds) *Medical Encounters: The Experience of Illness and Treatment*. London: Croom Helm.

Jones, E.E., Farina, A., Hastorf, A.H., Markus, H., Miller, D.T., Scott, R.A. and French, R.S. (1984) *Social Stigma: The Psychology of Marked Relations*. New York: WH Freeman.

Kassebaum, G.G. and Baumann, B.O. (1965) Dimensions of the sick role in chronic illness, *Journal of Health and Social Behavior*, 6, 16–27.

Kelleher, D. (1988) *Diabetes*. London: Routledge.

Kelly, M. (1986) The subjective experience of chronic disease: some implications for the management of ulcerative colitis, *Journal of Chronic Diseases*, 39, 653–66.

Kelly, M. (1991) Coping with an ileostomy, *Social Science and Medicine*, 33, 115–25.

Kelly, M. (1992) *Colitis*. London: Tavistock/Routledge.

Kelly, M. and May, D. (1982) Good patients and bad patients: a review of the literature and a theoretical critique, *Journal of Advanced Nursing*, 7, 147–56.

Kotarba, J.A. (1983) *Chronic Pain: Its Social Dimension*. Beverly Hills: Sage.

Lawler, J. (1991) *Behind the Screens: Somology and the Problem of the Body*. Edinburgh: Churchill Livinston.

Lawrence, P. (1958) Chronic illness and socio-economic status. In Jaco, E.G. (ed) *Patients, Physicians and Illness: Sourcebook in Behavioural Science and Medicine*. New York: Free Press.

Lemert, E.M. (1962) Paranoia and the dynamics of exclusion, *Sociometry*, 25, 2–20.

Locker, D. (1983) *Disability and Disadvantage: The Experience of Chronic Illness*. London: Tavistock.

Lorber, J. (1975) Good patients and problem patients: conformity and deviance in a general hospital, *Journal of Health and Social Behavior*, 16, 213–55.

McIntosh, J. (1977) *Communication and Awareness in a Cancer Ward*. London: Croom Helm.

Mercer, J. (1972) Who is normal? Two perspectives on mild mental retardation. In Jaco, E.G. (ed) *Patients, Physicians and Illness* (2nd Edition). Glencoe: Free Press.

Moos, R. and Tsu, V. (eds) (1977) *Coping with Physical Illness*. New York: Plenum.

Morris, J. (1993) *Independent Lives: Community Care and Disabled People*. London: Macmillan.

Navarro, V. (1978) *Class Struggle, The State and Medicine: An Historical and Contemporary Analysis of the Medical Sector*. London: Martin Robertson.

Oliver, M. (1990) *The Politics of Disablement*. Basingstoke: Macmillan.

Oliver, M. (1994) *Understanding Disability*. Basingstoke: Macmillan.

Parker, G. (1993) *With this Body: Caring and Disability in Marriage*. Buckingham: Open University.

Parsons, T. (1951a) *The Social System*. Glencoe Ill: Free Press.

Parsons, T. (1951b) Illness and the role of the physician: a sociological perspective, *American Journal Orthopsychiatry*, 21, 452–60.

Pinder, R. (1990) *The Management of Chronic Disease: Patient and Doctor Perspectives on Parkinson's Disease*. London: Macmillan.

Radley, A. (1993) (ed) *Worlds of Illness: Biographical and Cultural Perspectives on Health and Illness*. London: Routledge.

Robinson, I. (1988) *Multiple Sclerosis*. London: Tavistock/Routledge.

Rose, A.M. (1962) A social–psychological theory of neurosis. In Rose, A.M. (ed) *Human Behavior and Social Processes*. London: Routledge and Kegan Paul.

Scambler, G. (1989) *Epilepsy*. London: Tavistock.

Scambler, G. and Hopkins, A. (1986) Being epileptic: coming to terms with stigma, *Sociology of Health and Illness*, 8, 26–43.

Scheff, T.J. (1966) *Being Mentally Ill: A Sociological Theory*. Chicago: Aldine.

Schou, K.C. (1993) Awareness contexts and the construction of dying in the cancer treatment setting: 'micro' and 'macro' levels in narrative analysis. In Clark, D. (ed). *The Sociology of Death*. Oxford: Blackwell/The Sociological Review.

Schutz, A. (1970) *On Phenomenology and Social Relations*. Chicago: University of Chicago Press.

Scott, R. (1969) *The Making of Blind Men: A Study in Adult Socialisation*. New York: Russell Sage Foundation.

Shilling, C. (1993) *The Body and Social Theory*. London: Sage.

Strauss, A.L. *et al.* (1984) *Chronic Illness and the Quality of Life* (2nd Edition), St Louis: CV Mosby.

Turner, B. (1992) *Regulating Bodies: Essays in Medical Sociology*. London: Routledge.

Voysey, M. (1975) *A Constant Burden: The Reconstitution of Family Life*. London: Routledge and Kegan Paul.

West, P. (1986) The social meaning of epilepsy: stigma as a potential explanation for psychopathology in children. In Whitman, S. and Hermann, B.P. (eds) *Psychopathology in Epilepsy: Social Dimensions*. New York: Oxford University Press.

West, P. (1990) The status and validity of accounts obtained at interview: a contrast between two studies of families with a disabled child, *Social Science and Medicine*, 30, 1229–39.

Wiener, C. (1975) The burden of rheumatoid arthritis: tolerating the uncertainty, *Social Science and Medicine*, 6, 97–104.

Williams, G. (1984) The genesis of chronic illness: narrative reconstruction, *Sociology of Health and Illness*, 6, 175–200.

Chapter 21

Michael Bury

DEFINING AND RESEARCHING DISABILITY
Challenges and responses

From C. Barnes and G. Mercer (eds) *Exploring the Divide: Illness and Disability*, Leeds: Disability Press (School of Sociology and Social Policy, Leeds University) (1996)

Introduction

IT IS SOMETHING OF A CLICHÉ to say that we are living in a period of rapid social change. Yet it seems clear that a fundamental process of cultural as well as economic and social transformation is underway, and on a global scale. Arguments have proliferated as to the directions of such change. For some, the changes represent little more than cultural fragmentation, perhaps even degeneration; for others they represent renewal (Featherstone, 1992). What is less in doubt is that assumptions underpinning a range of social and intellectual activities are under strain. Nowhere is this more in evidence than in the health field. Not only is modern medicine being challenged on all sides, from managerialism to alternative medicine, but the very categories that have underpinned modern health and welfare systems are being severely scrutinised.

In this chapter, a preliminary sketch of change in one area of health and welfare is presented, namely that of disability. The chapter first examines the recent history of defining and researching disability, and identifies the emergence of a 'socio-medical' model, particularly in the British context. It then notes the development of a more explicit sociological view, which has emerged from these concerns and from more theoretical considerations. Second, the chapter examines recent arguments put forward by a number of 'disability theorists', that disability should be defined and researched primarily as a form of 'social oppression'. Critiques of the socio-medical model and sociological work which have been informed by these arguments will be examined. Finally, the chapter considers the impact this controversy is having on the field of disability studies, and on the relationship between researchers and researched.

The emergence of disability

In the immediate post-war world, at least in Britain, health care and social welfare in the disability area were characterised, in Topliss' terms, by a mixture of neglect and humanitarian concern (Topliss, 1979). The effects of war and industrial injury slowly gave way to the impact of chronic disease and disability in an ageing population. Though, of course, not all disability at this time was associated with chronic illness, and not all such illness involved disability, the relationship between the two was becoming increasingly evident (Taylor, 1976). In addition, disability in earlier stages of the life course, from the effects of congenital abnormalities, and from injuries caused by high risk sports and leisure activities was also becoming significant. The relationship between age, life course, disability and such factors as gender and ethnicity has subsequently received more attention, especially in social research (Arber and Evandrou, 1993).

During the same period medical specialties grew, and this has sometimes led to accusations, mentioned in more detail below, of the medicalisation of disability. Since then, areas such as rheumatology, stroke and rehabilitation services have grown rapidly, alongside the massive expansion of services for patients with a wide variety of other chronic disabling conditions. Specialist facilities for treating the effects of trauma, whether on the sports field or the roads, have also grown. Medical research on these conditions and on the general profile of disability has also expanded at a rapid rate.

In Britain, research on the social dimensions of chronic illness and disability began in earnest in the 1960s, though it has to be said, within a less theoretical framework than in the U.S. (Bury, 1991). Collaboration between public health oriented rehabilitation specialists such as Michael Warren, and sociologists such as Margot Jefferys, focused on the definition and assessment of motor impairment in prevalence studies (Jefferys et al., 1969). As Donald Patrick has pointed out, such work was linked to the task of estimating medical need and the possibility of developing preventive strategies (Patrick and Peach, 1989, p. 21).

This and other work culminated in the first OPCS national study of 'impairment and handicap' carried out by Amelia Harris and her colleagues, and published in 1971. This showed, for the first time, the extent of impairment in Britain, and suggested that just under 4% of the population aged 16–64 and just under 28% population over the age of 65 suffered from some form of impairment (Harris et al., 1971a). Importantly, gender differences were noted, with twice the level of impairment in women compared with men (Patrick and Peach, 1989, p. 22). Comparable studies were carried out in the U.S. at this time (ibid.).

Subsequently, in Britain, Wood and his colleagues sought to clarify the terminology that was being used in this research, especially in the light of confusion, present even in the Harris survey, where different definitions (e.g. of impairment and handicap) were evident, with the terms sometimes being used synonymously.

In 1980 the World Health Organisation published the results of this work in the form of the International Classification of Impairments, Disabilities and Handicaps (ICIDH) which provided a more consistent definition of the terms involved (WHO, 1980). In this classification, *impairment* referred to abnormality in the structure of the functioning of the body, whether through disease or trauma; *disability* referred to the restriction in ability to perform tasks, especially those associated with everyday life and self care activities; and *handicap* referred to the social disadvantage that could be associated with either impairment and/or disability. The latter term was particularly emphasised as a means of revealing needs created as a consequence of chronic illness interacting with a sometimes hostile social environment.

The widespread use of this schema helped focus the socio-medical model that earlier work had been building, and provided the basis for both developments and debate in the years that followed. Community based studies, such as that in Lambeth, South London, provided the framework for the exploration of prevalence of impairment, health care and rehabilitation needs in disability and social aspects of handicap, such as material hardship and the role of social support. This kind of research helped to explore the mediating relationship between the various planes of experience that the WHO schema described (Patrick and Peach, 1989).

National and local studies underlined, in particular, the economic dimensions of disability, and the hardship experienced by many, particularly in a period of growing recession. Though the Harris survey had been associated with the 1970 Chronically Sick and Disabled Persons Act, which for the first time obliged local authorities in Britain to estimate and meet the needs of the disabled, various research findings reinforced the view held by Mechanic and others in earlier U.S. work, that the consequences of disability were most obviously seen in financial hardship. In fact, a less well publicised volume of the Harris study revealed the extent of financial hardship among the disabled (Harris *et al.*, 1971b). Townsend's compendious work on *Poverty in the United Kingdom* gave additional weight to the link between disability and inequality (Townsend, 1979).

Though the socio-medical model provided the grounds for identifying and drawing attention to the various needs of disabled people, many problems remained. At the research level, it had long been recognised that the definition of disability, unlike disease, was less categorical and more 'relational' in character. It was pointed out that the term disability was conceptually 'slippery' and difficult to pin down (Topliss, 1979), and involved complex interactions between the individual and the social environment. Moreover, the boundaries between impairment, disability and handicap were recognised as less than clear cut in everyday settings, and difficult to operationalise in research, even though the distinctions remained important in directing attention to different planes of experience (Bury, 1987).

At the policy level, though the consequences of disability were being identified, financial compensation and greater emphasis on disabled people's own views was not much in evidence. In part this arose from the continuing part that medicine played, within administrative circles, in adjudicating access to benefits. In order to tackle this problem, and provide new estimates of disability based on a broader definition, a new national study was commissioned by the OPCS in 1984, and several surveys, including one on children, were carried out between 1985 and 1988. The main purpose of this new initiative was to inform a review of social security in the disability field, and pave the way for such benefits to be based on a more systematic appreciation of the relational character of disability.

As a result of this orientation, the OPCS developed an approach to measuring disability which would be more sensitive to the difficulties encountered in earlier work. By combining judgements of professionals, researchers and disabled people themselves, and by using the basic definition of disability as laid down in the WHO classification, the OPCS was able to operationalise a new approach that gave a wider picture. Scales were developed on key areas of disability ranging from problems with locomotion, through seeing, hearing and personal care, to difficulties with communication (Martin et al., 1988, p. 10). . . .

For present purposes, two main findings are of note. First, the association of disability with age was once more confirmed. This is of particular importance in the OPCS survey, which was innovatory in assessing the level of disability without, at the point of interview, an age reference; in other words, if a person could not perform a particular activity they were counted as disabled irrespective of age. However, when the data from the survey were analysed, they showed that of six million people living in Great Britain with at least one form of disability (based on the relatively low threshold used in the survey) almost 70% of disabled adults were aged 60 and over, and nearly half were aged 70 and over (Martin et al., 1988, p. 27). The very old emerged as those most likely to be affected, with 63% of women and 53% of men over the age of 75 being disabled. When severity is taken into account, the very old again predominate, with 64% of adults in the two highest categories aged 70 or over, and 41% aged 80 or over (Martin et al., 1988). I will return to the significance of some of these findings later in the chapter . . .

It is the predominance of chronic disease as the cause of disability, which is of particular note in the OPCS study. Many of the disorders associated with later life, especially arthritis, and hearing loss (the former helping to explain much of the gender difference in disability rates) were most frequently associated with disability, underlining the long term trend away from disabilities caused by trauma and medical conditions in early life, to disorders in later life. . . .

Some needs may, therefore, be condition specific, depending upon the particular illness or impairment concerned. A follow up study by the RNIB, for example, involving further interviews with a sample of visually impaired people from the OPCS survey, and a more detailed analysis of the relevant OPCS material, was able to provide a more in depth picture of the special needs of people with visual impairments, including their health needs (Bruce et al., 1991). The relationship between the general profile of disability and the specific needs of groups within the population clearly needs to be appreciated.

This issue, for sociologists, at least, has underpinned their growing concern with the meaning of disability, and not simply its definition or prevalence. Alongside work on the socio-medical model, therefore, a more independent sociological voice began to emerge. This set out a more distinctive research approach, in comparison with the medical and policy agendas, which had dominated the field until then. This approach began to apply more explicitly sociological concepts to the area.

In Britain, Mildred Blaxter's book The Meaning of Disability (Blaxter, 1976), and in the U.S., Strauss and Glaser's book, Chronic Illness and the Quality of Life (Strauss and Glaser, 1975) captured the spirit of these concerns. Using different methods, both books explored the range of problems encountered by people with disabilities. In the case of Blaxter's book, she showed that over time the impact of disability on social life was particularly marked, even when other more practical problems had been resolved. She also showed how the complicated relationship between health and welfare systems hampered individuals and their families in adapting to disability. Strauss and his colleagues looked particularly at the balance people sought to strike between the demands of illness and treatment regimens and the need to maintain a normal everyday life.

Since these pioneering studies, more sociological work on specific disabling illnesses have now been undertaken, documenting both the problems people face and the active steps they take to overcome them. The emphasis on meaning in this work has revealed, in more depth, the issues that people find most difficult in adapting to in disabling illness. Such studies have also highlighted the constraints of societal responses and the availability or the lack of resources needed to tackle them (Bury, 1991). The exploration of the contextual and emergent nature of disability in sociological work of this kind has acted as a counter point to the more formal definitions and assessments in the socio-medical model, as described above.

However, despite, or perhaps because of this wider body of work, in both the U.S. and U.K., new challenges have developed, not least from among people with chronic disorders and disabilities themselves. As services and research have expanded so the boundaries that have separated fields of activities, notably those between professionals and patients/clients, have shifted. And as numerous sources of information have emerged these have inevitably provided grounds for more critical perspectives to develop. Indeed, under conditions of information explosion and media interest, as Anthony Giddens has pointed out in a more general cultural context, experts and expert knowledge become 'chronically contestable' (Giddens, 1991).

Though the field of chronic illness and disability has long contained a large number of lay charitable and self help groups, whose interests and views have often departed from those in the medical and academic establishments, new forms of organisation and outlook have recently emerged. While some groups, especially those linked to specific chronic diseases, continue to concentrate on supporting medical and, to a lesser extent, social research, others have begun to adopt and develop a more critical position with respect to both the definition and study of disability.

The emergence of the 'disability movement', characterised by an increasingly challenging attitude to the discrimination and 'exclusionary practices' which have historically affected the disabled in modern society, has gained considerable momentum. New forms of political, educational and professional activities have proliferated as expressions of these developments. In addition, help lines, lobbyists, and rights activists, have provided numerous opportunities for challenges to existing policies and practices to gain ground. Many of these activities have drawn on a range of writings that seek to confront current research. For example, a special issue of *Disability, Handicap and Society* was given over to the topic in 1992, following a conference supported by the Rowntree Foundation. It is to the main lines of the criticisms found here and elsewhere that the chapter now, therefore, turns.

Following a brief outline of the definitional and theoretical issues addressed in these recent arguments, the implications for social research are then addressed.

Disability as a form of social oppression

Perhaps the sharpest challenge to existing ideas about disability is the argument that disability should be seen as a form of 'social oppression' (Oliver, 1990; 1992). Although this term is not clearly defined, the basic position is clear. In contrast to existing notions of disability, which, it is argued, portray it as a characteristic of individuals, 'disability' is seen, instead, as a wholly social phenomenon. Mike Oliver, whose writing may act as an exemplar in this context, states, for example, that 'disability as a category can only be understood within a framework, which suggests that it is culturally produced and socially constructed' (Oliver, 1990, p. 22). 'Disability' is seen to be a function of those practices and perceptions linked to certain bodily mental or behavioural states which are so designated. Here the ICIDH definition of 'disability' is rejected, in favour of an approach which at times is similar to that of the ICIDH definition of 'handicap', that is, the social disadvantage experienced by disabled people.

From the 'social oppression' viewpoint, disability is not the resulting limitations caused by chronic illness, impairment or trauma, but the way such matters are responded to and categorised by the wider society. Disability is the product of definitions and practices that seek to exclude individuals who might be seen to deviate from the socially constructed norms of the 'able bodied'. In short, 'disability' is what a 'disablist' society decides so to call. The links with labelling theory developed by sociologists in the 1960s are immediately apparent in such an argument. It is not the 'inherent' nature of disability that matters, but the labelling process, which categorises people by virtue of their position in relation to the dominant structures and values of the society.

The important starting point for 'oppression theory', is that 'disability' should not be conceptualised as an individual attribute, but as the result of 'exclusionary practices'. In a capitalistic society, these designate which attributes are seen as productive and acceptable and which are abnormal or deviant. Definitional questions, according to this argument, therefore flow not from the 'personal tragedy' of disability, but from the needs of the social system to distinguish between people in industrial and educational environments, and the need to decide who is to be excluded or segregated (Oliver, 1990, p. 28).

State involvement in people's lives, throughout the modern period, is seen to be preoccupied with the sorting and segregating of individuals, especially in terms of their abilities to meet the dictates of the work place, and, in general, to ensure that social order is maintained by regulating exclusions in matters such as eligibility for state benefits. Thus disability turns out to be a central rather than peripheral matter to the development and maintenance of modern welfare states (Stone, 1984; Albrecht, 1992).

In addition to the 'exclusionary practices' that result from this process, the tendency to portray disability as a feature of the individual, it is held, reinforces an 'ideology of individualism'. This, to stay with Oliver's argument, is held to be at the heart of our current concepts. In extending his 'political economy' view of disability, to cover this point, Oliver argues:

> It is not the ideological construction of property owning, self interested or rational individuals that is important (in discussing disability). Rather it is the construction of 'able bodied' and 'able minded' individuals which is significant. (Oliver, 1990, pp. 45–46).

The 'theory of medicalisation' is then added to this approach in order to explain the role of medicine in regulating and managing disability. Rather than accepting medicine as a means of meeting the needs of individuals, Oliver, again, casts medicine's role as essentially the handmaiden to the capitalist order. Referring to Zola's (1972) theory of medicalisation and social control, Oliver argues that medical labels 'stick to some groups and not others'. This process is held to be a function of the ideological and material needs of the system, rather than the health and welfare needs of individuals. Indeed the latter act as a screen behind which discriminatory practices take place. In this sense, the argument that medical knowledge is 'socially constructed' (Bury, 1986) is also invoked.

Given the apparent lack of effective treatment for many chronic disorders, the only explanation Oliver can find for medicine's involvement in disability is a regulatory and 'imperialistic' one. Though the expanding role of medicine, including surgery, in treating a variety of different 'impairments' is left unclear, Oliver echoes Finkelstein's employment of the idea of 'medical dominance' of disability to account for the development of specialisms such as rehabilitation medicine (Finkelstein, 1980). In so doing such writers draw on a range of medical sociology writings from the 1970s which, as Gerhardt (1989) has noted, portrayed medicine as the result of the (largely arbitrary) artful practices of the medical profession, rather than as the application of objective knowledge to the patient's condition. In an attempt to turn the tables on this process Oliver asks, 'who should be in charge of the rehabilitation process, disabled people or the professionals?' (Oliver, 1993, p. 61).

Researching disability

As has been stated, one of the purposes of this chapter is to trace how these critical ideas about disability are being applied to the area of research. Perhaps one of the first questions that arises, in this connection, is why 'disability theorists' should be particularly concerned with research in the first place. If disability, from a 'social oppression' viewpoint, is self evidently entirely 'social' and therefore 'political' in character (Oliver, 1992) a social movement espousing such a position might well be expected to concern itself primarily with political action against a 'disablist society' and use social research findings, wherever possible, for these purposes, rather than focus on the activities of research and researchers as such. Indeed, Oliver has done precisely that, using the OPCS study and its estimates (which, as I will show, has been severely criticised elsewhere by 'disability theorists') in support of disability rights (Barnes and Oliver, 1995).

In fact, disability groups have long adopted this approach, in their campaigning as the reference to the RNIB earlier in this chapter indicates. Others, such as the Disability Alliance, have long used the research findings of Townsend and others in pamphleteering, campaigning and advancing their case. Recent campaigns for 'disability rights' legislation in the British parliament have employed similar tactics. It could be argued that in such activity, challenging definitions and research approaches has not been a high priority. The majority of those arguing for disability rights seem more concerned with other, more substantive issues. The position of 'disabled people' has been advanced without the need for a radical 'deconstruction' of the term, as defined, for example, by WHO/OPCS. These 'second order' constructs have not been the focus of concern. It seems that appeals to generally accepted definitions of disability, rather than 'social oppression' theory, have been more than adequate for the political tasks in hand.

However, the role that medical and social research has played in the recent history of disability is often held by others, especially the 'disability theorists', to be negative and part of the problem to be addressed, rather than a potential (if limited) part of its solution.

As a result, 'disability theorists' have developed critiques both of the putative effects of recent research, and the research process itself. In so doing they have drawn links between their general critiques of the variety of professional discourses on disability, and recent research activities. Here, both medical and social research have become the focus of 'struggle', because they have been seen, like other professional activities, as largely self serving. As Oliver has stated:

> The idea that small groups of 'experts' can get together and set a research agenda for disability, is again, fundamentally flawed. (Oliver, 1992, p. 102)

This suggests that 'disability theorists' should extend their arguments to fashion a different research agenda and possibly a new methodology. Whilst this immediately opens up the possible counter charge that 'disability theorists' may be making a similar play to establish themselves as a group of 'experts' – especially as many now hold university posts, and run research projects and units – the main thrust is to argue a strong case against the activities of the present research community. . . .

The background to this takes us back to the underlying conception of disability discussed earlier. While critics such as Finkelstein and Oliver recognise that research endeavours such as Harris's 1971 survey, Wood's WHO classification and the OPCS survey contain a social component, they remain dismissive of them because, they argue, such 'research is based on the idea that disability and handicap arise as a direct consequence of individual impairments' (Oliver, 1990, p. 7). This argument is advanced despite the fact that the WHO approach expressly underlined the complexities of the relationships between the different dimensions, and that the disability movement's own conception of disability also begins with some form of underlying impairment, whether through disease or trauma. French (1993), for example, has made the point that though she agrees with 'the basic tenets of the ("disability theorists") model', she believes, 'that some of the most profound problems experienced by people with certain impairments are difficult, if not impossible, to solve by social manipulation' (French, 1993, p.17).

Here, French seems to recognise the dangers of an 'oversocialised' view of disability, creating a reductionist perspective in its zeal to exclude the role that different factors plays.

In fact, the idea that impairment and disability are closely related but distinct proves difficult to reject. Without some underlying initial problem, social responses would, so to speak, have nothing to respond to. If labelling theory is invoked, some form of 'primary deviation' is necessary, if societal reactions are to have any meaning. Labels have to be attached to a restricted range of phenomena if they are to be effective (positively or negatively) as labels at all. Moreover, while the role of impairment (especially as the result of chronic illness) was clearly conceptualised in the WHO approach, this was not the most important aspect of the schema. It was the emphasis on handicap which mattered most, in its attempt to point to the social disadvantage which may result from the social reactions and conditions within which disability is experienced.

As mentioned earlier, as a result of the 'relational' character of the processes at work, the distinctions between disability and handicap are inevitably problematic (Bury, 1987). Both disability and handicap can be seen as a product, from this viewpoint, *of the interaction of the individual and the social environment*. The distinction between them is simply designed to direct attention to the different dimensions of experience, that is, the difference between restricted activity (which, following French's comment, may be more or less 'socially produced' in character) and related social disadvantage. Without such a distinction, the ability to know that disadvantage has increased or reduced would be difficult indeed to establish. The 'disability theorists' critique, however, rejects this distinction and asserts that disability is wholly a product of social circumstances. . . .

The future of researching disability

The scene is set, therefore, for a lively period in both 'official' research and socio-logical work. It appears that this may involve a struggle for influence, and possibly control over the direction and funding of research in disability. Quoting Gollop (cited in Oliver, 1992), Oliver has argued that the new emancipatory paradigm should be based on 'reciprocity, gain and empowerment'. In effect this means that, 'researchers have to learn how to put their knowledge and skills at the disposal of their research subjects' (Oliver, 1992, p. 111). In this way a new research agenda will, apparently, be fashioned. Moreover, research relationships, as expressed in traditional social research methods, are likely to be the focus of considerable critical debate.

Partly as a result of these developing arguments and criticisms (though also for other reasons) researchers are already coming under greater pressure to examine their assumptions and methods. In many respects this is to be welcomed, and is already having the effect of bringing 'client' and patient groups into the research process. However, this chapter has said enough to suggest that there are also grounds for concern with the alternatives being argued. Two main reservations about their implications for research relationships may act as an appropriate conclusion to the present discussion.

First, this chapter has tried to show that the 'social oppression' approach to disability is open to the criticism of reductionism, especially as an 'over socialised' conceptualisation of the processes at work. If this is accepted, the models it seeks to replace may be of continuing use, both in research, and in the policy process. There is a danger, in adopting the 'social oppression' approach of caricaturing alternatives, and generating hostility where collaboration and rational debate would be of greater value. While the relationship between researchers and the researched is always a sensitive issue, and needs to be approached with care, it is difficult to sustain the argument that either survey methods or qualitative research in themselves are inherently 'alienating'.

Second, the idea that research should become a site for 'struggle' suggests a politicisation of research that may have a number of unintended consequences. While it may be taken as axiomatic that individuals have a unique insight into their own experiences, it does not logically follow that they are qualified or able to undertake research. Moreover, such a view also runs the risk that the status of being disabled should be the main criteria for carrying out research on the subject. This sits uneasily in an argument in which the very idea of 'disability', as a defining characteristic of individuals, is being challenged.

Taken to its logical conclusion this could also mean a direct threat to the independence of research. Given the political climate in which we now live, this argument needs to be approached with caution. The independence of research has long been guarded by researchers, and others, including the disabled. Independence in this context does not mean a lack of engagement with social issues, or a naive view of 'value free' research, or most importantly an unwillingness to work closely with those being researched (Bury, 1996). What it does mean, though, is that research findings need to be based on the use of 'publicly available methods' (Hammersley, 1992) if they are to withstand hostile scrutiny, especially by governments. Threats from neo-conservative sources to social research have seriously reduced this independence throughout the 1980s and 90s. Margaret Thatcher, in particular, was associated with a view that research should serve political interests. It would be an irony indeed if 'disability theorists' in emphasising empowerment and autonomy of people with disabilities were to add to this trend. Instead, a process of open debate and mutual tolerance would seem to offer a more productive way forward.

References

Albrecht, G. (1992) *The Disability Business*, London: Sage.

Arber, S. and Evandrou, M. (eds.) (1993) *Ageing, Independence and the Life Course*, London: Jessica Kingsley Publishers.

Barnes, C. and Oliver, M. (1995) 'Disability Rights: rhetoric and reality in the UK', *Disability and Society*, 10, 1, pp. 111–116.

Blaxter, M. (1976) *The Meaning of Disability*, London: Heinemann.

Bruce, I., McKennel, A. and Walker, E. (1991) *Blind and Partially Sighted People in Great Britain*, London: HMSO.

Bury, M. (1986) 'Social Constructionism and the Development of Medical Sociology', *Sociology of Health and Illness*, 8, 2, pp. 137–169.

Bury, M. (1987) 'The International Classification of Impairments, Disabilities and

Handicaps: A Review of Research and Prospects', *International Disability Studies*, 9, 3, pp. 118–122.

Bury, M. (1991) 'The Sociology of Chronic Illness: a review of research and prospects', *Sociology of Health and Illness*, 13, 4, pp. 451–468.

Bury, M. (1996) 'Disability and the Myth of the Independent Researcher: A Reply', *Disability and Society*, 11, 1, pp. 111–114.

Featherstone, M. (1992) 'The Heroic Life and Everyday Life', *Theory, Culture and Society*, 9, 159–182.

Finkelstein, V. (1980) *Attitudes and Disabled People: Issues for Discussion*, New York: World Rehabilitation Fund.

French, S. (1993) 'Disability, impairment or something in between?', in Swain, J., Finkelstein, V., French, S. and Oliver, M. (eds.) *Disabling Barriers – Enabling Environments*, London: Sage.

Gerhardt, U (1989) *Ideas About Illness: an intellectual and political history of medical sociology*, London: Macmillan.

Giddens, A. (1991) *Modernity and Self Identity*, Cambridge: Polity Press.

Hammersley, M. (1992) 'On Feminist Methodology', *Sociology*, 26, 2, 187–206.

Harris, A., Cox, E. and Smith, C. (1971a) *Handicapped and Impaired in Great Britain*, Vol. 1, London: HMSO.

Harris, A., Cox, E. and Smith, C. (1971b) *Handicapped and Impaired in Great Britain, Economic Dimensions*, London: HMSO.

Jefferys, M., Nullard, J. B., Hyman, M. and Warren, M. D. (1969) 'A set of tests for measuring motor impairment in prevalence studies', *Journal of Chronic Diseases*, 28, 303–309.

Martin, J., Meltzer, H. and Elliot, D. (1988) *The Prevalence of Disability Among Adults*, London: HMSO.

Oliver, M. (1990) *The Politics of Disablement*, London: Macmillan.

Oliver, M. (1992) 'Changing the Social Relations of Research Production', *Disability, Handicap and Society*, 7, 2, 101–114.

Oliver, M. (1993) 'Re-defining disability: a challenge to research', in Swain, J., Finkelstein, V., French, S. and Oliver, M. (eds.) *Disabling Barriers – Enabling Environments*, London: Sage.

Patrick, D. and Peach, H. (eds.) (1989) *Disablement in the Community*, Oxford: Oxford Medical Publications.

Stone, D.A. (1984) *The Disabled State*, London: Macmillan.

Strauss, A. L. and Glaser, B. (1975) *Chronic Illness and the Quality of Life*, St. Louis: C.V. Mosby and Co.

Taylor, D. (1976) *Physical Impairment: Social Handicap*, London: Office of Health Economics.

Topliss, E. (1979) *Provision for the Disabled* (2nd ed.), Oxford: Blackwell with Martin Robertson.

Townsend, P. (1979) *Poverty in the United Kingdom*, Harmondsworth: Penguin Books.

World Health Organisation (1980) *International Classification of Impairments, Disabilities and Handicaps*, Geneva: WHO.

Zola, I. (1972) 'Medicine as an Institution of Social Control', *Sociological Review*, 20, 487–504.

Chapter 22

Mike Oliver

DEFINING IMPAIRMENT AND DISABILITY
Issues at stake

From C. Barnes and G. Mercer (eds) *Exploring the Divide: Illness and Disability,* Leeds: Disability Press (School of Sociology and Social Policy, Leeds University) (1996)

Introduction

FOR THE PAST FIFTEEN YEARS the social model of disability has been the foundation upon which disabled people have chosen to organise themselves collectively. This has resulted in unparalleled success in changing the discourses around disability, in promoting disability as a civil rights issue and in developing schemes to give disabled people autonomy and control in their own lives. Despite these successes, in recent years the social model has come under increasing scrutiny both from disabled people and from others working in the field of chronic illness.

What I want to explore in this chapter are some of the issues that are at stake in these emerging criticisms and suggest that there is still a great deal of mileage to be gained from the social model and that we weaken it at our peril. I will do this by briefly outlining the two alternative schemes which have emerged in the articulation of conflicting definitions of chronic illness, impairment and disability. I will then discuss six issues that, I suggest, go to the heart of the debate as far as external criticisms from medical sociologists are concerned. These are: the issue of causality; the question of conceptual consistency; the role of language; the normalising tendencies contained in both schemas; the problem of experience; and finally, the politicisation of the definitional process.

Having identified the issues at stake externally, I will discuss a number of internal criticisms that have emerged from disabled people themselves around the place of impairment, the incorporation of other oppressions and the use and explanatory power of the social model of disability. While remaining sceptical about these criticisms, I will finally suggest that a start can be made towards resolving some of them by focusing on what disabled people would call impairment and medical sociologists would call chronic illness.

The problem of definitions

Since the 1960s there have been various attempts to provide and develop a conceptual schema to describe and explain the complex relationships between illness, impairment, disability and handicap. This has led to the adoption of the International Classification of Impairments, Disabilities and Handicaps (ICIDH) by the World Health Organisation (WHO) (Wood, 1980) which has been used as the basis for two national studies of disability in Britain (Harris, 1971; Martin *et al.*, 1988).

Not everyone has accepted the validity of this schema nor the assumptions underpinning it. Disabled people's organisations themselves have been in the forefront of the rejection of the schema itself (Driedger, 1988), others have rejected the assumptions which underpin it (Oliver, 1990) and the adequacy of it as a basis for empirical work has also been questioned (Abberley, 1993). This is not the place to discuss these issues in detail; rather I intend to look at some of the dimensions of the debate that is currently taking place. In order to facilitate this, I reproduce the two alternative schemas below for those who are not familiar with either or both:

The WHO International Classification of Impairments, Disabilities and Handicaps:

> IMPAIRMENT: In the context of health experience, an impairment is any loss or abnormality of psychological, physiological, or anatomical structure or function . . .

> DISABILITY: In the context of health experience, a disability is any restriction or lack (resulting from an impairment) of ability to perform an activity in the manner or within the range considered normal for a human being . . .

> HANDICAP: In the context of health experience, a handicap is a disadvantage for a given individual, resulting from an impairment or a disability, that limits or prevents the fulfilment of a role that is normal (depending on age, sex, social and cultural factors) for that individual. (Wood, 1980, pp. 27–29)

The Disabled People's International (DPI) definition:

> IMPAIRMENT: is the functional limitation within the individual caused by physical, mental or sensory impairment.

> DISABILITY: is the loss or limitation of opportunities to take part in the normal life of the community on an equal level with others due to physical and social barriers. (DPI, 1982)

The issue of causality

The search for causality has been a major feature of both the scientific and the social scientific enterprise. What is at stake for the disability schemas described above is how to explain negative social experiences and the inferior conditions under which disabled people live out their lives. For those committed to the WHO schema, what they call chronic illness is causally related to the disadvantages disabled people experience. For those committed to the DPI schema, however, there is no such causal link; for them disability is wholly and exclusively social. Hence each side accuses the other of being incorrect in causal terms.

These schemas appear to be incompatible and have led one medical sociologist critically to suggest:

> Sometimes, in seeking to reject the reductionism of the medical model and its institutional contexts, proponents of independent living have tended to discuss disablement as if it had nothing to do with the physical body. (Williams, 1991, p. 521)

Ironically that is precisely what the DPI definition insists, disablement is nothing to do with the body. It is a consequence of the failure of social organisation to take account of the differing needs of disabled people and remove the barriers they encounter. The schema does not, however, deny the reality of impairment nor that it is closely related to the physical body. Under this schema impairment is, in fact, nothing less than a description of the physical body.

The appearance of incompatibility however, may be precisely that: appearance. It may well be that this debate is in reality, the result of terminological confusion; that real similarities exist between chronic illness and impairment and that there is much scope for collaboration between supporters of both schemas if this confusion can be sorted out.

The question of conceptual consistency

This terminological confusion is not just a matter of agreeing to use the same words in the same way. It is also about understanding and appeared when a policy analyst attempted to relate her own experience to policy issues in the area of disability.

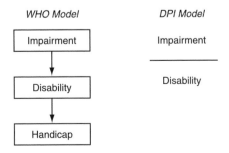

Figure 22.1 Causality in the two schemas

> I found myself puzzled by arguments that held that disability had nothing to do with illness or that belief in a need for some form of personal adaptation to impairment was essentially a form of false consciousness. I knew that disabled people argue that they should not be treated as if they were ill, but could see that many people who had impairments as a result of ongoing illness were also disabled. My unease increased as I watched my parents coming to terms with my mother's increasing impairments (and disability) related to arterial disease which left her tired and in almost continual pain. I could see that people can be disabled by their physical, economic and social environment but I could also see that people who became disabled (rather than being born with impairments) might have to renegotiate their sense of themselves both with themselves and with those closest to them. (Parker, 1993, p. 2)

The DPI schema does not deny that some illnesses may have disabling consequences and many disabled people have illnesses at various points in their lives. Further, it may be entirely appropriate for doctors to treat illnesses of all kinds, though even here, the record of the medical profession is increasingly coming under critical scrutiny. Leaving this aside, however, doctors can have a role to play in the lives of disabled people: stabilising their initial condition, treating any illnesses which may arise and which may or may not be disability related.

The conceptual issue underpinning this dimension of the debate, therefore, is about determining which aspects of disabled people's lives need medical or therapeutic interventions, which aspects require policy developments and which require political action. Failure to distinguish between these up to now has resulted in the medicalisation of disability and the colonisation of disabled people's lives by a vast army of professionals when perhaps, political action (i.e. civil rights legislation) would be a more appropriate response.

The role of language

Despite recent attempts to denigrate those who believe in the importance of language in shaping reality, largely through criticisms of what has come to be called 'political correctness', few would argue that language is unimportant or disagree that attempts to eradicate terminology such as cripple, spastic, wobbler and mongol are anything other than a good thing.

This role of language, however, is more complex than simply the removal of offensive words. There is greater concern over the way language is used to shape meanings and even create realities. For example, the language used in much medical discourse including medical sociology is replete with words and meanings which many disabled people find offensive or feel that it distorts their experiences. In particular the term chronic illness is for many people an unnecessarily negative term, and discussions of suffering in many studies have the effect of casting disabled people in the role of victim.

The disabling effect of language is not something that is unique to disabled people. Other groups have faced similar struggles around language. Altman in his study of collective responses to AIDS points out:

> . . . in particular the Denver Principles stressed the use of the term 'PWA' as distinct from 'victims' or 'patients', and the need for representation at all levels of AIDS policy-making 'to share their own experiences and knowledge'. (Altman, 1994, p.59)

The struggles around language are not merely semantic. A major bone of contention is the continued use of the term 'handicap' by the WHO schema. This is an anathema to many disabled people because of its connections to 'cap in hand' and the degrading role that charity and charitable institutions play in our lives.

The normalising tendencies of both schemas

Underpinning both schemas is the concept of normality and the assumption that disabled people want to achieve this normality. In the WHO schema it is normal social roles and in the DPI schema it is the normal life of the community. The problem with both of these is that increasingly the disability movement throughout the world is rejecting approaches based upon the restoration of normality and insisting on approaches based upon the celebration of difference.

From rejections of the 'cure', through critiques of supposedly therapeutic interventions such as conductive education, cochlea implants and the like, and on to attempts to build a culture of disability based upon pride, the idea of normality is increasingly coming under attack. Ironically it is only the definition advanced by the Union of the Physically Impaired Against Segregation (UPIAS) that can accommodate the development of a politics of difference. While its definition of impairment is similar to that of DPI, its definition of disability is radically different:

> DISABILITY: the disadvantage or restriction of activity caused by a contemporary social organisation which takes no or little account of people who have physical impairments and thus excludes them from the mainstream of social activities. (UPIAS, 1976)

Again, this is not just a matter of semantics but a concerted attempt to reject the normalising society. That some organisations of disabled people have not fully succeeded cannot be explained only as a matter of dispute between different political positions within the disability movement but also as evidence of just how ingrained and deep-rooted the ideology of normality is within social consciousness more generally.

The problem of experience

Recently, a number of sociologists working in the general area of medical sociology and chronic illness have expressed concern over the growing importance of the 'social oppression theory' of disability, associated research methodologies, and their implications for doing research in the 'chronic illness and disability fields' (Bury, 1992).

Whilst these writers feel the need to 'positively debate' these developments, the basis of their concern is similar to that expressed by Hammersley with respect to some aspects of feminist research, i.e. the tendency to 'privilege experience over sociological research methodology' (Hammersley, 1992). In short, this privileging of experience is perceived as a threat; firstly, to 'non-disabled' researchers doing disability research; secondly, to the traditional role of the sociologist giving 'voice to the voiceless' – in this case 'older' disabled people whose interests are said to be poorly served by 'social oppression theory'; and, thirdly, to the 'independence' of sociological activities within the 'medical sociology world'.

As a social researcher, I have some sympathy for these concerns but the problem is that most social research has tended to privilege methodology above experience and, as a consequence, does not have a very good track record in faithfully documenting that experience; whether it be the black experience, the experience of women, the experience of disability and so on. Additionally, scientific social research has done little to improve the quality of life of disabled people. Finally, it is difficult to demonstrate that so called 'independent research' has had much effect on policy, legislation or social change (Oliver, 1992).

The politicisation of the definitional process

By now it should be clear that defining impairment or disability or illness or anything else for that matter is not simply a matter of language or science; it is also a matter of politics. Altman captures this in respect of the definitional battles surrounding AIDS:

> How AIDS was conceptualised was an essential tool in a sometimes very bitter struggle; was it to be understood as a primarily bio-medical problem, in which case its control should be under that of the medical establishment, or was it rather, as most community-based groups argued, a social and political issue, which required a much greater variety of expertise? (Altman, 1994, p.26)

This battle is related to two political processes; exclusion and inclusion as far as disabled people and disability definitions are concerned. The ways in which disabled people have been systematically excluded from the definitional process has recently been described in one incident which captures the nature of this exclusion more generally.

> It is a hot summer day in London in the late 1980's. Gathered together in one of the capital's most venerable colleges is a large number of academics, researchers and representatives of research funding bodies. Their purpose? A symposium on researching disability comprising

presentations on a variety of different methodological and other themes, given and chaired by a panel of experienced disability researchers.

Those convening the seminar are proud that it will shine a spotlight on a usually neglected area of social science research. But some in the audience (and one or two others who have chosen not to attend) hold a different view. What credibility can such a seminar muster, they ask, when none of those chairing or presenting papers are themselves disabled? What does it say about current understanding of disability research issues that such an event has been allowed to go ahead in this form, when a symposium on researching gender issues given entirely by men, or race relations research given entirely by white people, would have been laughed out of court? (Ward and Flynn, 1994, p.29)

It should be pointed out that this exclusion has been systematic and disabled people have not been properly consulted by organisations such as WHO and the Office of Population Censuses and Surveys who have been most heavily funded in Britain to undertake such work. Where claims that this is not the case have been made, the reality is that research organisations have demonstrated that they don't even understand the difference between organisations *for* and organisations *of* disabled people and while they may have consulted the former, they have not consulted the latter.

However, disabled people have begun to resist this situation by producing their own research based upon their own definitions (Barnes, 1991; 1992), the British Council of Disabled People (BCODP) has established its own research sub-committee and in Canada disabled people have produced their own guidelines on what is acceptable and not acceptable research for disability organisations to be involved in (Woodhill, 1993).

These initiatives have begun to have some impact on not only the research community but on Government as well. Altman discusses the role of people with AIDS (PWAs) in AIDS research and argues that it is in everyone's interest to encourage such developments:

CRI (Community Research Initiative) has proved that a community model of research, involving PWAs themselves in decision making, could run effective trials – partly because it was able to successfully access suitable patients and encourage them to participate – and could resolve the complex ethical questions of such research successfully. (Altman, 1994, p.70)

At a recent meeting of disabled people from all over Europe, the group decided to reaffirm their own definition of disability and to spell out the implications of this for the WHO schema.

A Disabled Person is an individual in their own right, placed in a disabling situation, brought about by environmental, economic and social barriers that the person, because of their impairment(s), cannot overcome in the same way as other citizens. These barriers are all too often reinforced by the marginalising attitudes of society. It is up to society to eliminate, reduce or compensate for these barriers in order to enable each individual to enjoy full citizenship, respecting the rights and duties of each individual.

By supporting this resolution this meeting on human rights expresses its non-support for the current classification of impairment, disability and handicap operated by the World Health Organisation. We call upon the WHO to enter into a dialogue with disabled people's organisations to adopt a new definition in line with the above resolution. (DPI, 1994)

Developing a social model of impairment?

Whatever happens to this call for a dialogue between organisations of disabled people and the World Health Organisation, disabled people have begun their own internal dialogue around the social model of disability. It is to some of the dimensions of this dialogue that I now turn before considering some of the implications.

A major criticism that some disabled people have made of the social model concerns the way it connects, or rather doesn't connect with the experience of impairment. French (1993), for example, argues that her visual impairment imposes some social restrictions which cannot be resolved by the application of the principles of the social model. She cites as examples her inability to recognise people and read or emit non-verbal cues in social interactions.

Clearly, most disabled people can come up with similar examples. As a wheelchair user when I go to parties I am more restricted than some other people from interacting with everyone else and what's more, it is difficult to see a solution – houses are usually crowded with people during parties and that makes circulation difficult for a wheelchair user. But other people may find circulation difficult as well but for other reasons; they may simply be shy. The point that I am making is that the social model is not an attempt to deal with the personal restrictions of impairment but the social barriers of disability as defined earlier by DPI and UPIAS.

Other disabled people have criticised the social model for its assumed denial of 'the pain of impairment', both physical and psychological. In many ways some of these criticism mirror those made from without although they are not beset by the same terminological confusion between illness and impairment.

> . . . there is a tendency within the social model of disability to deny the experience of our own bodies, insisting that our physical differences and restrictions are entirely socially created. While environmental barriers and social attitudes are a crucial part of our experience of disability – and do indeed disable us – to suggest that this is all there is to it is to deny the personal experience of physical or intellectual restrictions, of illness, of the fear of dying. (Morris, 1991, p.10)

This denial of the pain of impairment has not, in reality been a denial at all. Rather it has been a pragmatic attempt to identify and address issues that can be changed through collective action rather than medical or other professional treatment.

> If a person's physical pain is the reason they are unhappy then there is nothing the disability movement can do about it. All that BCODP can do is facilitate the politicisation of people around these issues. Of course this politicisation is fairly difficult to make practical progress with – much easier to achieve anti-discrimination legislation than a total review of how society regards death and dying, I imagine. This might explain why these subjects haven't been made a priority, but their day will come. (Vasey, 1992, p.43)

These criticisms are taken further by Crow (1992) who argues that the way forward for the social model of disability is to fully integrate the experience of impairment with the experience of disability. However, up to now and for very important reasons, the social model has insisted that there is no causal relationship between impairment and disability.

> The achievement of the disability movement has been to break the link between our bodies and our social situation, and to focus on the real cause of disability, i.e. discrimination and prejudice. To mention biology, to admit pain, to confront our impairments, has been to risk the oppressors seizing on evidence that disability is 'really' about physical limitation after all. (Shakespeare, 1992, p.40)

Finally the social model of disability is criticised because it was written (if it ever was?) by healthy wheelchair users. According to one recent commentator:

> The social model of disability appears to have been constructed for healthy quadriplegics. The social model avoids mention of pain, medication or ill-health. (Humphrey, 1994, p.66)

The social model of disability does indeed avoid mention of such things, not because it was written by healthy quadriplegics, but because pain, medication and ill-health properly belong within either the individual model of disability or the social model of impairment.

Other internal criticisms of the social model of disability

A further internal criticism comes from other oppressed groups who feel that these other oppressions such as racism (Hill, 1994), sexism (Morris, 1991) and homophobia (Hearn, 1991) have not been incorporated into the social model. Again, it is certainly true that the social model of disability has not explicitly addressed the issue of multiple or simultaneous oppression but then such issues are only just beginning to be explored in respect of both impairment and disability (Begum *et al.*, 1994; Zarb and Oliver, 1993; Priestley, 1995).

This dissatisfaction has been expressed not simply because the social model does not adequately reflect experience of oppression of all disabled people but also because it may 'oversimplify' some of the issues raised in Disability Equality Training (DET).

> For some time I have been dissatisfied with the oversimplified 'social model' of disability we are obliged to use in Disability Equality Training and have read with interest the recent arguments re-introducing 'impairment' into that model.

> Although the 'social model' has for some time served us well as a way of directing attention away from the personal to the political, I feel now that the debate has been hampered by the rather rigid genealogy of disability thinking. My own literary, linguistic and therapeutic back-ground led me to post-modernist thinkers such as Foucault, Derrida, Barthes and Lacan in an attempt to make sense of the personal and political aspects of the disability debate. (Cashling, 1993, pp. 199–200)

While it is undeniably true that some DET trainers may have used the social model in an over rigid way, those like myself who draw on Marxist rather than post-modernist thinking call this reification; that is, the elevation of a concept into a thing, a social construction into reality. And it remains to be seen whether post-modernist explanations of the oppression of disabled people as simply a manifestation of society's hatred of us, will take us as far as the social model of disability in challenging that oppression. Cashling suggests they might but I have my doubts. For me our oppression is ultimately due to our continued exclusion from the processes of production, and not because of society's hatred (real or imagined) of us.

Such criticism, however, raises questions about the way the model is used, rather than the model itself. If we expect models to explain, rather than aid under-standing, then they are bound to be found wanting. Many of those arguing for the incorporation of impairment have confused models and theories. I suggest that the continuing use and refinement of the social model of disability can contribute to rather than be a substitute for the development of an adequate social theory of disability. As both Abberley (1987) and myself (Oliver 1990) have argued, an adequate social theory of disability must contain a theory of impairment.

A final criticism comes from one of the founding fathers of the social model, Vic Finkelstein, who is also critical of the adequacy of the social model's explanatory power. Recently he has questioned the ability of the social model to explain fully the social position of disabled people in modern society, and suggests that there are at least two variants: the social death model and the social barriers model (Finkelstein, 1993). He then goes on to suggest that the administrative model is the only one which has sufficient scope to fully explain societal responses to disabled people.

> In my view administrative approaches dominate all forms of helping services for disabled people in the UK, whether these are provided by

statutory agencies or voluntary bodies, or demanded by pressure group organisations. The cure or care forms of intervention are administered within the rehabilitation and personal-care services respectively. (Finkelstein, 1993, p.37)

For me, the administrative model is similar to the position I took in trying to locate disability historically within the rise of capitalist society.

> As the conditions of capitalist production changed in the twentieth century, so the labour needs of capital shifted from a mass of unskilled workers to a more limited need of skilled ones. As a result of this, the Welfare State arose as a means of ensuring the supply of skill, and in order to 'pacify' the ever increasing army of the unemployed, the under-employed and the unemployable. (Manning and Oliver, 1985, p.102)

While I think Finkelstein and I are basically saying the same thing, for me it is important not to stretch the explanatory power of models further than they are able to go. For me the social model of disability is concerned with the personal and collective experiences of disabling social barriers and how its application might influence professional practice and shape political action. It is not a substitute for social theory, it is not an attempt to provide a materialist history of disability and it is not an explanation of the failure of welfare state in respect of services to disabled people.

The social model of disability is alive and well

These are some of the major internal debates going on around the social model. One of the things they have in common is their concern to somehow integrate impairment into the social model of disability. Personally I have no interest in such attempts because, as Vasey (1992) has already pointed out, the collectivising of experiences of impairment is a much more difficult task than collectivising the experience of disability. Our own history has taught us this in the way in which we have been classified and segregated by our impairments and the way in which single impairment organisations have failed to provide an adequate basis for collective self-organisation amongst disabled people in the past (Campbell and Oliver, 1996).

Additionally there is still much mileage in the social model of disability. It has the power to transform consciousness in a way that a social model of impairment never will. David Hevey describes his own transformation:

> The second flash on this road to Damascus as a disabled person came when I encountered the disability movement. I had learnt to live with my private fear and to feel that I was the only one involved in this fight. I had internalised my oppression. As a working class son of Irish immigrants, I had experienced other struggles but, in retrospect, I evidently saw epilepsy as my hidden cross. I cannot explain how significantly all this was turned around when I came into contact with the notion of the

social model of disability, rather than the medical model which I had hitherto lived with. Over a matter of months, my discomfort with this secret beast of burden called epilepsy, and my festering hatred at the silencing of myself as a disabled person, 'because I didn't look it', completely changed. I think I went through an almost evangelical conversion as I realised that my disability was not, in fact, the epilepsy, but the toxic drugs with their denied side-effects; the medical regime with its blaming of the victim; the judgement through distance and silence of bus-stop crowds, bar-room crowds and dinner-table friends; the fear; and, not least, the employment problems. All this was the oppression, not the epileptic seizure at which I was hardly (consciously) present. (Hevey, 1992, pp. 1–2)

While it has the power to transform consciousness in the way described above, its demise is surely premature.

Finally, the hegemony of the individual model of disability may have begun to be challenged by the social model, but it has not yet replaced it. Hence, engaging in public criticism may not broaden and refine the social model; it may instead breathe new life in the individual model with all that means in terms of increasing medical and therapeutic interventions into areas of our lives where they do not belong.

Despite my reservations about the project, the development of a social model of impairment to stand alongside a social model of disability appears inevitable. This being the case, those disabled people concerned may wish to develop a dialogue with medical sociologists working on the experience of chronic illness. In so doing, the issues identified earlier in this chapter may well help the dialogue to develop. In any case, our understandings of the experience of impairment may well be enhanced and the enterprise of medical sociology enriched.

Conclusions

In this chapter I have looked at some of the definitional issues involved in impairment and disability. Subsequently, my argument has centred on three key points. Firstly, we must not assume that models in general and the social model of disability in particular can do everything; that it can explain disability in totality. It is not a social theory of disability and it cannot do the work of social theory. Secondly, because it cannot explain everything, we should neither seek to expose inadequacies, which are more a product of the way we use it, nor abandon it before its usefulness has been fully exploited. Finally, if a social model of impairment is to be developed, a dialogue between disabled people and medical sociologists may enrich the process.

References

Abberley, P. (1993) 'The Significance of the OPCS Disability Surveys', in Oliver, M. (ed.) *Social Work: Disabled People and Disabling Environments*, London: Jessica Kingsley Publishers.

Altman, D. (1994) *Power and Community: Organisational and Community Responses to AIDS*, London: Taylor and Francis.

Barnes, C. (1991) *Disabled People in Britain and Discrimination*, London: Hurst and Co.

Barnes, C. (1992) *Disabling Imagery and the Media: An Exploration of the Principles for Media Representation of Disabled People*, Derby: Ryburn Publishing and BCODP.

Begum, N., Hill, M. and Stevens, A. (eds.) (1994) *Reflections: Views of black disabled people on their lives and community care*, London: Central Council for Education and Training in Social Work.

Bury, M. (1992) 'Medical Sociology and chronic illness: A Comment on the Panel Discussion', *Medical Sociology News*, 18, 1, pp. 29–33.

Campbell, J. and Oliver, M. (1996) *Disability Politics in Britain: Understanding Our Past, Changing Our Future*, London: Routledge.

Cashling, D. (1993) 'Cobblers and Song-birds: the language and imagery of disability', *Disability, Handicap and Society*, 8, 2, 199–206.

DPI (1982) *Proceedings of the First World Congress*, Singapore: Disabled People's International.

DPI (1994) 'Agreed Statement', at Human Rights Plenary Meeting in Support of European Day of Disabled Persons, London: Disabled People's International.

Driedger, D. (1989) *The Last Civil Rights Movement*, London: Hurst and Co.

Finkelstein, V. (1993) 'Disability: a social challenge or an administrative responsibility', in Swain, J. et al. (eds.) *Disabling Barriers – Enabling Environments*, London: Sage.

French, S. (1993) 'Can you see the rainbow?', in Swain, J. et al. (eds.) *Disabling Barriers – Enabling Environments*, London: Sage.

Hammersley, M. (1992) 'On Feminist Methodology', *Sociology*, 26, 2, pp.187–206.

Harris, A. (1971) *Handicapped and Impaired in Britain*, London: HMSO.

Hearn, K. (1991) 'Disabled Lesbians and Gays Are Here to Stay', in Kaufman, T. and Lincoln, P. (eds.) *High Risk Lives: Lesbian and Gay Politics After the Clause*, Bridport: Prism Press.

Hevey, D. (1992) *The Creatures Time Forgot: Photography and Disability Imagery*, London: Routledge.

Hill, M. (1994) 'Getting things right', *Community Care* 'Inside', 31 March, p.7.

Humphrey, R. (1994) 'Thoughts on Disability Arts', *Disability Arts Magazine*, 4, 1, pp. 66–67.

Manning, N. and Oliver, M. (1985) 'Madness, Epilepsy and Medicine', in Manning, N. (ed.) *Social Problems and Welfare Ideology*, Aldershot: Gower.

Martin, J., Meltzer, H. and Elliot, D. (1988) *OPCS Surveys of Disability in Great Britain: Report 1 – The prevalence of disability among adults*, London: HMSO.

Morris, J. (1991) *Pride against Prejudice*, London: Women's Press.

Oliver, M. (1990) *The Politics of Disablement*, Basingstoke: Macmillan and St Martins Press.

Oliver, M. (1992) 'Changing the social relations of research production', *Disability, Handicap and Society*, 7, 2, pp. 101–114.

Parker, G. (1993) *With This Body: Caring and Disability in Marriage*, Milton Keynes: Open University Press.

Priestley, M. (1995) 'Commonality and Difference in the Movement: an association of Blind Asians in Leeds', *Disability and Society*, 10, 2, pp. 157–70.

Shakespeare, T. (1992) 'A Response to Liz Crow', *Coalition*, September 1992, pp. 40–42.

Vasey, S. (1992) 'A Response to Liz Crow', *Coalition*, September 1992, pp. 42–44.

Ward, L. and Flynn, M. (1994) 'What Matters Most: Disability, Research and Empowerment', in Rioux, M. C. and Bach, M. (eds.) *Disability Is Not Measles: New Research Paradigms in Disability*, Ontario: Roeher Institute.

Williams, G. (1991) 'Disablement and the Ideological Crisis in Health Care', *Social Science and Medicine*, 33, 4, pp. 517–524.

Wood, P. (1980) *International Classification of Impairments, Disabilities and Handicaps*, Geneva: World Health Organisation.

Woodhill, G. (1993) *Independent Living and Participation in Research*, Toronto: Centre for Independent Living in Toronto (CILT).

Zarb, G. and Oliver, M. (1993) *Ageing with a Disability: What do they expect after all these years?* London: University of Greenwich.

Chapter 23

Danièle Carricaburu and Janine Pierret

FROM BIOGRAPHICAL DISRUPTION TO BIOGRAPHICAL REINFORCEMENT
The case of HIV-positive men

From *Sociology of Health and Illness,* 17 (1) 1995: 65–88

Introduction

RESEARCH IN THE SOCIOLOGY of illness has mainly focused on chronic illnesses, which develop over time, acute phases alternating with periods of relief. The chronically ill are usually confronted with a solidly established, though still evolving, corpus of medical knowledge about their illness (at least about diseases such as poliomyelitis or cancer). They must live with the new situation resulting from their condition and cope with the consequences on everyday life. With regard to the onset of a serious illness and its unsettling consequences, sociologists have studied the biographical accommodations made in everyday life as well as changes in self-conceptions and personal relationships. Concepts such as 'biographical disruption', 'biographical work' and 'identity reconstitution' have been used to shed light on how illness affects a person's identity or construction of a biography (see, in particular, Bury 1982, 1991; Corbin and Strauss 1987, 1988; Charmaz 1987). Herein, the concepts of biographical disruption and biographical work will be used to analyse the particular situation of asymptomatic carriers of the Human Immunodeficiency Virus (HIV).

Being HIV-positive is not a chronic illness of the sort sociology has investigated. Instead, it corresponds to what we have called 'a situation at the risk of illness' (Carricaburu and Pierret 1992). Being infected with HIV is not the same as having AIDS. What it does mean is that those infected will eventually come down with a fatal disease. No medical prognosis can predict when they will actually fall sick. As a consequence, asymptomatic HIV-positive persons must manage an apparently healthy life in conditions of uncertainty. For many of them, having a low CD_4 count or taking AZT for the first time is a signal that they are entering a new phase; but even then, they know neither when they will fall ill nor with what disease. At present, only one thing is sure: they have every chance of eventually dying from an AIDS-related disease. A further source of uncertainty has to do with medicine and science. Scientific knowledge and medical know-how about AIDS, much of it experimental, is still being developed. This has a direct bearing on people's prospects and everyday lives. In this very special situation, even more than during chronic illness, medical and scientific uncertainty itself shatters certitude: any 'sure' knowledge may be invalidated.

This situation has another particularity: AIDS has, especially through the mass media, been constructed 'live' as a social phenomenon. This has strongly, sometimes violently, affected the lives of those concerned. The latter have been forced to see themselves in terms of 'public discourses' about AIDS. Life as an HIV-positive person means that one's private experiences as an infected individual become part of the collective experience of an infectious illness associated with ideas of contagious diseases and epidemics. Given how this virus is transmitted, many of the HIV-positive come from groups with their own collective histories, notably of haemophilia and homosexuality.

After describing the method used in this research, we shall analyse the data in terms of concepts such as: biographical disruption, contextualisation, biographical work and preferred identity. We shall then comment on the major consequences of HIV-infection in everyday life: managing the secret, mobilising resources and constructing hope. In conclusion, the relations between these various theoretical concepts will be reviewed; and their pertinence, pointed out. This research can help broaden approaches adopted by the sociology of illness.

Method

This qualitative research project is based on in-depth interviews with HIV-positive men infected through either homosexual relations or medical products used to treat haemophilia. We chose to centre our study on HIV-positive, homosexual or haemophilic, men with jobs who had learned about their infection at least two years beforehand. By selecting persons who had known they were HIV-positive for this length of time, we hoped that interviewees would no longer be in shock from learning about their immune status. We asked two private medical practitioners and five teams of hospital doctors (two of them specialising in haemophilia) to help us meet men of the sort just described who might be willing to take part in our survey. This procedure helped us obtain a group with more varied social backgrounds than had we recruited interviewees through associations or networks of friends. The advantage of selecting interviewees through medical practitioners – bound by professional secrecy – was that privacy and anonymity would be respected. It took nearly a year to overcome doctors' reluctance and obtain enough men who were willing to be interviewed. . . .

From January 1990 to June 1991, in-depth interviews, each lasting an average of two hours, were conducted with 44 HIV-positive men: 24 homosexual and 20 haemophilic men. None of them was a drug-user. All of them lived in the Paris region; and all were under medical supervision. Most had known about their immune status for at least five years; and three of them, for as long as seven years.

Interviews, which were recorded and then transcribed in full, were conducted as follows. Focusing on their illness condition, we asked the haemophilic men:

> Could you tell me what everyday life is like for a haemophilic person? I'd like to understand what happens during the major phases of life (childhood, adolescence, adulthood . . .) and in various fields of life (at work, during leisure time, in the family, with doctors, and with friends).

With homosexual men, interviews were centered around HIV-infection:

> Could you tell me about being infected with the HIV? How did it happen to you? Tell me about everyday life, about what happens in various fields of life (at work, during leisure time, in relationships, in the family, with doctors, and with friends . . .).

Since all men in the latter group spontaneously introduced themselves as being homo-sexual, we shall refer to them as gay. We kept interviews as open-ended as possible while gradually broaching topics one after another. As doctors requested, we interviewed the haemophilic men in the hospital, whereas the gay men chose the place of meeting: we interviewed half of them in their homes, and the other half either at the hospital or in our office.

Conceptual background

Sociological research, mainly in English-speaking lands, has been conducted on the personal and social repercussions of chronic illnesses. In a recent article, M. Bury (1991:453) recalled how he came up with the idea of biographical disruption:

> Following Strauss and Glaser's (1975) pioneering work, this idea brings into focus the meaning of illness as well as the setting in which it occurs, including in the latter case, the resources available to the individual.

Strauss and Glaser have shown the importance of centring study on the patient and the management of chronic illness in everyday life. The sociology of illness would no longer focus exclusively on the doctor–patient relationship. Attention was drawn to the social and psychological aspects of living, day after day, with chronic illness. As Strauss and Glaser (1975:viii) asked, 'How is the *quality of life* affected by having a chronic illness?'

Criticising interactionism for being too descriptive and inadequately grounded in theory, Bury conceptualised chronic illness as a biographical disruption. He intended to show that it causes a break in people's lives, what Giddens (1979: 123) has called 'a critical situation':

> We can learn a good deal about day-to-day situations in routine settings from analyzing circumstances in which those settings are radically disturbed.

Bury (1982:169), too, defended the idea that chronic illness

> is precisely that kind of experience where the structures of everyday life and the forms of knowledge which underpin them are disturbed.

It wreaks havoc in people's everyday lives and their 'forms of knowledge'. Bury (1982:169–70) pointed out three aspects of this disruption:

> First, there is the disruption of taken-for-granted assumptions and behaviors; the breaching of commonsense boundaries [. . .] Second, there are more profound disruptions in explanatory systems normally used by people, such that a fundamental rethinking of the person's biography and self-concept is involved. Third, there is the response to disruption involving the mobilization of resources in facing an altered situation.

This everyday-life approach has been pursued in studies of illnesses as different as epilepsy (Schneider and Conrad 1983), diabetes (Kelleher 1988), multiple sclerosis (Robinson 1988) and polyarthritis (Bury 1982; Locker 1983).

While reviewing 'research and prospects', Bury (1991:453) tried to work out the concept of biographical disruption by taking into account the context, a notion missing till then:

> The notion of biography suggests that meaning and context in chronic illness cannot easily be separated.

By placing chronic illness in its social context, attention can be turned to factors such as social policies, patients' associations, charitable organisations, consumerism and the mass media. In particular, two types of meaning can be distinguished (Bury 1991:453):

> In the first place, the 'meaning' of illness lies in its consequences for the individual. The effects of the onset of disruptive symptoms on everyday life at home or at work, including, for example, giving time to managing symptoms or regimens (Locker 1983) may be uppermost [. . .] Second, the meaning of chronic illness may be seen in terms of its *significance*. By this, I mean that different conditions carry with them different connotations and imagery. These differences may have a profound influence on how individuals regard themselves, and how they think others see them.

. . .

The consequences of HIV-infection for everyday life

All interviewees had been deeply disturbed by their HIV-infection and its menace to their health. But reactions to a positive immune status differed significantly. Some interviewees made thoroughgoing changes in their lives whereas others seemed to maintain the status quo. Changes might or might not have been visible. In general, interviewees had to organise everyday life around three issues:

- For all of them, managing the secret was the central issue in, and the starting point for, reorganizing their lives.
- Although being HIV-positive is not a chronic illness in the ordinary sense, it always entailed constraints (given the nature of HIV-infection) and self-restraints (owing to uncertainty about the future).
- An interviewee's ability to find and use resources, pursue a palliative strategy and build up hope depended on how he had assessed his situation since being infected. This assessment fluctuated as a function of medical, personal and social factors. It also varied depending on when, in life, and how infection had occurred.

Managing the secret: to tell or not to tell

Managing the secret was based on decisions about whether or not to tell others about being HIV-positive, whom to tell, and when. This was the central issue all interviewees, regardless of how they had been infected, had to face. As R. Weitz (1989), K. Siegel and B. Krauss (1991), and D. Silverman (1989) have shown, secrecy about AIDS is linked to stigma. In effect, a social discourse took shape before there were any widespread, collective or individual, experiences of AIDS itself (Herzlich and Pierret 1989, 1993). In France as in many other lands, the HIV-positive have, if haemophilic, been presented as the 'innocent victims' of medical and governmental mismanagement of blood products but, if gay, been seen as 'guilty' because of 'their choice'. Significantly, all interviewees – regardless of the cause of infection – decided to tell no one save a few close, carefully chosen persons. For R. Frankenberg (1986), an anthropologist, society always produces and imposes metaphors to talk about the illness experience. The patients of Weitz's (1990) study, when they asked themselves 'Why am I sick?', responded by referring to divine punishment. Our interviewees did not often allude to this sort of interpretation. This can probably be ascribed to cultural differences between the United States and France. In France, HIV-infection is not generally seen as a divine punishment. Nonetheless, it is still not an easy topic to discuss.

Since all interviewees were asymptomatic, their immune status was not directly visible. For this reason, they could decide whether or not to reveal their immune status to others. In general, both the haemophilic and the homosexual men kept it secret, a secret shared with only a few people to whom they were, or came to be, close. The quandary about revealing one's immune status followed from public discourse about AIDS, wherein this 'shameful sickness' was presented as a stigma. To be infected by HIV, even though one is not yet sick, is both an 'enacted' and 'felt' stigma, to borrow two phrases Scambler and Hopkins (1988:156–7) used when studying epilepsy:

> Enacted stigma refers to instances of discrimination against people with epilepsy based on the perception of them as somehow unacceptably different or inferior [. . .] Felt stigma refers principally to the fear of meeting with enacted stigma, although it also embraces a sense of shame that frequently attends 'being epileptic'.

All interviewees strongly experienced a 'felt stigma', because their bodies were both infected and, we might say, 'infectious'. The notion of an 'enacted stigma' refers to social discourse about AIDS.

But the decision to say nothing bore different meanings depending on the social situation wherein silence was kept. The fear of rejection or of dismissal from work motivated those interviewees who abstained from telling colleagues, as a 26-year-old haemophilic atomic engineer said, 'What's the use of looking for the switch to be spanked with?' Interviewees who did not inform family or friends mostly justified their silence by stating that they did not want to be pitied or did not want to hurt those they loved. A 36-year-old homosexual aeronautics engineer said,

> I don't want the others to look at me any differently. I don't want any condescension, and even less pity. I want to have the same relations with people, especially since, for now, there's no need to talk about it.

Keeping the secret entailed constant vigilance. It amounted to real 'work' in A. Strauss et al.'s (1982) sense. This work was all the harder whenever others knew the interviewee was haemophilic or gay, as a 43-year-old biologist pointed out:

> Since they know I'm haemophilic, as soon as I catch one thing or another, I feel them looking at me, wondering. But I don't want to say anything, so I stick in my office.

As time went on, the least sign – whether a preventive treatment or the appearance of certain symptoms (shingles, herpes, etc.) – could make the potential stigma visible. This stressful situation forced interviewees to draw up strategies for dissimulating the sign's origins. A 35-year-old homosexual public relations employee preferred, since he often had to go to the hospital, saying he was diabetic. All interviewees knew they would have more and more trouble keeping the secret over time. In the words of a 46-year-old homosexual secondary school teacher:

> If I fall sick, I'll probably change my mind. But for the time being, it's my secret, and I'm keeping it.

Being HIV-positive is a 'discreditable stigma' whereas coming down with AIDS is a 'discredited stigma' (Goffman 1963) that can no longer be kept a secret. In Scambler and Hopkins' words (1986:38):

> The fear of enacted stigma leads to a policy of nondisclosure, a policy which remains feasible for as long as they are 'discreditable' rather than 'discredited'.

For all interviewees, not revealing their HIV-positive immune status meant that they wanted to be treated like anyone else, not like someone with limited prospects. A 37-year-old homosexual librarian put this into words,

> It's true that telling my friends would change their attitude, whether they wanted it to change or not. Not that they're going to think of me as being a sick person, a potential fatality. But inevitably, in their subconscious, something will change.

We can conclude that secrecy is a central way of managing everyday life, for one's self and for others. It was necessary to keep the secret in order to live as normally as possible while also reorienting one's life and mobilising resources. The way secrecy was managed can be used to relate the consequences of infection on everyday life to the social meanings of this illness condition. . . .

Mobilising resources

Despite the disruption resulting from infection, interviewees tried to give a sense of continuity to their lives. To this end, each of them had begun reviewing his personal situation – his love life, family, job and history of infection. This process could, in turn, be affected by any new events, fortunate or unfortunate, that occurred. The person's capacity for mobilising resources depended on the outcome of this review process.

For Bury (1982), cognitive and material resources are tapped to deal with biographical disruption. In people's experiences in concentration camps, Pollak (1990:289) discerned

> physical and corporal (body-related) resources, relational resources [. . .] and cognitive resources (certified qualifications and practical know-how).

But understanding how and why resources are mobilised is more important than classifying them. Whatever means are already at hand may be used to mobilise resources; or new means may be developed. In our survey, interviewees mobilised resources to attain two objectives: to reorganise everyday life and augment the capacity to deal with an uncertain future. We observed significant differences among interviewees. Many haemophilic men fell back on what was already being used to manage everyday life, whereas the gay men, while also using the means at hand, more often tried to tap new resources.

When inquiring about the resources the *haemophilic men* had already tapped to deal with their haemophilic condition, we found that most of them developed diversified strategies and worked out concrete arrangements to cope with their illness condition in everyday life. They had spent considerable energy in order to be seen, especially at the workplace, as 'normal' instead of 'handicapped'. When faced with AIDS, however, they no longer felt as combative. They did not seek out new resources, and they even tended to abandon those that had helped them organise their lives as persons with haemophilia. They withdrew into work, family and friends.

Furthermore, these haemophilic interviewees had misgivings about medicine, since they had been infected through medical products. A 38-year-old assistant accountant explained,

> Despite their good will, how can doctors possibly help me? I can't take my mind off it: they're responsible for what's happening to me.

AIDS upset their life plans and disrupted the biographies they had constructed. They were unable to cope with their immune status so as to allow room for hope. In the words of a 40-year-old computer programmer,

> HIV-positive and AIDS, for me, they're the same thing. I've had too many encounters with sickness. I know how things are going to end.

For these interviewees, infection meant death. This pervasive idea kept them from planning for the future.

In contrast, most *gay* interviewees tried to maintain the status quo by using existing resources and/or finding new ones. First of all, jobs and relations with friends or family took on more importance, especially when infection was kept a secret. A 46-year-old secondary school teacher commented.

> I've recentered my life around close relationships. I mean I devote more time to the people I like, whether ex-lovers who are now friends or straight friends. Simply put, we see each other more often. I'm more available. I'm more interested in them, in what they're doing, what they think. I have the impression my life has lost in diversity but gained in intensity.

These men looked for material, emotional and relational support from various sources so as to remain integrated in their affective environment and in society. A 39-year-old bank manager said,

> I'm more attentive and sensitive if something happens to my friends. I get more involved in their troubles than I could have before. I live more intensely whatever happens. I try to be closer to my family in the provinces, and I phone more often.

Secondly, gay interviewees developed a strong relationship with medicine. This provided them with a cognitive resource. These interviewees thought it important to follow up on appointments and treatments. Relations with medical care-givers became a source of emotional support, as for this 44-year-old antique-dealer,

> Going to the hospital isn't a hassle. Besides, I'm telling you, it's friendly over there. The personnel's friendly too. And the room's been redone. I trust them a lot. I had no experience with hospitals before, didn't know anything about them. I realise it's great, from the nurse to the chief doctor. The dedication is extraordinary.

For these interviewees, such relationships were a source of emotional support that helped them exercise control over their bodies and cope with the current situation.

For a few of these gay interviewees, activism in associations provided emotional involvement and affective support. But all the gay men recognised that associations were an important source of knowledge and information.

A last point: gay interviewees believed in their ability to find resources so as to reinforce their psychological well-being and physical health and, thereby, delay the onset of illness. A 35-year-old journalist made this very point:

> Now I have a test every three months, because my T4 count had dropped and I'd refused to take AZT. At that time, you had to take huge doses, but I waited for the next blood test and, thank God, it improved. It improved by itself. That's when I noticed something. It's a personal tip, but I don't know whether I should tell the doctor: when I stop taking vitamin C and magnesium, I feel a little weaker. Yeah, from the position where I am, I think vitamin C, magnesium, vitamins do work. They suit me to a T. They reassure me, make me feel safer. The test every three months is my race against the clock, a way of keeping an eye on myself. I think you take responsibility for your own body. It's a decision. The doctor can't do anything.

In effect, these interviewees adopted a wide variety of means to cope with HIV-infection: new eating habits, 'vitamin therapy', psychotherapy or even spirituality. Besides fighting against the passage of time, all this kept them from being passive and helped them take responsibility for themselves so as to go on living like everyone else for as long as possible.

Pursuing palliative strategies and constructing hope

Although HIV-infection means a limited future, some interviewees, regardless of how they had been infected, struggled against uncertainty by, paradoxically, taking risks. They were all the more capable of doing this insofar as they felt freed of certain social constraints and, therefore, free to do things they could not have before being infected. The risks thus taken figured in the 'palliative strategies' adopted to 'reopen the doors closed by AIDS'.

Citing a few examples of these strategies will show how diverse they were and how imaginative, and inventive, these men were. Several of the gay men had changed occupations or even their line of work, despite losing job security. In addition to his job, one gay interviewee, who lived with another man, started breeding pedigree cats despite the risk of toxoplasmosis. After counting how long he had left to live, one haemophilic man borrowed a large amount of money in order to travel as much as he wanted. Another asked his father to donate sperm so that if he and his wife were to want a child, the baby would be 'of the same blood' but without any risk of infection. These calculated risks can be interpreted as the will to keep some control over one's life. Indeed, being active, doing things, is a way to project one's life into the future and to refuse being taken prisoner by illness.

When faced with an illness that cannot – at least not yet – be cured, how does one keep the will to live alive? Looking after one's body so as to postpone as long as possible the onset of illness is essential for what Pollak (1990:259) called 'constructing hope'. This hope is fully turned toward medical science and research: 'you have to last as long as possible' in the hope that 'they will find something'. This hope is the expectancy of a vaccine or treatment being developed that will, if not cure AIDS, at least help suffers go on living. Once again, the temporal aspect of this illness condition crops up.

Among interviewees, this hope had three grounds: the attention they paid to their bodies and health; confidence in the medical sciences and research; and the conviction that illness could be avoided. Events with repercussions on any of these three grounds could upset hope's fragile balancing act. Such an event might be new, less favourable test results, the swelling of ganglions, a feeling of being more tired than usual or disappointing medical news in the mass media. The work of constructing hope was constantly imperilled.

Understandably, most interviewees were deeply disturbed when they had to start taking AZT or DDI, even though doctors presented these drugs as means of helping the immune system defend itself. A 38-year-old musician told us,

> Thrice a day, I take two 100 mg capsules. I don't often forget. That's pretty good. But it reminds me, necessarily in some way or another, that I'm HIV-positive. It brings my haemophilia back up. It's a kind of chain you can't break out of since it's all around.

Such a prescription amounted to a full-scale assault on the deep personal conviction that illness could be avoided. The previously quoted public relations employee emphasised,

> AZT has changed me a lot more psychologically than being HIV-positive. It upset me a lot because, without actually falling sick, it means I'm getting closer to it.

The work of constructing hope was jeopardised.

At this point, illness had to be accepted as part of the biography so that hope could be rebuilt on other grounds. This entailed a thorough reworking of one's identity. For this reason, as several interviewees pointed out, denying the difference between being HIV-positive and having AIDS impeded the work of constructing hope, which, however precariously built or however hard to build, was indispensable for the will to live. . . .

Conclusion

For these asymptomatic haemophilic or homosexual men, the consequences for everyday life of being HIV-positive cannot be separated from how they interpreted their situation. This interpretation entailed reconstructing individual and collective pasts. The individual's life story could not be separated from his reference group's history. At this point, the characteristic of AIDS and of HIV-infection must be borne in mind: this illness, having reached epidemic proportions, is transmitted in specific, identifiable ways not just to isolated individuals but to individuals who are part of certain groups. By relating the reinterpretation and reconstruction of their individual and collective pasts to the current situation, interviewees recomposed a sense of identity and tried to give continuity to their biographies.

Whether or not biographical disruption occurred, all interviewees had to rework their sense of identity. This complex process entailed what we have called biographical reinforcement, i.e., a reinforcement of the components of identity that, prior to HIV-infection, had already been built around haemophilia or homo-sexuality. Although a 'positive illness identity' (Herzlich and Pierret 1991:274) has been hypothesised, we did not observe any such identity being worked out around being HIV-positive. The haemophilic men considered their immune status to mean they already had AIDS. Despite their efforts to live normal lives as persons with haemophilia, their way of interpreting their situation had always been based on an illness logic. In contrast, gay interviewees insisted on distinguishing between AIDS and the immune status. Even when under medical supervision, they did not consider being HIV-positive to be an illness state. It was a phase in their lives during which they could reorganise their biographies and construct the hope necessary to go on. Maintaining the distinction between AIDS and a positive immune status provided gay interviewees with a resource for building hope.

In line with Charmaz's thesis that the ill have an 'identity hierarchy', we can conclude that asymptomatic HIV-positive persons develop this hierarchy around components of their identity that existed prior to infection. Out of these already existing components, the preferred identities are – at least in a context where infection can be linked to either medical treatment or a way of life – those having to do with haemophilia or homosexuality. HIV-infection is collective: it affects a group, not just an isolated individual, since the transmission of the virus takes place through individual and collective practices. As a consequence, interviewees recontextualised their haemophilia or homosexuality as they introspectively worked on their pasts. Although it would be tempting to compare Charmaz's 'restored self' to our notion of biographical reinforcement, the two ideas are not the same. Interviewees, whether haemophilic or homosexual, mainly mentioned the com-ponents of their identity from before HIV-infection that had to do with their bodies and with the idea of being different. These components had direct links to the origin of infection. Identities were not simply reconstructed, they were systematically reinforced.

This return to, and reinforcement of, former components of identity bring to mind what Goffman (1963) has pointed out about managing stigmata. But Goffman, when mentioning this return to former components of identity, focused on social identity, whereas we are dealing with personal identity. At the level of social identity – the affirmation of the self in relation to others – haemophilic and homosexual interviewees differed significantly. Fearing AIDS stigmata, the former went so far as to hide their haemophilia – which they had never done before being infected with HIV. On the contrary, the gay men tended to assert, even claim, that homosexuality was something 'ordinary'.

Further research is needed to examine how AIDS affects the collective identities of homosexual and haemophilic men. Such research could provide us with a close-up view of a much broader phenomenon. AIDS and its consequences for everyday life raise problems that are faced by the chronically ill in general: dealing with uncertainty, coping with stigmatisation, managing illness trajectories, doing biographical work and recomposing a sense of identity. Such research would help us better understand what it means to live with an uncertain prognosis and handle its consequences for everyday life. These questions will become more acute as 'predictive medicine' develops and earlier diagnoses are made.

By drawing our attention to the interrelations between the individual's experience of infection, his life story and the history of his reference group, sociological research on AIDS sheds light on a little explored aspect of the illness experience: its shared, collective dimension. Being HIV-positive is not just a matter of being individually infected: it is also a question of being affected as part of a group that has its own history and has been decimated by AIDS. This experience bears little comparison with what happened during past epidemics, which felled victims more randomly (Herzlich and Pierret 1991). By observing *in situ* the evolution of the AIDS epidemic and its collective impact, we should advance our understanding, on the one hand, of the relations between micro- and macro-levels of social analysis and, on the other, of the feedback between individual experiences, cultural factors and macrosocial structures.

References

Bury, M. (1982) Chronic illness as a biographical disruption, *Sociology of Health and Illness*. 4, 167–82.

Bury, M. (1991) The sociology of chronic illness: a review of research and prospects, *Sociology of Health and Illness*. 13, 451–68.

Carricaburu, D. and Pierret, J. (1992) *Vie quotidienne et recompositions identitaires autour de la séropositivité*, a research report. Paris: CERMES-ANRS.

Charmaz, K. (1987) Struggling for a self: identity levels of the chronically ill, *Research in the Sociology of Health Care*. 6, 283–321.

Corbin, J. and Strauss, A. (1987) Accompaniments of chronic illness changes in body, self, biography and biographical time, *Research in the Sociology of Health Care*. 6, 249–81.

Corbin, J. and Strauss, A. (1988) *Unending Work and Care*, San Francisco: Jossey-Bass Publishers.

Frankenberg, R. (1986) Sickness as cultural performance: Drama, trajectory and pilgrimage, root metaphors and the making social of disease, *International Journal of Health Services*. 16, 603–26.

Giddens, A. (1979) *Central Problems in Social Theory*. London: Macmillan.

Goffman, E. (1963) *Stigma*. Englewood Cliffs, NJ: Prentice-Hall.

Herzlich, C. and Pierret, J. (1989) The construction of a social phenomenon: AIDS in the French press, *Social Science and Medicine*. 29, 1235–42.

Herzlich, C. and Pierret, J. (1991) *Illness and Self in Society*, translation by E. Forster of the first edition (1984) of *Malades d'hier, malades d'aujourd'hui*. Baltimore: Johns Hopkins University Press, 1987.

Herzlich, C. and Pierret, J. (1993) From epidemic to modern illness: the social construction of AIDS in France. In Albrecht, G. and Zimmerman, R. (eds.) *Advances in Medical Sociology*, Vol. 3: *The Social and Behavioral Aspects of AIDS*. Greenwich, Conn: JAI Press.

Kelleher, D. (1988) Coming to terms with diabetes: coping strategies and non-compliance. In Anderson, R. and Bury, M. (eds.) *Living with Chronic Illness*. London: Unwin Hyman.

Locker, D. (1983) *Disability and Disadvantage: The Consequences of Chronic Illness*. London-New York: Tavistock Publications.

Pollak, M. (1990) *L'expérience concentrationnaire*. Paris: A.M. Métailié.

Robinson, I. (1988) *Multiple Sclerosis*. London: Routledge.

Scambler, G. and Hopkins, A. (1986) Being epileptic: coming to terms with stigma, *Sociology of Health and Illness*, 8, 26–43.

Scambler, G. and Hopkins, A. (1988) Accommodating epilepsy in families. In Anderson, R. and Bury, M. (eds.) *Living with Chronic Illness*. London: Unwin Hyman.

Schneider, J. and Conrad, P. (1983) *Having Epilepsy: The Experience and Control of Illness*. Philadelphia: Temple University Press.

Siegel, K. and Krauss, B. (1991) Living with HIV-infection: adaptive tasks of seropositive gay men, *Journal of Health and Social Behavior*. 32, 17–32.

Silverman, D. (1989) Making sense of a precipice: constituting identity in an HIV Clinic. In P. Aggleton, G. Hart, P. Davies (eds.) *AIDS: Social Representations, Social Practices*. London-Philadelphia: The Falmer Press.

Strauss, A. and Glaser, B. (1975) *Chronic Illness and the Quality of Life*. St. Louis-Toronto: Mosby.

Strauss, A., Fagerhaugh, S., Suczek, B. and Wiener, C. (1982) The work of hospitalized patients, *Social Science and Medicine*. 16, 977–86.

Weitz, R. (1989) Uncertainty and the lives of persons with AIDS, *Journal of Health and Social Behavior*. 30, 270–81.

Weitz, R. (1990) Living with the stigma of AIDS, *Qualitiative Sociology*, 13, 23–38.

Chapter 24

Arthur Frank

WHEN BODIES NEED VOICES

From *The Wounded Story Teller: Body, Illness and Ethics,* Chicago: University of
Chicago Press (1997)

"**THE DESTINATION AND MAP** I had used to navigate before were no
longer useful." These words were in a letter describing chronic fatigue syndrome. Judith Zaruches wrote of how, after an illness that is never really finished,
she "needed . . . to think differently and construct new perceptions of my relationship to the world."[1]

Serious illness is a loss of the "destination and map" that had previously guided
the ill person's life: ill people have to learn "to think differently." They learn by
hearing themselves tell their stories, absorbing others' reactions, and experiencing
their stories being shared. Judith's story not only stated her need for a new map
and destination; her letter itself was an experimental performance of the different
thinking she called for. Through the story she was telling me, her new map was
already taking shape.

Even though we did not know each other, Judith needed to write to me—she
had read my own story of cancer and seen a video tape of a lecture I gave—for me to
witness her story and her personal change. As she told me her story, she discovered
"new perceptions of [her] relationship to the world." That my response would
only come later, in another letter, perhaps made it easier. Seeing herself write, like
hearing herself speak, was the major threshold.

Judith's distinctiveness as a storyteller is her illness. Illness was not just the topic
of her story; it was the condition of her telling that story. Her story was not just
about illness. The story was told *through* a wounded body. The stories that ill people
tell come out of their bodies. The body sets in motion the need for new stories when

its disease disrupts the old stories. The body, whether still diseased or recovered, is simultaneously cause, topic, and instrument of whatever new stories are told.[2] These embodied stories have two sides, one personal and the other social.

The *personal* issue of telling stories about illness is to give voice to the body, so that the changed body can become once again familiar in these stories. But as the language of the story seeks to make the body familiar, the body eludes language. To paraphrase Martin Buber, the body "does not use speech, yet begets it."[3] The ill body is certainly not mute—it speaks eloquently in pains and symptoms—but it is inarticulate. We must speak for the body, and such speech is quickly frustrated: speech presents itself as being about the body rather than of it. The body is often alienated, literally "made strange," as it is told in stories that are instigated by a need to make it familiar.

The alternative to this frustration is to reduce the body to being the mere topic of the story and thus to deny the story's primary condition: the teller has or has had a disease. That the teller's diseased body shapes the illness story should be self-evident. Only a caricature Cartesianism would imagine a head, compartmentalized away from the disease, talking about the sick body beneath it. The head is tied to that body through pathways that science is only beginning to comprehend, but the general principle is clear: the mind does not rest above the body but is diffused throughout it.[4]

But actually hearing traces of the body in the story is not easy. Observing what stories say *about* the body is a familiar sort of listening; describing stories as told *through* the body requires another level of attention. This book attempts to evoke this other level of attention: How can we make sense of illness stories as being told *through* the diseased body?

The ill body's articulation in stories is a personal task, but the stories told by the ill are also *social*. The obvious social aspect of stories is that they are told *to* someone, whether that other person is immediately present or not. Even messages in a bottle imply a potential reader. The less evident social aspect of stories is that people do not make up their stories by themselves. The shape of the telling is molded by all the rhetorical expectations that the storyteller has been internalizing ever since he first heard some relative describe an illness, or she saw her first television commercial for a non-prescription remedy, or he was instructed to "tell the doctor what hurts" and had to figure out *what* counted as the story that the doctor wanted to hear. From their families and friends, from the popular culture that surrounds them, and from the stories of other ill people, storytellers have learned formal structures of narrative, conventional metaphors and imagery, and standards of what is and is not appropriate to tell. Whenever a new story is told, these rhetorical expectations are reinforced in some ways, changed in others, and passed on to affect others' stories.[5] . . .

Postmodern illness

The prefix "post" is not quite right; I do not propose any strict periodization of the modern and the postmodern. I do believe that over a period of time, perhaps the last twenty years, how people think about themselves and their worlds has changed enough to deserve a label, and the most accepted label—increasingly diffused in journalism and popular culture—is postmodernism.[6] Because of the number of intellectual agendae that employ some version of this label, I prefer "postmodern times." The times that contemporary illness stories are told in, which are also the times I am writing in, have changed fairly recently.

Albert Borgmann's title *Crossing the Postmodern Divide*[7] provides a particularly useful metaphor. Journeys cross divides. Once on the other side, the traveler remains the same person, carrying the same baggage. But on the other side of certain divides, the traveler senses a new identity; that same baggage now seems useful for new purposes. Fundamental assumptions that give life its particular meaning have changed. Postmodernity is such a crossing, occurring when the same ideas and actions are overlaid with different meanings. Sometimes these differences of having crossed the divide are clear, but more often they are subtle: things just feel different. Illness has come to feel different during the last twenty years, and today the sum of those differences can be labeled postmodernism. I make no attempt to define postmodernism; the utility of that term lies only in thick descriptions of the feel of the differences.

A useful, if simplified, evocation of the shift from the *premodern* experience of illness to modernity is provided by a North African woman quoted by Pierre Bourdieu in his anthropological research. That Bourdieu recorded this quotation from a living person is a reminder of the proximity and overlap of the premodern, modern, and postmodern. "In the old days," the woman said, "folk didn't know what illness was. They went to bed and they died. It's only nowadays that we've learned words like liver, lung, stomach, and I don't know what!"[8]

Of course premodern people had rich descriptors for disease and its remedies; ethnomedicine was and is highly specific. But I interpret the speaker's closing exclamation as indicating being overwhelmed: she literally doesn't know what. The specialized medical terms that the woman claims her people have only recently learned overwhelm her experience because they *come from elsewhere*. The shift to modernity crosses a divide into a medical culture that is foreign to this woman's experience of illness.

The *modern* experience of illness begins when popular experience is overtaken by technical expertise, including complex organizations of treatment. Folk no longer go to bed and die, cared for by family members and neighbors who have a talent for healing. Folk now go to paid professionals who reinterpret their pains as symptoms, using a specialized language that is unfamiliar and overwhelming. As patients, these folk accumulate entries on medical charts which in most instances they are neither able nor allowed to read; the chart becomes the official story of the illness. Other stories proliferate. Ill people tell family and friends versions of what the doctor said, and these others reply by telling experiences that seem to be similar: both experiences they have had themselves and ones heard from others. Illness becomes a *circulation of stories*, professional and lay, but not all stories are equal.

The story of illness that trumps all others in the modern period is the medical narrative. The story told by the physician becomes the one against which others are ultimately judged true or false, useful or not. I will discuss Talcott Parsons's theory of the "sick role" in later chapters. What is relevant here is Parsons's observation, made about 1950, that a core social expectation of being sick is surrendering oneself to the care of a physician. I understand this obligation of seeking medical care as a *narrative surrender* and mark it as the central moment in modernist illness experience. The ill person not only agrees to follow physical regimens that are prescribed; she also agrees, tacitly but with no less implication, to tell her story in medical terms. "How are you?" now requires that personal feeling be contextualized within a secondhand medical report. The physician becomes the spokesperson for the disease, and the ill person's stories come to depend heavily on repetition of what the physician has said.

Times have come full circle from Bourdieu's North African informant when we read of a patient whose running joke with his surgeon involves reporting his symptoms in an overdone version of medical obscurity. For example, "If you will diligently investigate the pilar projections rising sparsely from the vertext of my cranial ossification, you will detect a macular callosity which may have malignant potential."[9] If modern medicine began when physicians asserted their authority as scientists by imposing specialized language on their patients' experiences, the post-modern divide is crossed when patients such as this one can mimic this language in a send-up of medicine that is shared with the physician. But lay familiarity with medical terms and techniques, even to the point of parody, is only one potential of the postmodern experience of illness.

The *postmodern* experience of illness begins when ill people recognize that more is involved in their experiences than the medical story can tell. The loss of a life's map and destination are not medical symptoms, at least until some psychiatric threshold is reached. The scope of modernist medicine—defined in practices ranging from medical school curricula to billing categories—does not include help-ing patients learn to think differently about their post-illness worlds and construct new relationships to those worlds. Yet people like Judith Zaruches express a self-conscious need to think differently.

Both the divide that was crossed from the premodern to the modern and that from modern to postmodern involve issues of voice. The woman reported by Bourdieu seems to perceive that medicine has taken away her voice: medicine assails her with words she does not want to know and leaves her not knowing what. But this woman does not perceive a need for what would now be called *her own voice*, a personal voice telling what illness has imposed on her and seeking to define for herself a new place in the world. What is distinct in postmodern times is people feeling a need for a voice they can recognize as their own.

This sense of need for a personal voice depends on the availability of the means—the rhetorical tools and cultural legitimacy—for expressing this voice. *Postmodern times are when the capacity for telling one's own story is reclaimed.* Modernist medicine hardly goes away: the postmodern claim to one's own voice is halting, self-doubting, and often inarticulate, but such claims have enough currency for illness to take on a different feel.

Voices tell stories. Stories are premodern; Bourdieu's informant suggests that the coming of modern medicine took away a capacity for experiencing illness in her folk's traditional stories. In the modern period the medical story has pride of place. Other stories become, as non-medical healers are called, "alternative," meaning secondary. The postmodern divide is crossed when people's own stories are no longer told as secondary but have their own primary importance.[10] Illness elicits more than fitting the body into traditional community expectations or surrendering the body to professional medicine, though both community traditions and professional medicine remain. Postmodern illness is an experience, a reflection on body, self, and the destination that life's map leads to.

The remission society

The possibility, even the necessity, of ill people telling their own stories has been set in place by the same modernist medicine that cannot contain these stories. At the end of the story that I wrote about my own experience of having cancer, I used the term "remission society" to describe all those people who, like me, were effectively well but could never be considered cured.[11] These people are all around, though often invisible. A man standing behind me in an airport security check announces that he has a pacemaker; suddenly his invisible "condition" becomes an issue. Once past the metal detector, his "remission" status disappears into the background.

Members of the remission society include those who have had almost any cancer, those living in cardiac recovery programs, diabetics, those whose allergies and environmental sensitivities require dietary and other self-monitoring, those with prostheses and mechanical body regulators, the chronically ill, the disabled, those "recovering" from abuses and addictions, and for all these people, the families that share the worries and daily triumph of staying well.

Cathy Pearse writes in middle-age about having a bleeding cerebral aneurysm— a stroke—when she was twenty.[12] During the operation, a cranial nerve was damaged. She still suffers from double vision, which she reports is "an ever present reminder" of her near-death experience. Her body is now beginning to feel the long-term effects of muscle asymmetry and favoring her "good side." But her illness history would be invisible to most people she meets, and she is long since considered "cured" by medicine. Cathy is a member of the remission society. Years after her hospitalization and treatment, she can still describe what happened in exquisite detail; she recalls the hurt caused by a nurse's casual comment as if it had been spoken yesterday. She refers to being a "recovered stroke patient" as one aspect of her "ethnicity," a word suggesting an irrevocable identity.

The physical existence of the remission society is modern: the technical achievements of modernist medicine make these lives possible. But people's self-consciousness of what it means to live in the wake of illness is postmodern. In modernist thought people are well *or* sick. Sickness and wellness shift definitively as to which is foreground and which is background at any given moment. In the remission society the foreground and background of sickness and health constantly shade into each other. Instead of a static picture on the page where light is separated from dark, the image is like a computer graphic where one shape is constantly in process of becoming the other.

Parsons's modernist "sick role" carries the expectation that ill people get well, cease to be patients, and return to their normal obligations. In the remission society people return, but obligations are never again what used to be normal. Susan Sontag's metaphor of illness as travel is more subtle than Parsons's sick role. We are each citizens of two kingdoms, Sontag writes, the kingdom of the well and that of the sick. "Although we all prefer to use only the good passport, sooner or later each of us is obliged, at least for a spell, to identify ourselves as citizens of that other place."[13] Sontag's notion of dual citizenship suggests a separation of these two kingdoms. The remission society is left to be either a demilitarized zone in between them, or else it is a secret society within the realm of the healthy.

To adapt Sontag's metaphor, members of the remission society do not use one passport *or* the other. Instead they are on permanent visa status, that visa requiring periodic renewal. The triumph of modernist medicine is to allow increasing numbers of people who would have been dead to enjoy this visa status, living in the world of the healthy even if always subject to expulsion. The problem for these people is that modernist medicine lacked a story appropriate to the experience it was setting in place. People like Judith Zaruches were left needing a new map for their lives.

The postmodernity of the remission society is more than a self-consciousness that has not been routinely available to the ill. Many members of the remission society feel a need to claim their visa status in an active voice. Those who work to express this voice are not only postmodern but, more specifically, *post-colonial* in their construction of self. Just as political and economic colonialism took over geographic areas, modernist medicine claimed the body of its patient as its territory, at least for the duration of the treatment. "When we're admitted to a hospital or even visiting a doctor," writes Dan Gottlieb, who as a quadriplegic has extensive experience with such visits, "the forms ask for 'Patient Name.' We stop being people and start being patients . . . Our identity as people and the world we once knew both are relinquished; we become their patients and we live in their hospital."[14] Gottlieb's anger reflects a widespread resentment against medical colonization.

For those whose diseases are cured, more or less quickly and permanently, medical colonization is a temporary indignity. This colonization becomes an issue in the remission society when some level of treatment extends over the rest of a person's life, whether as periodic check-ups or as memories. The least form of treatment, periodic check-ups, are not "just" monitoring. "The fear comes and goes," writes Elizabeth Tyson, a breast cancer survivor, "but twice a year, at checkup time, it's ferocious."[15] For the person being checked, these check-ups represent the background of illness shading back into the foreground. Even for those whose visa is stamped expeditiously, the reality of lacking permanent citizenship is reaffirmed.

Colonization was central to the achievement of modernist medicine. Claudine Herzlich and Janine Pierret describe the "sick person" emerging as a recognizable social type in the early modern period, during the eighteenth century. The condition necessary for the emergence of this type was that "the diversity of suffering be reduced by a unifying general view, which is precisely that of clinical medicine."[16] This reducing of the particular to the general provided for scientific achievements, but the clinical reduction created a benevolent form of colonialism.

The ill person who plays out Parsons's sick role accepts having the particularity of his individual suffering reduced to medicine's general view. Modernity did not question this reduction because its benefits were immediate and its cost was not yet apparent. The colonization of experience was judged worth the cure, or the attempted cure. But illnesses have shifted from the acute to the chronic, and self-awareness has shifted. The post-colonial ill person, living with illness for the long term, wants her own suffering recognized in its individual particularity; "reclaiming" is the relevant postmodern phrase.

In postmodern times more and more people, with varying degrees of articulation and action, express suspicion of medicine's reduction of their suffering to its general unifying view. Members of the remission society, who know medicine from the inside out, question their place in medical narratives. What they question can be clarified by drawing an analogy to people who were politically colonized. Gayatri Chakravorty Spivak speaks of colonized people's efforts "to see how the master texts need us in [their] construction . . . without acknowledging that need."[17] What do the master texts of medicine need but not acknowledge?

I met a man who had a cancer of the mouth that required extensive reconstructive surgery to his jaw and face. His treatment had been sufficiently extraordinary for his surgeon to have published a medical journal article about it, complete with pictures showing the stages of the reconstructive process. When he told me about the article and offered to show it to me, I imagined the article might actually be about *him*: his suffering throughout this mutilating, if life-saving, ordeal. As I looked at the article I realized his name was not mentioned. Probably the surgeon and the journal would have considered it unethical to name him, even though pictures of the man were shown. Thus in "his" article he was systematically ignored as anyone—actually anything—other than a body. But for medical purposes it was not his article at all; it was his surgeon's article. This is exactly the colonization that Spivak speaks of: the master text of the medical journal article needs the suffering person, but the individuality of that suffering cannot be acknowledged.

Most ill people remain willing to continue to play the medical "patient" game by modernist rules without question, and almost all do so when required. But post-colonial members of the remission society are demanding, in various and often frustrated ways, that medicine recognize its need for them. Refusing to be reduced to "clinical material" in the construction of the medical text, they are claiming voices.

Because illness, following medicine, is effectively privatized, this demand for voice rarely achieves a collective force. Feminist health activists are a major exception. Susan Bell writes about the attempts by members of the Cambridge Women's Community Health Center (WCHC) to change the role played by women who were recruited by Harvard Medical School to serve as paid "pelvic models" for medical students to learn to perform gynecological examinations.[18] Bell tells of the women's escalating demands to participate in a full teaching role rather than serve as inert bodies to be taught upon. Women negotiated for their own class time with medical students, they sought to demonstrate how women could perform their own gynecological examinations using a mirror, and they injected political issues into the medical curriculum.

The medical school finally rejected WCHC demands that teaching be limited to women (since the experience of being examined should be, in principle, reciprocal), that non-student hospital personnel and other consumers be included in the teaching sessions, and that more political discussion contextualize the medical teaching. The specifics of the WCHC demands are less important than their basic post-colonial stance: women wanted to have their necessity acknowledged in the construction of medical knowledge and practice. They claimed an active voice in that knowledge and practice.[19]

Post-colonialism in its most generalized form is the demand to speak rather than being spoken for and to represent oneself rather than being represented or, in the worst cases, rather than being effaced entirely. But in postmodern times pressures on clinical practice, including the cost of physicians' time and ever greater use of technologies, mean less time for patients to speak.[20] People then speak elsewhere. The post-colonial impulse is acted out less in the clinic than in stories that members of the remission society tell each other about their illnesses.[21]

The post-colonial stance of these stories resides not in the content of what they say about medicine. Rather the new feel of these stories begins in how often medicine and physicians do *not* enter the stories. Postmodern illness stories are told so that people can place themselves outside the "unifying general view." For people to move their stories outside the professional purview involves a profound assumption of personal responsibility. In Parsons's sick role the ill person as patient was responsible only for getting well; in the remission society, the post-colonial ill person takes responsibility for what illness means in his life. . . .

Notes

1   Personal communication. All attributed quotations are used by permission. Unattributed quotations, where the speaker/writer was not available to give permission, may be altered to preclude identification.

2   Here and below I seek to adhere as much as possible to established usage that differentiates the "disease" as a physiological process from the "illness" as a social experience of that disease. Yet my attempt to consider illness stories as embodied also deconstructs the distinction: the illness experience is an experience in and of a diseased body. This book is about the precariousness of the accepted thinking, as well as of the professional and institutional practices, that too strictly separate disease from illness.

3   Martin Buber, *I and Thou*, trans. Ronald Gregor Smith (New York: Scribners, 1958), 6.

4   An excellent popularization of scientific research is found in the interviews with Candace Pert (177–93) and David Felton (213–37) in Bill Moyers, *Healing and the Mind* (see Preface, n. 2). The social implications of what can be called mind–body research have been developed furthest in cognitive science, in particular: George Lakoff and Mark Johnson, *Metaphors We Live By* (Chicago: University of Chicago Press, 1980), Mark Johnson, *The Body in the Mind: The Bodily Basis of Meaning, Imagination, and Reason* (Chicago: University of Chicago Press, 1987), George Lakoff, *Women, Fire, and Dangerous Things: What Categories Reveal about the Mind* (Chicago: University of Chicago Press, 1987), and Mark Johnson, *Moral Imagination: Implications of Cognitive Science for Ethics* (Chicago: University of Chicago Press, 1993).

5   Another point of usage: I have tried to use *story* when referring to actual tales people tell and *narrative* when discussing general structures that comprise various particular stories. But since narratives only exist in particular stories, and all stories are narratives, the distinction is hard to sustain.

6   On the distinction of "postmodernity," as a time period, and "postmodernism," as a style, see Mike Featherstone, "In Pursuit of the Postmodern: An Introduction," *Theory, Culture & Society* 5 (1988): 195–215. Below I use the adjective "modernist" to remind readers that I mean the modern period, not simply what is contemporary. My usage, however, is informed less by academic debates than by popular usage: "postmodernism" is the term I read in my daily paper.

7   Albert Borgmann, *Crossing the Postmodern Divide* (Chicago: University of Chicago Press, 1992).

8   Pierre Bourdieu, *Outline of a Theory of Practice* (Cambridge: Cambridge University Press, 1977), 166.

9   George S. Bascom, "Sketches From a Surgeon's Notebook," in Spiro et al., *Empathy and the Practice of Medicine*, 29 (see Preface, n. 3).

10   The complementary change that marks this side of the postmodern divide is that the medical story is increasingly trumped by the administrative story, but that postmodern trend is the topic for a different book than this one.

11   Arthur W. Frank, *At the Will of the Body: Reflections on Illness* (Boston: Houghton Mifflin, 1991), 138ff.

12   Personal communication.

13   Susan Sontag, *Illness as Metaphor* (New York: Vintage, 1978), 3.

14   Dan Gottlieb, "Patients must insist that Doctors see the Face behind the Ailment," *The Philadelphia Inquirer*, July 4, 1994.

15   Elizabeth Tyson, "Heal Thyself," *Living Fit*, Winter 1994, 38.

16   Claudine Herzlich and Janine Pierret, *Illness and Self in Society* (Baltimore: Johns Hopkins University Press, 1987), 23. Stanley Joel Reiser quotes the seventeenth-century physician Thomas Sydenham, "Nature, in the production of disease is uniform and consistent; so much so, that for the same disease in different persons the symptoms are for the most part the same; and the self-same phenomena you would observe in the sickness of a Socrates you would observe in the sickness of a simpleton." The unavoidable implication is that all patients, for diagnostic purposes, might as well be simpletons. Reiser's conclusion is more moderated: "Thus the symptoms that combine patients into populations have become more significant to physicians than the symptoms that separate patients as individuals." ("Science, Pedagogy, and the Transformation of Empathy in Medicine," in Spiro et al., *Empathy and the Practice of Medicine*, 123–24.)

17   Gayatri Chakravorty Spivak, *The Post-Colonial Critic: Interviews, Strategies, and Dialogues*, ed. Sarah Harasym (New York: Routledge, 1990), 73.

18   Susan Bell, "Political Gynecology: Gynecological Imperialism and the Politics of Self-Help," in Phil Brown, ed., *Perspectives in Medical Sociology* (Prospect Heights, Ill: Waveland Press, 1992), 576–86.

19   For another story of lay narratives achieving a collective voice in opposition to orthodox medicine, see Martha Balshem, *Cancer in the Community: Class and Medical Authority* (Washington: Smithsonian Institution Press, 1993).

20   Physicians, who certainly have their own stories, express their version of post-colonialism when they object to having their experiences of caring for patients taken away from them. A physician employed by an HMO says, "I don't want to *manage clients*, I want to *care for patients*. I don't want to hide behind bureaucratic regs and physician assistants. I want to do the caring." Quoted by Kleinman, *The Illness Narratives*, 219 (see Preface, n. 2).

21   One indicator of the need for storytelling about illness are "grass roots" publications

such as *Expressions: Literature and Art by People with Disabilities and Ongoing Health Problems* (Sefra Kobrin Pitzele, editor; P.O. Box 16294, St. Paul, Minn. 55116–0294) and *Common Journeys* (Leslie Keyes, editor; 4136 43rd Avenue South, Minneapolis, Minn. 55406). Storytelling also takes place in numerous journal writing workshops conducted in all illness support centers I have visited or received information from. The truly postmodern form of storytelling among the ill are electronic messages exchanged in media such as the Internet. An increasing number of specialized "nets" exist for illness stories. On Internet stories, see Faith McLellan, "From Book to Byte: Narratives of Physical Illness," *Medical Humanities Review* 8 (Fall 1994): 9–21.

PART FIVE

Evaluation and politics of health care

THE FINAL PART OF THE READER provides examples of sociological perspectives on the evaluation and politics of health care. There is at present a great deal of applied 'health services research' being carried out which draws on social science perspectives. One obvious area is in the evaluation of quality of life following intervention, using either quantitative or qualitative methods, or a combination of the two. However, there are broader issues at stake as well. The advent of 'evidence-based health care' has brought with it a new set of issues. In part these are political in character, and relate to the way evidence may be used to deal with resource issues, and to bring a new discipline to bear on professional practice. But they are also sociological in the sense that unintended social consequences may follow, for example in the professional–client relationship.

The first extract in this part, by Gabe, takes a broad view of recent changes in the British National Health Service (NHS). The introduction of managerial structures and a plethora of quality assurance and performance indicators have arguably eroded the autonomy of doctors and other health professionals. As shown elsewhere in this Reader, the original postulates of a 'Freidsonian' approach to the medical profession in particular – in which medical dominance, autonomy and power are emphasised – need to be reconsidered in the light of such developments. In addition, Gabe points to the growth of consumerism in health care, underpinned by government edicts and charters, through which a more assertive patient body may develop. Both managerialism and consumerism are two sides of the same coin in Gabe's analysis, namely that a form of 'internal market' within the NHS has developed, decentralising and fragmenting the service. Gabe also analyses the shifting balance in the public–private mix, both inside the NHS itself, and between the NHS and private providers. These developments, in turn, are seen to be part of a wider agenda to emphasise self-provision and to reduce collective responsibilities.

In the second extract, Harrison examines the more recent turn in managing the NHS, towards the development of evidence-based practice. The idea that medical procedures and treatments should be properly evaluated, especially in terms of their outcomes, appears self-evidently to be a positive move, as does the idea of clinicians basing their actions on the best possible evidence. However, Harrison shows that this is not a disinterested policy. It is, he argues, part of a cost control drive, such that those procedures or treatments that cannot be shown to be cost effective may be threatened. Underpinning this move is a strong commitment to a particular form of research and evidence base, epitomised in the randomised controlled trial (RCT). By emphasising the need to carry out evaluations in which patients are randomly allocated to intervention groups and control groups, two consequences follow. First, decisions about the allocation of resources can be seen to be increasingly 'scientific' in character. If research is carried out by the profession on different treatment modalities, then politicians can distance themselves from unpopular decisions about such treatments, especially where cost is the overriding factor. Second, although evidence-based medicine appears to give new sources of power to the profession, this is less to the ordinary practitioner, and more to an elite of academic/epidemiological research doctors. Harrison concludes his article by pointing to some of the difficulties in implementing an evidence-based approach in practice, given these dynamics.

In the next extract by Light and Hughes, the question of resource allocation and rationing is tackled directly. Light and Hughes set out to examine common assumptions about rationing, and the value of a sociological perspective. One of the main assumptions they challenge is that rationing is 'inevitable'. In fact, the degree of provision and choice in health care systems varies widely, and for many years, they argue, modern health care systems have met most health care needs in a timely manner. Light and Hughes call for a more empirical approach to claims about rationing, including the need to examine the preferences of different groups of actors – lay people, organisations, governments – and what degree of consistency exists in such claims. A sociological view would seek to throw light on the interactions, power and perspectives held by the various parties, and how these work through in specific contexts. Such a perspective would also examine the consequences, intended and unintended, of implicit and explicit rationing. In answer to those writers that suggest more explicit rationing would drag health policy into the mire, Light and Hughes suggest that implicit rationing, already being carried out by doctors, produces large variations and uneven quality in service provision. Light and Hughes show that a sociological view of rationing in all its dimensions has been long overdue.

The next article, by Fitzpatrick and Boulton, shifts attention to the methodological issues involved in a sociological approach to evaluation, especially those associated with qualitative research. If the 'black box' of health care is to be opened, and the issues identified above, among others, are to be examined in depth, then clarity about what is involved in qualitative research is particularly needed. It is not enough, as is sometimes thought, that small-scale research involving a few respondents is, by definition, the basis of qualitative research. Fitzpatrick and Boulton distinguish different kinds of qualitative methods, and provide examples of health services research where such methods have been appropriately used. For example they compare interviews and focus groups, and suggest reasons why one or other of these should be used. They then discuss the use of 'nominal groups' where more structured discussions and thus data collection are pursued. In this form of research, tasks or vignettes are given to participants, and this may provide the basis for qualitative discussion or more quantitative assessments, or both. Fitzpatrick and Boulton also examine observational studies, where ethnographic techniques are employed, and cases studies where a particular area of activity may be studied using a variety of methods. The previous discussion of rationing within a particular service would be a case in point. Here, interviews and focus groups might be combined. Finally, Fitzpatrick and Boulton outline the main steps involved in data analysis and those that need to be taken to ensure good practice in qualitative research.

The last two articles of this final Part of the Reader provide examples of qualitative research which reveal critical features of evaluation and evidence-based practice, and also relate to some of the themes of earlier articles. The article by Howitt and Armstrong is based on a study of patients suffering from a heart condition known as atrial fibrillation. These patients had been identified as being at risk from stroke, and were drawn from a large urban practice in the South East of England. Fifty-six patients consented to be interviewed and were asked if they were aware that they were at increased risk of stroke. The patients were then offered warfarin, which has been shown to be effective in reducing stroke. However, twenty of the patients refused the new treatment. Interviews with these patients showed that lay beliefs about medicine, and values that cut across health as an overriding consideration, limited the uptake of the treatment. For some of the older men in the study, perceptions of being at risk and of the seriousness of their condition were such that they did not think it worth starting a new drug. Howitt and Armstrong draw a number of important conclusions from the discrepancies between lay and professional views of 'evidence', including the fact that the effectiveness of a treatment may be exaggerated unless the willingness or otherwise of patients actually to take up the treatment is built into its evaluation.

The final article, by Featherstone and Donovan, deals with the critical issue of patient involvement in evidence-based medicine, but this time in relation to participating in research rather than in the up-take of treatment. In this study a sub-sample of patients from a large randomised controlled trial, which was comparing different treatments for benign prostatic disease, were interviewed. The main purpose of the interviews was to gain insight into the men's understanding of randomisation, and thus their involvement in the trial. While most of those interviewed showed that they understood the nature of randomisation, and the need for research, many found aspects of it difficult to square with their experience as patients. For research doctors, randomisation represents a statistical device that ensures that each patient in the trial has an equal chance of being allocated to one of the different treatment 'arms' of the study. For the men in this study, however, randomisation (signalling a process without logic) clashed with their expectation that the doctor would tailor their treatment to their condition. In RCTs there is an added problem, in that doctors and patients are supposed to achieve 'equipoise' before the beginning of the trial, where prior clinical judgement about the patient by the doctor is minimised. Importantly, this study showed that differences in the meaning of research terms and procedures between doctors and patients could lead to confusion and a breakdown in trust, with patients sometimes becoming resentful about the way they were treated. Featherstone and Donovan cast doubt as to whether improved information on trials for patients would lessen or worsen patient acceptance. The potential damage to the doctor–patient relationship of both evidence-based practice and a heavily research-oriented health service are thus underlined. Research on patient beliefs, interactions in health service settings, and questions of power and knowledge continue to be high on the medical sociology agenda.

Chapter 25

Jonathan Gabe

CONTINUITY AND CHANGE IN THE BRITISH NATIONAL HEALTH SERVICE

From P. Conrad (ed.) *The Sociology of Health and Illness: Critical Perspectives* (5th edition), New York: St Martin's Press (1997)

. . .

The restructuring of the National Health Service

1 The new managerialism

POOR NHS MANAGEMENT, in one form or another, has long been blamed by governments of all political persuasions for shortcomings in the service. The Conservative administrations of the 1980s, however, attached particular weight to this assessment as it coincided with their ideological attachment to the New Right with its emphasis on monetarism, political liberalism, professional deregulation and the application of private sector business principles to the public sector as a way to control expenditure. Moreover . . . it also served the political function of distancing the Conservatives from the impact which the application of monetarist principles to public spending would have on the level of service. As Klein put it, "to decentralize responsibility is also to disclaim blame."[1]

In 1983 the Conservatives decided to institute change by appointing a business-man, Roy Griffiths—then the managing director of Sainsbury's supermarket chain—to review the management of the NHS. His proposed solution was to alter the organizational culture of the service by introducing features of business management, along the lines suggested particularly by US management theorists.[2] Previously management had been based on consensus teams involving representatives from medicine, nursing and administration each of whom had the power of veto. Griffiths recommended the creation of general managers at each level of the service, in place of consensus teams, who would take responsibility for developing management plans, ensuring quality of care, achieving cost improvements and monitoring and rewarding staff.[3] At the same time the managers were to be appointed on short term contracts and to be paid by performance as a spur to good management, as happened in the private sector.[4]

The proposals, which were accepted wholesale by the Government, were designed to alter the balance of power in favor of managers, at the expense of other professionals, especially doctors, whose clinical freedom to make decisions about individual patients regardless of cost had previously been a major determinant of the level of expenditure. In the new system doctors were to be more accountable to managers who had stricter control over professional and labor costs through a system of management budgets which related workload objectives to the resources available.[5]

Doctors were encouraged to participate in this micromanagement system and help secure and oversee the most effective use of resources. While some doctors applied for and were appointed as general managers and a few experiments were set up involving the delegation of budgetary responsibility to doctors, many were reluctant to give their unequivocal support to these developments.[6] As a result doctors continued to exercise considerable autonomy and managers continued to lack real control over medical work.

Not to be put off, in 1989 the government published a White Paper, *Working for Patients*, subsequently enacted through the 1990 NHS and Community Care Act, which attempted, amongst other things, to shift the balance of power more forcefully in the direction of managers. The White Paper recommended that managers should have greater involvement in the specification and policing of consultants' contracts.

At the same time a plethora of new techniques of managerial evaluation were developed. Quality assurance and performance indicators, made possible by advances in information technology, increased opportunities for the managerial determination of work content, productivity, resource use and quality standards.[7] In addition, managers now had available a growing body of evidence from the NHS Research and Development program regarding clinical effectiveness and health outcomes which could be used to challenge clinical autonomy.[8]

Such developments would seem to have given managers the opportunity to constrain British doctors as never before, along the lines identified in the proletarianization thesis. Advocates of this position argue that doctors are being deskilled, are losing their economic independence and are being required to work in bureaucratically organized institutions under the instruction of managers, in accordance with the requirements of advanced capitalism.[9] However, as Freidson[10] indicates, the widespread adoption of new techniques for monitoring the efficiency of performance and resource allocation does not on its own illustrate reduced professional autonomy. What really matters is whose criteria for evaluation and appraisal are adopted and who controls any actions which are taken.[11] Moreover, doctors are perfectly capable of transforming themselves into managers while exerting themselves in such a way that no fundamental challenge is mounted to their view of the health service.[8] It is quite conceivable that the increasing devolution of budgets to clinicians will provide the opportunity for new forms of autonomy for consultants.[6]

In sum, while doctors in the NHS now have to account for their actions in ways which were unthinkable a decade ago it is far from certain that the new managerialism in the NHS will result in a victory for the "corporate rationalizers" over the "professional monopolists."[12] What is certain, however, is that the policy changes outlined above have been good for the managers themselves. Their number increased by 53% between 1975 and 1991 while their total salaries have risen by £380 million over the decade since the Griffiths reforms were introduced.[13] This is somewhat ironic given that Conservative governments responsible for this new managerialism have consistently maintained that reducing bureaucracy was an important policy objective.

2 The internal market in health care

In addition to enhancing the role of management, *Working for Patients* and the 1990 NHS and Community Care Act also introduced a market system to the NHS, while reaffirming the principle of providing health care free at the point of use. Premised on the assumption that competition enhances efficiency, it was proposed that the NHS should be divided into providers and purchasers of services; purchasers, it was assumed, would shop around for the cheapest health care while providers would minimize their price in order to remain competitive in the market.

The idea for an internal market apparently originated with the US economist, Alain Enthoven, who, on a visit to Britain in 1985, declared that the NHS was in a state of "gridlock" or general rigidity and inflexibility and that this could only be broken if the most efficient providers were rewarded with economic incentives.[14] Enthoven's solution, based on experience with US Health Maintenance Organizations,[15,16] proved to be attractive to New Right "think tanks" such as the Centre for Policy Studies, but the government did not take up the idea until the winter of 1987/8 when it faced a political crisis as a result of mounting public and professional concern about the financial problems facing the health service.[17] It was this set of circumstances which triggered Prime Minister Margaret Thatcher's decision to review the NHS, the outcome of which was *Working for Patients*.

The White Paper and the subsequent Act turned District Health Authorities (DHAs) into purchasers (or commissioning agencies), with capitation budgets, who were responsible for assessing local needs, determining priorities and buying community services. These services could be bought from either the public or private sector. Larger general practices could also opt to become purchasers, known as fundholders.

Providers of care such as large hospitals and community units were given the opportunity to become self governing Trusts with the promise of increased financial freedom and greater autonomy. They were to be allowed to set the rate of pay for their staff, invest in capital projects and alter their service according to the needs of the market. The idea was that self government would encourage a greater sense of ownership and pride, or corporatism, on the part of those providing services, as well as encouraging local initiative and greater competition.

The reforms were implemented within two years of the publication of *Working for Patients*. Purchasers found some opportunities for cost savings but were constrained by the lack of choice between service providers (e.g., only one district general hospital in the area) and the need to provide services locally, whatever the savings to be achieved by contracting further afield.[2]

On the supply side, the formation of hospitals and community units into Trusts seems to have provided certain benefits for the service and for patients. Costs seem to have been kept down and the number of patients waiting over a year for hospital treatment has been reduced. At the same time the Trusts' attempts to create a corporate spirit have not been entirely successful and there is a danger that they will respond to purchasing power at the expense of social need and concentrate on more profitable areas of work to the detriment of certain categories of patient.[2]

Overall, the internal market would seem to have produced a decentralized and fragmented system with numerous buyers and sellers, in place of a centrally planned, uniform, top down approach. There have been certain benefits for patients from this most radical of recent reforms but these appear to have been offset by a series of problems stemming from a system which puts efficiency before equity. It seems likely that these will be dealt with by regulating rather than replacing the market. The new commercial culture and the vested interests of those who have benefited from the reforms will make it extremely difficult for any government to put this "genie back in the bottle."[18]

3 Empowering the consumer

Another strand of the health service reforms has involved greater emphasis on consumer choice and redress. The application of consumerist principles to the NHS was given a major impetus with the publication of the 1983 Griffiths Report on management.[19] In line with New Right thinking with its emphasis on individuals exercising choice through the market, Griffiths stated that managers should give pride of place to "patient," or as they were renamed "consumer," preferences when making health care decisions. He argued that they should try and establish how well the service for which they were responsible was being delivered by employing market research techniques and other methods to find out the views of their customers. They were then to act on this information by amending policy and monitoring subsequent performance against it. Thereafter, this management-led consumerist approach was promoted vigorously, with Directors of Quality Assurance appointed to Health Authorities to establish users' views, and staff sent on customer relations courses and encouraged to follow newly established "mission statements" outlining their organizations' common goals. However, the benefits to patients seems to have been limited, with managers being mainly concerned with hotel aspects of care such as cleanliness and food rather than with patients' views of clinical effectiveness.[19]

Further policy initiatives to enhance consumer choice followed in the 1990s. The 1990 NHS and Community Care Act required Health Authorities, as purchasers, to discuss services with community groups, amongst others, before drawing up contracts. This policy was reinforced in *Listening to Local Voices*, published by the

NHS Management Executive in 1992, which stressed that purchasing authorities should listen to the views of local people about their priorities for health care before making rationing decisions.[3]

The 1990 Act also required GP fundholders to purchase services on their patients' behalf. As Paton states, however, "the fact that the individual was not the purchaser meant that any new consumerism in the NHS was not to be based on the individual's purchasing rights."[20] Rather, GP fundholders, along with Health Authorities, were to be proxy consumers. It was assumed that these fundholders had the incentive to fulfil this role effectively as otherwise their patients would simply switch to a competing practice.[21] However, as patients lack the necessary knowledge or inclination to shop around in the medical market place and often do not have a great choice of alternative GPs with which to register, there is little evidence that this aspect of the reforms has markedly increased consumer choice.[21] Moreover, for those patients who remain with nonfundholding GPs the 1990 reforms may have had the perverse effect of actually restricting choice. These patients' GPs are no longer free to refer their patients to a consultant of their choice but instead must refer them to providers with whom the District has a contract (unless they can obtain special permission to do otherwise from their local DHA manager).

In addition, consumerism has been promoted by the introduction in 1992 of a Patient's Charter, one of a number intended to transform the management of the public services. Taking its lead from the first of the charters, the Citizen's Charter, introduced by Prime Minister Margaret Thatcher's successor, John Major, the Patient's Charter was intended to make the health service more responsive to consumers by setting the rights and service standards which they could expect. These standards were to provide the basis for targets against which the performance of managers could be measured. In addition to seven existing rights, for example the right to change doctor, three new rights were established. These were the right to: detailed information on local health services, including quality standards and waiting lists; guaranteed admission to hospital within two years of being put on the waiting list; and having any complaint about the service fully investigated and promptly dealt with. Subsequently, doubt has been expressed about whether these rights will be realized in practice as they are not legally binding.

Despite the rhetoric of consumerism over the last decade there is some doubt as to whether the quality of the service provided to NHS patients has greatly increased. Certainly the number of people complaining has increased substantially since the early 1980s. For example, while 3.1 written complaints per 100,000 of the population were made about community services in England in 1981, there were 9.9 per 100,000 in 1989–90, an increase of almost 220%.[22]

As these developments reveal, the model of consumerism employed in the reform of the NHS is concerned with promoting the self-interest of individual users of the service rather than with enhancing patients' collective representation or involvement in service planning.[23] Given the attachment of the Conservatives to the business ethic and individual choice this is not surprising and reflects a belief in a supermarket approach to consumerism. In this approach the consumer is confined to purchasing what is on the shelf or complaining when a product is faulty, and has no direct voice in determining what appears on the shelf in the first place.[19]

As Nettleton and Harding[22] recognize, this supermarket model presupposes a certain type of citizenship in which citizen rights are reduced to consumer rights and the social right to representation and participation in decision making is downplayed.

The Conservative government's emphasis on empowering the individual consumer also reflects a distrust of professionals, another tenet of New Right ideology.[11] The restrictive practices and collegiate control of the medical profession were seen to have resulted in an unresponsive service which could only be improved if power was shifted to users of the service by giving them sufficient information to participate in the market. But to what extent have users been empowered at the expense of the medical profession? Have the reforms contributed to the deprofessionalization of medicine.[24-5] As noted above no attempt was made in the reforms explicitly to empower individual patients by giving them direct purchasing power. Nor was consideration given to the differences in ability of particular social groups to use the information newly available to shop around for medical services. Consequently, much will depend on where people live as this will determine the choice of doctor or hospital available to them.[26] It would thus seem that the power of the individual patient has changed relatively little as a result of these reforms, leaving doctors with their specialized knowledge and skills still largely in control.

Finally, it should be noted that some commentators[22,27] have argued that the emphasis on consumerism in the health service reforms parallels more general socio-economic changes from a society based on Fordist principles (mass production, universalization of welfare, mass consumption) to one based on post-Fordism (flexible production techniques designed to take account of rapid changes in consumer demand and fragmented market tastes). In a post-Fordist society it is the consumers rather than the producers who call the tune. While this approach has some value in placing the health policy changes under consideration in a broader context, it fails to distinguish between surface changes in appearance and underlying social relations. As we have seen, while the rhetoric has been about enhanced consumer power, producers in the form of the medical profession continue to dominate the users of the service.

4 Promoting welfare pluralism

A further principle underpinning the NHS reforms is welfare pluralism. While the health services in Britain, like all others in the developed world,[28] have long been pluralist in the sense of having both public and private funding, planning and provision, the reforms of the 1980s and 1990s have attempted to shift the balance profoundly in favour of greater private sector involvement.[29-30] Again this is in line with New Right thinking which abhors monopoly and lack of choice. Changing the balance of provision has the attraction of providing the desired levels of services without the need for extra government spending. The latter would be anathema for a government wedded to cutting or at least controlling public expenditure in order to reduce the tax burden on individuals.[30]

One strategy for shifting the balance between the public and private sector has involved the development of policies to encourage the growth of private medicine.

Planning controls have been relaxed on private hospital development,[31] NHS consultants' contracts have been revised so that they have greater scope to undertake private practice in addition to their NHS commitments,[32] and tax changes have been introduced to encourage higher levels of private health cover.[33] These changes have created the climate for private hospital development and provided opportunities which have been fully exploited by the private sector. Between 1979 and 1989 the number of private hospitals increased by 30% and the number of private beds by 58%.[33] Many of these hospitals were located in the prosperous South East of England, compounding rather than eliminating geographical inequalities in the distribution of resources.

Shifting the balance between the public and private sector has also been enhanced by those reforms which have encouraged greater collaboration between the two sectors. An early attempt was the government's policy of requiring NHS District Health Authorities to introduce competitive tendering for domestic, catering and laundry services in 1983. The intention was to challenge the monopoly of the in-house providers of services in the expectation that costs would be reduced and greater "value for money" would be achieved. In practice the financial benefits proved relatively modest, at least initially, and the savings that have been achieved seem to have been at the expense of quality of service.[13] More recently, the NHS has been encouraged to contract out patient care to the private sector. Such cooperative arrangements were initially undertaken on a voluntary basis by individual Health Authorities faced with no in-house alternatives, for example as a result of capacity constraints.[32] Subsequently, HAs were directed by the government to use private hospitals as a way of reducing NHS waiting lists for non-urgent cases and those waiting more than one year.

While the reforms introduced by the Conservatives have generally been advantageous to the private sector they have not all been beneficial. In particular, the government's willingness to encourage the NHS to expand their pay-bed provision has served to sharpen competition for private patients and threaten the private providers' profit margins.

Originally introduced in 1948 as a concession to hospital consultants, pay-beds were in decline when the Conservatives came to power in 1979 and their number continued to fall subsequently. In the late 1980s, however, the government decided to revitalize this provision in the face of increasingly severe financial constraints. It was also in line with its belief in generating competition between providers so as to enhance consumer choice and maximize efficiency. In 1988 it therefore used the Health and Medicines Act to relax the rules governing pay-bed charges so that hospitals could make a profit rather than simply cover costs. As a result pay-bed income increased dramatically between 1991–2 and 1993–4 from just over £32 million to nearly £116 million.[34] The NHS now has 16% of the private market and is set to become the biggest provider of private health care in the UK by 1997.

These three examples illustrate the shift to a new public/private mix of services, a mixed economy of health care. The policy has been driven by ideological considerations and by economic and political calculations. The goal seems to have been to increase the role of the private sector and limit that of the public sector while improving its performance. As such it arguably represents an attempt to "privatize from within."[35]

It has also been suggested that these policies illustrate a shift towards post-Fordism in the sense that Health Authorities have become "flexible firms," concentrating on core functions and buying in peripheral services from outside.[36] While this argument is superficially attractive, it ignores the extent to which the reforms have been the result of deliberate political decisions in the face of external economic considerations and ideological preferences.[13] Rather than simply mirroring structural developments in the economy, the policy of welfare pluralism is best seen as an attempt to erode services that people experience collectively and persuade them to act instead in terms of their own immediate self interest.

Conclusion

This chapter has provided an account of the development of the British National Health Service in the 1980s and 1990s. Over this period, the Conservatives have embarked on a series of policy changes which have had the effect of radically restructuring the NHS while keeping the service free at the point of use. Driven by a deep ideological attachment to the New Right and faced with a financial crisis and public disquiet they have introduced managerialism and an internal market into the health service, along with a Patient's Charter and policies to encourage welfare pluralism. While these changes have seen certain benefits such as increasing the accountability of the medical profession, reducing hospital waiting times for patients, making rationing decisions explicit and creating a more responsive service, there have also been serious disadvantages. Of these perhaps the most significant is the possibility that a two tier system will develop with the wealthy paying for private care and the NHS providing a safety net for those who cannot afford it. The growth of the private health care sector, the regeneration of NHS pay beds, and the development of GP fundholding along the lines of HMOs all make this a realistic prospect. Indeed they could be seen to reflect a policy of Americanizing health care in the UK[33, 37–8] at a time when the US has been looking at the old style NHS as one possible alternative model of health care. This reference to convergence illustrates the extent to which the NHS has changed in recent times and makes it unlikely that the clock will ever be turned back.

References

1   Klein, R. *The Politics of the NHS*. Harlow: Longman, 1983, 141.
2   Ranade, W. *A Future for the NHS?* Harlow: Longman, 1994.
3   Allsop, J. *Health Policy and the NHS*. Second Edition. London: Longman, 1995.
4   Cox, D. Crisis and opportunity in health service management. In *Continuity and Crisis in the NHS*. Eds. Loveridge, R., and Starkey, K. Buckingham: Open University Press, 1992.
5   Hunter, D. Managing medicine: A response to the crisis. *Social Science and Medicine* 32, 4, 441–9, 1991.
6   Cox, D. Health service management—a sociological view: Griffiths and the non-negotiated order of the hospital. In *The Sociology of the Health Service*. Eds. Gabe, J., Calnan, M., and Bury, M. London: Routledge, 1991.

7   Flynn, R. *Structures of Control in Health Management*. London: Routledge, 1992.

8   Hunter, D. From tribalism to corporatism: The managerial challenge to medical dominance. In *Challenging Medicine*. Eds. Gabe, J., Kelleher, D., and Williams, G. London: Routledge, 1994.

9   McKinlay, J., and Arches, J. Towards the proletarianization of physicians. *International Journal of Health Services* 15, 161–95, 1985.

10 Freidson, E. *Medical Work in America: Essays in Health Care*. New Haven: Yale University Press, 1989.

11 Elston, M. A. The politics of professional power: Medicine in a changing health service. In *The Sociology of the Health Service*. Eds. Gabe, J., Bury, M., and Calnan, M. London: Routledge, 1991.

12 Alford, R. *Health Care Politics*. Chicago: University of Chicago Press, 1975.

13 Mohan, J. *A National Health Service? The Restructuring of Health Care in Britain since 1979*. Basingstoke: Macmillan, 1995.

14 Enthoven, A. *Reflections on the Management of the NHS*. London: Nuffield Provincial Hospitals Trust, 1985.

15 Allsop, J., and May. A. Between the devil and the deep blue sea: Managing the NHS in the wake of the 1990 Act. *Critical Social Policy* 38, 5–22, 1993.

16 The British reforms however parted company with the HMOs by splitting purchasers/insurers and providers. See Paton, C. *Competition and Planning in the NHS: The Danger of Unplanned Markets*. London: Chapman and Hall, 1992.

17 Baggott, R. *Health and Health Care in Britain*. Basingstoke, Macmillan, 1994.

18 Baggott, R. *op. cit.*, p. 200.

19 Seale, C. The consumer voice. In *Dilemmas in Health Care*. Eds. Davey, B., and Popay, J. Buckingham: Open University Press, 1993.

20 Paton, C. *op. cit.*

21 Klein, R. *The Politics of the NHS*. Third edition. London: Longman, 1995.

22 Nettleton, S., and Harding, G. Protesting patients: A study of complaints submitted to a Family Health Service Authority. *Sociology of Health and Illness* 16, 38–61, 1994.

23 Hughes, D. The reorganization of the National Health Service: The rhetoric and reality of the internal market. *The Modern Law Review* 54, 88–103, 1991.

24 Haug, M. Deprofessionalisation: An alternative hypothesis for the future. *Sociological Review Monograph*, 20, 195–211, 1973.

25 Haug, M. A re-examination of the hypothesis of deprofessionalisation. *Milbank Quarterly*, 66 (Suppl. 2), 48–56, 1988.

26 Walsh, K. Citizens, charters and contracts. In *The Authority of the Consumer*. Eds. Keat, R., Whiteley, N., and Abercrombie, N. London: Routledge, 1994.

27 Nettleton, S. *The Sociology of Health and Illness*. Cambridge/Oxford: Polity in association with Blackwell Publishers, 1995.

28 Klein, R. Private practice and public policy: Regulating the frontiers. In *The Private/Public Mix for Health*. Eds. McLachlan, G., and Maynard, A. London: Nuffield Provincial Hospitals Trust, 1982.

29 Davies, C. Things to come: The NHS in the next decade. *Sociology of Health and Illness* 9, 302–17, 1987.

30 Harrison, S., Hunter, D., and Pollitt, C. *The Dynamics of British Health Policy*. London: Unwin Hyman, 1990.

31   Mohan, J., and Woods, K. Restructuring health care: The social geography of public and private health care under the British Conservative government. *International Journal of Health Services* 15, 197–215, 1985.

32   Rayner, G. Lessons from America? Commercialization and growth of private medicine in Britain. *International Journal of Health Services* 17, 197–216, 1987.

33   Calnan, M., Cant, S., and Gabe, J. *Going Private: Why People Pay for Their Health Care.* Buckingham: Open University Press, 1993.

34   Higgins, J. Goldrush. *Health Service Journal* 23 November 24–6, 1995.

35   Ranade, W., and Haywood, S. Privatizing from within: The National Health Service under Thatcher. *Local Government Studies* 15, 19–34, 1989.

36   Kelly, A. The enterprise culture and the welfare state: Restructuring the management of health and personal social services. In *Deciphering the Enterprise Culture.* Ed. Burrows, R. London: Routledge, 1991.

37   Navarro, V. The relevance of the US experience to the reforms in the British National Health Service: The case of general practitioner fund holding. *International Journal of Health Services* 21, 381–7, 1991.

38   Hudson, D. Quasi-markets in health and social care in Britain: Can the public sector respond? *Policy and Politics* 20, 131–42, 1992.

Chapter 26

Stephen Harrison

THE POLITICS OF EVIDENCE-BASED MEDICINE IN THE UNITED KINGDOM

From *Policy and Politics,* 26 (1) 1998: 15–31

. . .

AT ITS SIMPLEST, the doctrine of evidence-based medicine (EBM) holds that the appropriate criterion for the provision of an intervention, either in the NHS generally or in the treatment of an individual patient, is its effectiveness (or efficacy; see Harrison and Long, 1989 for a discussion) as demonstrated by bio-medical research evidence. This is now manifest in formal policy for the NHS; in 1993 health authorities were asked to begin to identify interventions of which they would in future purchase more or less, on grounds of effectiveness and ineffectiveness respectively (NHS Management Executive, 1993). Some authorities chose the insertion of grommets (a treatment for children with otitis media – 'glue ear'), and dilatation and curettage ('D and C': a treatment for dysfunctional uterine bleeding) for women under the age of 40 as their candidates for the 'purchase less' category (see also Klein et al, 1996). Both procedures had been the subject of well-publicised academic reviews questioning their value (Effective Health Care, 1992; 1995). Current official policy on EBM holds that,

> The overall purpose of the NHS is to secure, through the resources available, the greatest possible improvement in the physical and mental health of the people . . . In order to achieve this, we need to ensure that decisions about the provision and delivery of clinical services are driven increasingly by evidence of clinical and cost-effectiveness, coupled with the systematic assessment of actual health outcomes. (NHS Executive, 1996a: 6)

This line of policy has been supported, at some expense, by two types of related development in the NHS. First, there has existed since 1991 a national research and development (R and D) strategy for the NHS, involving the creation of national and regional directors of R and D, the establishment of national and local research budgets to be the object of competitive bidding, and reorganisation of the flow of research funds through NHS hospitals (Department of Health, 1991; Task Force on R and D Funding, 1994; for a general review, see Baker and Kirk, 1996). The central objective of this strategy was to disaggregate the large proportion of health interventions stated never to have been the subject of proper evaluation into two categories: the effective and the ineffective. Second, a range of specialist institutions has been funded as the means of reviewing, collating and disseminating the findings of effectiveness research to the NHS; these include the Cochrane Centre at the University of Oxford; Effective Health Care bulletins coordinated from the University of Leeds, the NHS Centre for Reviews and Dissemination at the University of York and the Outcomes Clearing House at the University of Leeds.

Two key theories underlie this whole strategy. The first defines 'sound evidence', that is, that which may be relied upon to contribute to the classification of an intervention as effective or ineffective, as evidence derived from studies conducted in a certain way held to be 'scientific'. This approach is typified in the influential 'hierarchy of evidence' proposed by Canadian academics (and later modified in various ways) but widely cited as an authoritative definition of the soundness of scientific research purporting to demonstrate the effectiveness of medical and similar interventions. The hierarchy is displayed in Table 26.1.

The principle which underpins this hierarchy is *validity*, that is the elimination from research findings of bias arising from any differences between patients treated by means of the intervention being researched and patients not so treated (that is, treated with other interventions or simply not treated). The pinnacle of the

Table 26.1 The hierarchy of evidence

Level of validity of findings	Type of research
I	Strong evidence from at least one systematic review of multiple well-designed randomised controlled trials
II	Strong evidence from at least one properly designed randomised controlled trial of appropriate size
III	Evidence from well-designed non-randomised trials, single group pre-post, cohort, time series or matched case-controlled studies
IV	Evidence from well-designed non-experimental studies from more than one centre or research group
V	Opinions of respected authorities, based on clinical evidence, descriptive studies or reports of expert committees

Source: Canadian Task Force, 1979

hierarchy is occupied by the randomised controlled trial (RCT) in which patients are conscientiously allocated randomly (and with the patient's informed consent) between the group which will receive the intervention under investigation and whatever group(s) with which they will be compared: 'control' groups receiving perhaps placebos, or no treatment, and/or existing conventional treatment, as the case may be. Ideally, it is held, RCTs should be 'double blind', that is neither the treating clinician nor the patient should know which intervention they are receiving. This ideal cannot of course always be met; for instance it is hardly possible to conceal whether or not surgery is occurring or ethically to perform a dummy operation. Special methods, described as 'meta-analysis', have been developed in order to aggregate the results of several RCTs (Mulrow, 1994). Other research methods are ranked lower in the hierarchy, with other types of *controlled* study second to the RCT and uncontrolled methods a poor third: in practice, advocates of RCTs tend to regard uncontrolled methods as suitable only for hypothesis-building with a view to an eventual controlled study.

The second key theory upon which EBM is based is that the most useful, though not necessarily exclusive, method for disseminating sound research evidence as defined above to practising clinicians is the 'clinical guideline' (NHS Executive, 1996b); clinicians can clearly not be expected to read every research study relevant to their practice as it is published. The logic of guidelines is essentially algorithmic, that is, it guides its user to courses of (diagnostic or therapeutic) action, dependent upon stated prior conditions: 'if . . . then' logic. The logic is also normative, that is it tells the clinician what *ought* to be done. In general, guidelines do not claim to determine clinical action completely, and degrees of discretion are left.

The doctrine of EBM is of course by no means new and indeed the attempted popularisation in the UK of the notion that randomisation between comparison groups is a crucial means of avoiding bias in biomedical outcomes research dates from Professor A.L. Cochrane's seminal Rock Carling Lecture of 1971, published the following year as *Effectiveness and efficiency: random reflections on health services* (Cochrane, 1972). As is often the case with ideas, Cochrane's central insight took a long time to become officially, or widely, accepted. As also is often the case, it was probably changes in social and political context which were more important in allowing the wide-spread acceptance of the idea than any intrinsic 'rightness' (Kingdon, 1984). It seems unlikely that in the early 1970s, a time when NHS resources underwent rapid growth in real terms (Klein, 1983: 67–8), Cochrane had any concern to provide the tools to solve a policy problem of rationing. Indeed his main concerns were for what he saw as the genuine progress of science towards truth and for the avoidance of subjecting patients to ineffective (and therefore in his analysis, unnecessary) interventions. He was fiercely critical of the NHS in this second respect:

> I once asked a worker at a crematorium, who had a curiously contented look on his face, what he found so satisfying about his work. He replied that what fascinated him was the way in which so much went in and so little came out. I thought of advising him to get a job in the NHS, it might have increased his job satisfaction.
>
> (Cochrane, 1972: 12)

Cochrane's ideas, 20 years on, serve both to provide criteria for health services rationing and to legitimate those criteria. Of this process we can ask the traditional question of political analysis, *cui bono?* Who benefits?

First, as is clear from what has been said above, EBM offers a solution to the particularly difficult political question of how to manage supply and demand for healthcare. The state (or the government, depending on one's theoretical presuppositions) is therefore a potential beneficiary. Although it is logically possible, as advocates of EBM regularly point out, that EBM might reveal the effectiveness of interventions and thereby *increase* demand, policymakers do not in practice seem to believe this to be likely; the retiring national NHS Director of R and D has been quoted as claiming that the implementation of research findings in clinical practice might save £1 billion per annum (Timmins, 1996). Not only does EBM offer a solution, but a solution which diffuses the responsibility for potentially unpopular decisions (Klein, 1983: 140) by their delegation to doctors. This is important for the political acceptability of rationing: in line with the general occupational status of doctors and the high public esteem in which they are held (for opinion poll data on these matters, see Harrison, 1988: 88–9; MORI, 1993), several studies have shown that the medical profession is seen by the public as by far the most legitimate actor in making rationing decisions. It is also the case that the NHS R and D strategy is in part a response to a report by a parliamentary Select Committee which saw medical research as an important component of the UK economy (House of Lords Select Committee on Science and Technology, 1988); there is therefore an implied economic benefit in EBM.

Second, the medical profession also benefits in that it retains a monopoly of clinical decision making, thus helping to protect itself from managerial challenges. It does however entail a shift of influence between different sections of the profession: away from the clinical practitioner and towards the academic/epidemiologist/health services researcher; see also Harrison, 1997.) It is also clear that the pursuit of EBM is defensible in the terms of traditional medical ethics; only a minority of clinicians seem to claim that they regularly undertake *every* healthcare intervention that might benefit the patient (Harrison et al, 1984). Moreover, although some commentators (for instance, Williams, 1985) have sought to extend its scope into the *cost-effectiveness* of healthcare interventions, its most prominent advocates insist that it is only concerned with effectiveness (see for instance, Sackett et al, 1996). There is a sense, therefore, in which EBM offers an accommodation between Alford's (1975) most powerful 'structural interests': the 'professional monopolists' and the 'corporate rationalisers'. The rationalisation is delegated to the monopolists, a tendency which may perhaps be read as the beginnings of a restructuring of the health policy field into new divisions.

Third, EBM can be made to appeal to the public and to potential patients. The approach draws on 'science' and all its modernist trappings of truth, progress and so on; it can therefore be presented as rational and politically neutral. Moreover, and despite the science, the rather neat thought experiment on this proposed by Evans shows that it can also be presented as common sense: what is the point of ineffective healthcare?

Overall, EBM and the interpretive flexibility which it offers provide an elegant resolution of the problem of matching demand for healthcare technologies to the level of resources available. Like clinical autonomy (Harrison, 1997), the main actors can all see something in it (albeit different things) for themselves.

Some current issues for evidence-based medicine

However, any policy has problems of its own and this section reviews two that are central to EBM: the weakness of the assumptions which underpin the use of guidelines as the main mode of implementing EBM; and the existence of epistemologies (theories of knowledge) which rival the one upon which RCTs are based.

Implementing evidence-based medicine

The choice of clinical guidelines as the main vehicle for implementing EBM is, at one level, a logical one; it is obviously unrealistic to expect the average busy clinician to read and understand all research papers relevant to their own sub-specialty, discriminate between acceptable and inadequate research methods, interpolate findings with existing knowledge, and modify routine clinical practice accordingly. At another level, however, it is an assumption which is extraordinarily naive; it is hard to imagine another policy arena in which what amount to a set of bureaucratic rules (the phrase is used in a technical, not pejorative sense) would be thought to be self-implementing. Yet this is effectively the approach which has been taken in most research to date on this topic: essentially as an issue of communication with studies mainly focused upon dissemination strategies.

There are substantial, and highly consonant, research findings available (for reviews, see Mugford et al, 1991; Haines and Feder, 1992; Russell and Grimshaw, 1992; Greco and Eisenberg, 1993; Grimshaw and Russell, 1993; Effective Health Care, 1994). In summary, these conclude that most effective in changing behaviour is likely to be the patient-specific reminder aimed at the specific clinician (perhaps through casenote markers or on-line prompts) at the time of treatment. Less, though still positively, effective is patient-specific feedback (perhaps through audit, continuing education, or 'preceptorship') from an educationally influential person or 'product champion'. The less clinician-specific and patient-specific the communication, the less effective it is likely to be in changing behaviour; general mailings and academic papers fall into this category.

Communication is, of course, a necessary condition for implementation of a policy such as EBM, but it is not a sufficient condition. Drawing on the logical approaches to the administration and implementation of public policy proposed by Hood (1976) and Gunn (1978), it is possible to outline a number of other necessary, though individually insufficient, conditions. These are as follows. (For a fuller account, see Harrison, 1994.)

Adequate resources   implementation clearly depends on the clinician's access to the material resources required for conformity to the guideline: drugs, equipment and so on. But non-material resources are essential too. Critical examples are skill and time and I shall give just one example to cover both. In the surgical treatment of rectal cancer, there is substantial evidence (MacFarlane et al, 1993) that the success of curative (as opposed to palliative) operations, measured in terms of non-recurrence locally, is heavily dependent on surgical technique. 'Total mesorectal excision', that is the precise sharp dissection of a specific plane of tissue, requires both particular surgical skills and substantially more theatre time than the standard operation. More generally, time requires trade-offs against other activities and it is not surprising that there is some evidence that clinicians consider time involved in audit activity to be less effective than seeing more patients (Black and Thompson, 1993). Even more generally, there is a recurrent theme in the sociology of the caring professions which explains 'corner cutting' behaviour, such as hasty diagnosis or the 'labelling' of clients, as an inherent and inevitable response to scarcity of time (Lipsky, 1980).

Incentives   it is clear that one cannot simply assume that communication of a guideline provides sufficient incentive for a clinician to comply with it. *Intrinsic* incentives might include the source of the guideline's being seen as authoritative; there is some evidence that locally determined guidelines are more likely to be seen as such (Brook, 1989; Russell and Grimshaw, 1992), even though it might be expected that nationally determined ones would be the most technically expert. Otherwise, little seems to be known about intrinsic incentives, though there are, at the time of writing, a number of ongoing studies into the role of 'opinion leaders' and into the possible impact of 'academic detailing' (that is, marketing preferred clinical practice to individual doctors in much the same way that drug companies market their products by face-to-face contact). *Extrinsic* incentives such as economic rewards can also be considered. UK experience with target payments for general practitioners (GPs) suggests that payment does affect behaviour, though Hughes and Yule's (1991) study of GPs' work–wage relationship suggests caution in assuming that doctors will do more in response to monetary incentives; indeed there is some evidence of a 'target income' phenomenon and hence a backward-sloping supply curve.

Disincentives   whatever incentives exist for compliance with guidelines may, of course, be wholly or partly offset by disincentives. Again there is little systematic knowledge, though it seems that covert organisational imperatives can often subvert ostensible policy (for an example from industry, see Brewster et al, 1981). Thus one UK study found that clinicians were prepared to manipulate audit results by modifying casenote entries to maintain the appearance of reaching targets, as well as a pervasive view that audit would have adverse consequences for the practice of medicine by routinising it and destroying both initiative and the ability to think through the logic of treatment (Black and Thompson, 1993). Melia's (1987) well-known study of nurses' work on the wards showed that they might actually be punished for practising what they had been taught in the school of nursing!

Coordination   a good deal of the literature about clinical guidelines makes the implicit assumption that what matters is the diagnostic and therapeutic behaviour of individual clinicians. Given the intellectual origins of much guidelines work in the puzzle of *medical* practice variations (Andersen and Mooney, 1990), this is not surprising. Yet it may be misleading; in practice the success of healthcare can depend on whole teams or chains of health workers performing the correct tasks correctly. This is particularly true in nursing care, where the 24-hour commitment multiplies the scope for error and omission, and community care, where multi-agency, multi-professional working has the same effect. The formal mathematics are gloomy; on the relatively optimistic assumptions that a chain of 10 health workers is involved in flowing a guideline for a particular patient, and that there is 0.95 probability that each will fully comply, the total probability of the patient getting precisely the care specified is 0.95 to the power 10, or little better than evens! This calculation, however, departs from what occurs in the real world in that it assumes that the compliance probabilities for each individual worker are independent. This is unlikely to be the case; people's behaviour is usually affected by the social (in this case, workplace) context in which they find themselves. Expressed differently, an important factor in guideline compliance is likely to be organisational or workplace 'culture', a concept which has been widely analysed in general (see, for instance, Allaire and Firsirotu, 1984; Meek, 1988) but not so far applied to the particular question under discussion.

Overall, the attention which has so far been paid to the problem of implementing EBM has been partial. It is clearly not sufficient to treat it as solely a matter of communication. . . .

Rival epistemologies

The epistemological underpinnings of randomised controlled trials and meta-analyses which, as we have seen above, form the basis of the EBM movement are in fact not necessarily identical with the way working clinicians think about evidence of effectiveness. This has recently been examined in a small-scale, but important American study of clinicians (Tanenbaum, 1994). In her study, Tanenbaum contrasts the traditional biomedical model of research, which is based in laboratory methods, with that entailed by RCTs. This contrast is summarised in Table 26.2.

For the sake of contrast Table 26.2 presents the two epistemologies as ideal types, though in the real world it seems unlikely that many clinicians are not influenced by elements of both. The point, however, is that *in the last analysis* it is the traditional model that predominates in medical decision making. (In contrast, as Table 26.1 above makes clear, the health services research model places clinical observations at the bottom of the hierarchy of evidence.) The traditional model, taught to and espoused by clinicians, relies on the discovery of cause–effect mechanisms by the observation of the way in which disease processes develop over time and impact upon normal physiological processes. Treatment is therefore very much a *logical* process of intervening in the aetiology (natural history) of a disease so as to arrest, reverse or retard it. Expressed in more philosophical/technical terms, the model is *deterministic* (that is, it assumes that clinical events necessarily have causes which can be identified and, in principle, modified) and *realist* or *naturalist* (that is, it entails a belief in a world of objectively real entities whose nature can be observed).

The outcomes/RCT model is the foundation of epidemiology and the relatively new discipline of health services research. It consists primarily of the *inference* of cause–effect relationships from past statistical relationships between treatment and outcomes. It is therefore less concerned with disease processes than with establishing what interventions are *likely to be effective, irrespective of why*. In technical/ philosophical language, the model is therefore *probabilistic* (that is, one where the

Table 26.2 Alternative epistemologies in medicine and research

Traditional biomedical laboratory research	*Outcomes research / randomised controlled trials*
Reveals cause–effect mechanisms (via aetiology pathology, etc.)	Demonstrates statistical relationships from past experience
Provides knowledge of what *ought to be* effective	Provides knowledge of what is *likely* to work, irrespective of how and why
Based on deterministic models	Based on probabilistic models
Underpinned by realist/naturalist epistemology	Underpinned by empiricist/positivist epistemology
Espoused by working clinicians	Espoused by epidemiologists and health services researchers

Source: Adapted from Tanenbaum, 1994.

cause–effect relationships are inherently uncertain) and *empiricist* (that is, one where knowledge can only justifiably be derived from past experience).

A very practical consequence of these apparently rather abstruse observations is that clinical doctors are more likely to be influenced in their practice by their own (and close colleagues') experience with similar types of patient, and by their own reasoning about treatment logic, than by the publication of meta-analyses of large numbers of cases. This, of course, is highly consonant with the individualistic ethic of the practice of medicine and the habit of doctors of being influenced by their own experience of single cases, a habit that is reflected by the occasional column in the *British Medical Journal* entitled 'A memorable patient'.

Concluding remarks: meso- and macro-level perspectives

The above analysis has been mainly concerned with the meso-level of politics, with occasional references to the micro. It might be summarised as having identified three main areas of naivety built into current policy for EBM. First, the attention so far paid to the problem of implementing EBM has been partial; it is clearly not sufficient to treat it as solely a matter of communication. Second, it is not uncommon to find disputes about what is the probability of an intervention's being effective, and about who is authorised to determine it; EBM is as much a social and political artefact as a scientific or technical one. Finally, it is not the outcomes/RCT model of knowledge, but rather the biomedical/laboratory one which is consonant with the individualistic ethic of the practice of medicine and the habit of doctors of being influenced by their own experience of single cases. The outcome of the policy of EBM remains to be discovered empirically. From a meso perspective, its chances look slim; all the above naiveties amount to the assumption of a consensus where there is none. From a more macro perspective, there is a sense in which EBM looks like a project which runs against the tide of the times: a late flowering of Fordism in a post-Fordist world, a blossoming of rationalism in a postmodern world. To address whether this is the case requires separate consideration of these two viewpoints.

First, post-Fordism: it has been argued elsewhere (Harrison, 1988: 110–1) that, whilst elements of the welfare state such as the NHS are important legitimators of the capitalist state, one should not assume a linear relationship between expenditure and the degree of legitimacy which it provides. Thus, 'cutting out waste' by means of the managerialist solutions applied to the NHS during the 1980s (Harrison et al, 1992) can be seen as one method for sustaining its legitimation function whilst controlling expenditure: a Fordist labour process applied, as it were, to the production of legitimacy and hence constituting a Fordist mode of regulation (Lipietz, 1992). Whether seen as labour process or mode of regulation (Jessop, 1992), post-Fordism does not however seem to entail the complete abandonment of Fordist methods; Hoggett (1990: 4) cites the familiar example of McDonald's, and Harrison et al (1992: 14–5) have noted the strong Fordist elements in the Griffiths general management reforms of the NHS which began in the mid-1980s, and have argued that they may well be a necessary condition for the more obviously post-Fordist developments of the purchaser–provider split. Rather, as Hoggett also notes, the core of post-Fordism is its rejection of the notion that there is a single 'best way' of production: mass production by an integrated organisation. In its place is 'the progressive decentralisation of production under conditions of rising flexibility and centralised strategic control' (Hoggett, 1990: 5; see also Hirst and Zeitlin, 1992). Given that the production of personal medical/health services is necessarily decentralised to individual clinicians (and, as noted above, that flexibility has already been enhanced by the creation of the purchaser–provider split), it might be expected that post-Fordist change in the NHS would entail the assertion of greater strategic control over medical production. Indeed, as the NHS becomes more flexible, with production increasingly delegated to general practice and similar settings (the so-called 'primary care-led NHS'; NHS Executive, 1995), such control may be seen as even more inevitable. Moreover, in principle at least, the algorithmic guidelines which, as has been seen, form a core element of EBM are capable of computerisation, a key strategy of post-Fordist control. Without assuming that it represents the only possible dimension of such strategic control, it is nevertheless clear that EBM is comprehensible as an element of the post-Fordist mode of regulation, and is in this sense not out of its time.

Whilst post-Fordism and postmodernism have a number of insights and observations in common (flexibility and the rejection of single 'best ways' are key examples) they imply fundamentally different epistemologies, a factor which makes the postmodern perspective much more inimical to EBM than is post-Fordism. Postmodernism's strong element of constructivism or epistemological relativism (Fox, 1993) is radically different from the philosophical realism which underpins both the naturalist and the positivist epistemologies outlined above. Postmodernism implies rejection of the unique truth claims of EBM. Indeed, it is often seen as a threat to medicine as a whole (see, for instance, Hodgkin, 1996), or more broadly to science as a whole. The proponents of the latter, unsurprisingly, have begun to defend their enterprise against this threat, for example, by the proliferation of academic posts in the 'public understanding of science' (Levinson and Thomas, 1997). EBM therefore has the prospect of becoming an additional component in this defence of science, thereby adding a further dimension of dissensus to an ostensibly commonsense policy.

References

Alford, R.R. (1975) *Healthcare politics*, Chicago, IL: University of Chicago Press.

Allaire, Y. and Firsirotu, M.E. (1984) 'Theories of organisational culture', *Organisation Studies*, vol 5, no 3: 193–226.

Andersen, T.F. and Mooney, G. (1990) *The challenge of medical practice variations*, Basingstoke: Macmillan.

Baker, M.R. and Kirk, S. (eds) (1996) *Research and development for the NHS: evidence, evaluation and effectiveness*, Oxford: Radcliffe Medical Press.

Black, N. and Thompson, E. (1993) 'Obstacles to medical audit: British doctors speak', *Social Science and Medicine*, vol 36, no 7: 849–56.

Brewster, C.J., Gill, C.G. and Richbell, S. (1981) 'Developing an analytical approach to industrial relations policy', *Personnel Review*, vol 10, no 2: 15–18.

Brook, R.H. (1989) 'Practice guidelines and practising medicine', *Journal of the American Medical Association*, vol 262, no 23: 3027–31.

Canadian Taskforce on the Periodic Health Examination (1979) 'Taskforce report: the periodic health examination', *Canadian Medical Association Journal*, vol 121, no 9: 1139–254.

Cochrane, A.L. (1972) *Effectiveness and efficiency: random reflections on health services*, London: Nuffield Provincial Hospitals Trust.

Department of Health (1991) *Research for health*, London: DoH.

Effective Health Care (1992) *The treatment of persistent glue ear in children*, Leeds: University of Leeds.

Effective Health Care (1994) *Implementing clinical practice guidelines*, no 8, Leeds and York: University of Leeds Nuffield Institute for Health and University of York Centre for Reviews and Dissemination.

Effective Health Care (1995) *The management of menorrhagia*, no 9, Leeds and York: University of Leeds Nuffield Institute for Health and University of York Centre for Reviews and Dissemination.

Fox, N. (1993) *Postmodernism, sociology and health*, Buckingham: Open University Press.

Greco, P.J. and Eisenberg, J.M. (1993) 'Changing physicians' practices', *New England Journal of Medicine*, vol 329, no 17: 1271–3.

Grimshaw, J. and Russell, I.T. (1993) 'Achieving health gain through clinical guidelines I: developing scientifically valid guidelines', *Quality in Healthcare*, vol 2: 243–8.

Gunn, L.A. (1978) 'Why is implementation so difficult?', *Management Services in Government*, vol 33, no 4: 169–76.

Haines, A. and Feder, G. (1992) 'Guidance on guidelines: writing them is easier than making them work', *British Medical Journal*, vol 305: 785–6.

Harrison, S. (1988) *Managing the National Health Service: shifting the frontier?* London: Chapman and Hall.

Harrison, S. (1994) 'Knowledge into practice: what's the problem?', *Journal of Management in Medicine*, vol 8, no 2: 9–16.

Harrison, S. (1997) 'Clinical autonomy and UK health policy: past and futures' in M. Exworthy and S. Halford (eds) *Professionals and managers in the public sector: conflict, compromise and collaboration*, Buckingham: Open University Press.

Harrison, S. and Long, A.F. (1989) 'Concepts of performance in medical care organisations', *Journal of Management in Medicine*, vol 3, no 3: 176–92.

Harrison, S., Pohlman, C.E. and Mercer, G. (1984) *Concepts of clinical freedom amongst English physicians*, Paper presented at EAPHSS Conference on Clinical Autonomy, King's Fund Centre, 8 June.

Harrison, S., Hunter, D.J., Marnoch, G. and Pollitt, C.J. (1992) *Just managing: power and culture in the National Health Service*, London: Macmillan.

Hirst, P. and Zeitlin, J. (1992) 'Flexible specialisation versus post-Fordism: theory, evidence and policy implications' in M. Storper and A.J. Scott (eds) *Pathways to industrialisation and regional development*, London: Routledge.

Hodgkin, P. (1996) 'Medicine, postmodernism and the end of certainty', *British Medical Journal*, vol 313: 1568–9.

Hoggett, P. (1990) *Modernisation, political strategy and the welfare state: an organisational perspective*, Bristol: SAUS Publications.

Hood, C. (1976) *The limits of administration*, London: Wiley.

House of Lords Select Committee on Science and Technology (1988) *Third report: priorities in medical research*, HL Paper 54–1, London: HMSO.

Hughes, D. and Yule, B. (1991) *Incentives and the remuneration of general practitioners*, HERU Discussion Paper 02/91, Aberdeen: University of Aberdeen Health Economics Research Unit.

Jessop, B. (1992) 'Fordism and post-Fordism: a critical reformulation' in M. Storper and A.J. Scott (eds) *Pathways to industrialisation and regional development*, London: Routledge.

Kingdon, J.W. (1984) *Agendas, alternatives and public policy*, Boston, MA: Little Brown.

Klein, R.E. (1983) *The politics of the National Health Service*, London: Longman.

Klein, R.E., Day, P. and Redmayne, S. (1996) *Managing scarcity: priority setting and rationing in the National Health Service*, Buckingham: Open University Press.

Levinson, R. and Thomas, J. (eds) (1997) *Science today: problem or crisis?* London: Routledge.

Lipietz, A. (1992) *Towards a new economic order: post-Fordism, ecology and democracy*, Cambridge: Polity Press.

Lipsky, M. (1980) *Street-level bureaucracy*, New York, NY: Russell Sage Foundation.

MacFarlane, J.K., Ryall, R.D.H. and Heald, R.J. (1993) 'Mesorectal excision for rectal cancer', *The Lancet*, vol 341: 457–60.

Meek, V.L. (1988) 'Organizational culture: origins and weaknesses', *Organization Studies*, vol 9, no 4: 453–73.

Melia, K.M. (1987) *Learning and working: the occupational socialisation of nurses*, London: Tavistock.

MORI (1993) *British public opinion*, December, London: MORI.

Mugford, M., Banfield, P. and O'Hanlon, M. (1991) 'Effects of feedback of information on clinical practice: a review', *British Medical Journal*, vol 303: 398–402.

Mulrow, C. (1994) 'Rationale for systematic reviews', *British Medical Journal*, vol 309: 597–9.

NHS Executive (1995) *Developing NHS purchasing and GP fundholding: towards a primary care-led NHS*, London: Department of Health.

NHS Executive (1996a) *Promoting clinical effectiveness: a framework for action in and through the NHS*, London: Department of Health.

NHS Executive (1996b) *Clinical guidelines: using clinical guidelines to improve patient care within the NHS*, London: Department of Health.

NHS Management Executive (1993) *Improving clinical effectiveness: executive letter* (93)115, Leeds: Department of Health.

Russell, I. and Grimshaw, J. (1992) 'The effectiveness of referral guidelines: a review of the methods and findings of published evaluations', in M. Roland and A. Coulter (eds) *Hospital referrals*, Oxford: Oxford University Press.

Sackett, D.L., Rosenberg, W.M.C., Gray, J.A.M., Haynes, R.B. and Richardson, W.S. (1996) 'Evidence-based medicine: what it is and what it isn't', *British Medical Journal*, vol 312: 71–2.

Tanenbaum, S.J. (1994) 'Knowing and acting in medical practice: outcomes research', *Journal of Health Politics, Policy and Law*, vol 19, no 1: 27–44.

Task Force on Research and Development Funding (1994) *Supporting research and development in the NHS* (Culyer Report), London: Department of Health.

Timmins, N. (1996) 'NHS "wastes £1bn" on ineffective treatments', *Independent*, 2 January:.

Williams, A. (1985) *Medical ethics: health service efficiency and clinical freedom*, Nuffield/York Portfolio no 2. London: Nuffield Provincial Hospitals Trust.

Chapter 27

Donald W. Light and David Hughes

A SOCIOLOGICAL PERSPECTIVE ON RATIONING
Power, rhetoric and situated practices

From D. Hughes and D. W. Light (eds) *Rationing: Constructed Realities and Professional Practices*, Oxford: Blackwell (2002)

T HE ANALYTIC POWER of sociology stems from examining closely the deep structures and power relations that underlie the rhetorics and practices of individuals, groups and organisations, by assuming a radical disengagement from them. Such is the analytic promise of sociological research into rationing, where unexamined rhetoric prevails and detailed empirical studies are thin on the ground. Intellectuals and policy makers, as well as those who pay the bills – be they governmental bodies, employers, insurers, or individuals – need the unclouded gaze of the sociological eye more than ever, as the rhetorics of rationing swirl around them. For rationing has become a predominant issue in the economic, moral and political discourses on health care. Yet as Conrad and Brown (1993: 3) observed, 'rationing has received little sociological attention'.

The sociological perspective has much to offer. At a time when scholarly thinking about rationing is dominated by the discipline of economics, sociology can help us to understand how economic transactions are embedded in social relations (Granovetter, 1985), which place limits on calculative rationality. Rationing provides a valuable array of social practices for exploring power relations in health care systems, particularly the linkage between resource allocation, rhetoric and the interests of different parties. Sociological studies can also complement and extend philosophical and ethical work on rationing by providing empirical case material grounded in the practical circumstances of real-world decision making, and investigating whether the ethical issues recognised by actors in the health care system correspond with those described in the scholarly literature . . .

The fallacy of inevitable rationing

As rationing has gained prominence in intellectual and policy circles, one increasingly hears that it has always been there, like Monsieur Jourdain in Molière's *Le Bourgeois Gentilhomme*, who learns that he has been speaking prose all his life. For example, a widely read article on the subject begins by stating that: 'Medical care has always been rationed by the supply available, by its distribution, and by the public's ability to pay' (Mechanic 1995: 1655). But what, exactly, does this mean? Was it rationed even in the decades when numerous studies documented in the United States surpluses of doctors and hospital beds, as well as large portions of excessive and unnecessary tests, prescriptions, operations, hospital admissions and bed days? (We will get to the uninsured later.) Still more broadly, a leading moral philosopher writes, 'Whenever we design institutions that distribute these goods, and whenever we operate those institutions, we are involved in rationing' (Daniels 1994; 27). If rationing always takes place, does that mean one cannot imagine a state in which medical care is not rationed? . . .

Arguably, rationing is not simply a product of an imbalance between supply and demand, but is also shaped by a layering of cultural beliefs and social organisation. David Hunter (1997: 20) hints at what we have in mind when he writes: 'So, given how politicians and public conceive of the issue, rationing, priority-setting, making choices, or whatever term is preferred, is inevitable at least to *some* degree.' Arguably, 'conceptions' are crucial. Rationing is not an invariant economic fact (although there are circumstances where it may be inescapable), but rather a central component of contemporary political and social discourses on the allocation of health care resources.

We argue that the concept of rationing is to a large extent a rhetorical construction: it formulates a particular linkage between allocative decisions and resources which can work to support certain interests against others. It is a way of framing reality that came to prominence in Western countries in the late 20th century, and which constructs the nature of resource allocation processes differently from the discourses of the past . . . A sociological research agenda must incorporate many previously neglected questions: what different stakeholders mean by 'rationing', what criteria they invoke when they say it is happening, what agenda they have in advancing their arguments, and what practitioners actually do and how they understand the reality they construct. We will first examine some of the prominent rhetorics, and then show how deeply 'rationing' is a socially constructed reality . . .

Parsing the rhetorics of rationing

Behind the increasing prevalence of statements that 'rationing is inevitable' lies the world view of economic theory and the degree to which it is being taken up by political scientists, moral philosophers, policy makers and politicians without sufficient examination. Economics is based on the assumption of scarcity: there is never enough of anything and therefore rationing is ubiquitous. Thus many economists equate rationing with choice, and assume that scarcity always exists and that priority-setting is an inherent part of rational choice (Begg *et al.* 1987). This too is a model-driven rhetoric, a mental construct that needs empirical examination and appears to be highly contestable, even within its own terms of reference.

Consider the basic model of modern microeconomics, taught around the world. That model assumes that all resources and services are scarce. Further, it asserts a 'principle of non-satiation', stating that people are never satisfied (Katz and Rosen 1991: Chapter 1). This guarantees scarcity, even of things that are abundant. Economic behaviour therefore focuses on how to deal with scarcity. The standard model assumes that people deal with scarcity by having preferences and by trying to maximise their preferences in rank order of priority (1991: Chapter 2). That is, rational choice is complete (one's preferences are clearly ranked and complete) and transitive (one prefers in rank order). Within the constructed world of the micro-economic model of reality, this leads to defining which combinations of trade-offs are equivalent so that one can plot an 'indifference curve' of points at which a person is indifferent about one combination or another. In short, rationing is inherent in all choices. If you choose to see a friend, whether you think about it or not (a sign of irrationality), you are choosing it over other things you would like to do and over seeing other friends in the same time-slot. Thus, maximising one's preferences, given their rankings and ratios, means maximising one's indifference curve until one reaches 'equilibrium', which is defined as reaching one's highest indifference curve within one's financial constraints or time constraints. Otherwise, one is wasting resources (time, money) and is acting irrationally.

So far, this model cannot predict or rank because no values have been assigned. This shortcoming is overcome by assigning 'utilities' to one's preferences. This allows one to calculate 'opportunity costs' which are the value of all the alternatives one might have chosen. It also allows one to write all the basic equations of microeconomics, their constants and slopes, so as to measure and predict all the choice/rationing trade-offs inherent in the model.

There are intuitive and experiential reasons to question this model that under-lies much modern economic policy analysis. Let us consider pure choice with no rationing consequences for others, choices with indirect consequences, and choices with direct consequences. If you go to a restaurant and choose the grilled bass, is this rationing? Clearly yes, says the dismal science. You have just foregone other entrées. Indeed we often weigh the choices offered by a menu and are very aware of what we have not chosen. What does the concept mean in these circumstances?

Now suppose you are at a family barbeque and you choose the pork chop, not the chicken or the burger, because you prefer it. The dismal science would point out that in choosing the chop, no one else can have it, a decision that has direct rationing consequences for others. Or does it? Suppose the other two did not want the pork chop in the first place?

'Would you like an aisle or window seat?' the airline reservationist asks. You like a window, but you don't like to climb over others to stretch or go to the toilet; so you choose an aisle seat. So far, this is like choosing the grilled bass, but suppose aisle seats are popular? Then your choice has indirect rationing consequences for others. Sociologically, how shall we understand such situations? Usually, they are more complex. For example, a number of patients on surgical waiting lists report that they pay privately for a consultation and then the consultant jumps them up and operates on them the next week. This is the low-cost way to get quick elective surgery, and of course it pushes everyone else back. Is this 'rationing' and if so in what sense, with what organisational dynamics?

The assumption of non-satiation needs examination. There is a five-day holiday coming up; shall we fly to a sun-dappled beach or go visit Grandma who lives across the country? Shall the government allocate more for education, or more for health care? Does it matter that we have been able both to visit Grandma and get away to a beach in the past several months? Does it matter how big the budget is for education and for health care? The implication is that calling these 'rationing' is based on thinking, 'But the budget could always be bigger' or 'You can't do everything all at once'. Priority setting need not be considered rationing, unless so declared.

Is enough never enough, by definition, even when people seemed quite satisfied? For example, a number of countries seem to have provided virtually all the health care that patients want or need in a timely manner for decades (Light 1997b). There is a bottom to the so-called bottomless pit of demand for health care, because people do have other things they like to do with their lives besides go to doctors and enter hospitals. In fact, many people shun them. To say that rationing 'always exists' or is 'inevitable', then, must be true by definition. As stated in a *British Medical Journal* round-up on rationing, 'Scarcity leads to a need to choose what to purchase and what not to purchase (that is, rationing)' (Donaldson 1996). 'I'll take the pork chop.' Thus 'rationing is inevitable' could be replaced with 'choice is inevitable' without missing a logical beat. Yet what a difference! The fallacy of defining a term as referring to nearly everything and being pervasive and inevitable is that it tells us nothing. The world is ready, in short, for a more differentiated, grounded and empirical account of what 'rationing' means and how it is carried out.

A sociological approach would be radically empirical about the claims of the microeconomic model. What preferences do people, or organisations or governments have, and how do they employ them in making choices with economic consequences? To what extent do they weigh and rank their preferences, or jump around, or use different frames in intermingled ways? To what extent do they estimate, or even think about, the 'opportunity costs' of what they have chosen not to do as they choose what to do? (Planners may point out that paying for a new costly drug that helps 2 per cent of patients could be used for a prevention programme in heart disease that would benefit 22 per cent, but are budgetary discussions carried on this way?) To the extent that people do not weigh and rank within a consistent frame, the concept of rationing has no logical basis and invocations of 'rationing' need to be understood in other ways.

Continua and rationing decisions

One possible solution to this definitional problem is to reframe rationing as a form of collective planning that suppresses individual choice. We might say that rationing happens when people are denied scarce resources, which they would have chosen if given the opportunity, and which would have been of benefit to them. Many scholars maintain that health care rationing only occurs when a person is denied a treatment or service that s/he needed and/or which would have been of benefit. How far does this rescue the argument about the economic inevitability of rationing?

The immediate problem that one encounters is that need or benefit must be measured on multiple dimensions, which generally do not share a common pattern. For example, Norman Daniels (1994), one of the most prominent moral philosophers of justice and rationing, argues that justifiable health care is limited to services that patients need and that are effective. In theory, this eliminates large volumes of demand, the growing number of drugs and operations that enhance normal capacities, and scores of ineffective tests or procedures. Yet each key term is surrounded by a continuum of ambiguity.

The need–demand continuum

The demand for most needed tests, drugs or procedures can be characterised as a triangle in which need fills the upper peak, demand fills the broad base and both become increasingly intermingled as one moves towards the middle. However, the picture is not static. The concept, or at least practice, of professionally certified need shifts as more services become available. No natural cut-off point is evident between rationing and non-rationing. One cannot identify a change in the pattern of need that allows one to draw a line where treatment should cease to be provided. Further, any plausible cut-off point will change as volume increases and expectations change. A good example would be the 'need' for hip or knee replacements. Even if clinical criteria for need are developed, it is the sociological dynamics of this process, the social construction of eligibility criteria and local practices that will shape real allocative decisions.

The effective–ineffective continuum

Effectiveness, however defined, is relative and a continuous variable with no clear cut-off. Different parties may define 'rationing' in different ways amongst themselves, and between different modes of production or service. Adverse and side effects add further complexity to determining what is 'effective'. There is no point at which 'rationing' begins, and therefore, any claim of rationing is a socially or politically constructed reality. Most continua of effectiveness or cost-effectiveness are unlikely to be linear. The question remains, where does 'rationing' begin? and thus what medical care is 'necessary?'

Nor is this question answered by recent attempts to make rationing 'rational' by recasting it as a set of systematic techniques to guide allocative decisions. Two tools, which have been subjected to considerable study and refinement and aim to allocate resources so that the greatest benefit is enjoyed by the greatest number of people, are quality adjusted life years and its cousin, disability adjusted life years. QALYs and DALYs, however, pose a number of problems. For example, they discriminate against people with chronic conditions who are unlikely to get better or are even getting worse (Alzheimer's disease comes to mind), and they presume to compare apples, oranges and pears on the grounds that they are all fruit. Or, to put it more formally, it is not 'feasible to collapse the multifaceted phenomena of life and its quality on to a single valid scale' (Hunter 1997: 72). Any attempt to quantify the quality of people's lives will be biased in its measures and sample. There are a number of practical and technical problems as well (Hunter 1997: 70–73). The point at which taking away more or fewer QALYs from an individual or population constitutes rationing cannot be resolved by a technical formula. Does rationing begin when the first QALY is taken away from a population? Most of the time health decision makers do not even know if it is happening.

Much more significant in practice are the large-scale efforts to ground clinical practices in scientific medicine – the movement known as evidence-based medicine (EBM). Enthusiasts believe that EBM will minimise rationing, because all ineffective tests, drugs and procedures will be stopped and the money saved will pay for effective interventions (for example, Roberts *et al.* 1996). This theory sounds fine, though even at its best EBM will produce evidence of marginal gains, trade-offs between benefits and complications or harms, and evidentiary ambiguity. The problem of how benefits are measured, like measuring improved quality of life, arises again, as does the problem of transposing different kinds of benefits into one scale. How, for example, does one weigh reduced risk of death against increased chances of impotence in the treatment of cancer, and how does one scale what these trade-offs mean for different men? Further, women favour reduced risk of death over less sex, while male partners favour sexual activities more heavily. Such problems point to internal forms of rationing embedded in methods used, samples drawn, and scales constructed – all by a technological élite that is usually invisible and not accountable to the patients affected. If one surmounts these difficulties, one comes again to a spate of practical problems of implementing evidence-based medicine, starting with the low priority that doctors and even purchasers give to such evidence, and ending with the complexities of applying epidemiological evidence to individual cases (Tanenbaum 1994, Frankford 1994, Hunter 1997). In terms of rationing, EBM poses the same problems as those posed by 'effectiveness'. In the absence of natural cut-off points in much of the data on effectiveness and costs, it is unclear conceptually where rationing begins to occur or, if rationing is framed as a technical exercise, where different decision tools indicate that treatments should cease to be provided.

Does rationing happen in voluntary markets?

One anomaly in economic theories of scarcity occurs when rationing is claimed to be inevitable, yet price competition is not considered to be 'rationing'; for 'rationing' is used to refer to non-price ways of allocating scarce resources. Such decisions may be made by politicians or clinicians at either the micro or macro level (through writing national protocols), but their nature is economic. Further, such conscious and planned forms of allocation, through QALYs or clinical protocols, are presumed to be just and fair. When forms of rationing are advocated in favour of 'just letting things happen' or leaving doctors to make their autonomous decisions, it is usually provoked by evidence of mischief or untrustworthy behaviour. To put this in the terms of David Hume and his modern interpreter, Julian LeGrand (1997), rationing aims to eliminate knavish behaviours towards pawns and supplant them with knightly schemes. Indeed, rationing presumes paternalism and trust in the knights, while markets presume people are knaves and aim to curb their clever knaveries by pitting them against each other so that self-seeking behaviours work for the common good.

Especially in the United States, many regard the notion of 'rationing by price' as a contradiction in terms. If allocations occur through prices and markets, that is regarded as 'natural'. Somehow, the choice-is-rationing argument gets dropped, so that allocating scarce resources by price is acceptable, while planned mechanisms which restrict access to care are not, and rationing per se is an unnatural, contrived way of allocating scarce resources.

This argument is central to whether health-care rationing can be said to exist at all in the United States or other systems that lack a mechanism for providing universal access to health care. Some claim that it does, as when Conrad and Brown (1993:11) write: 'one of the most disturbing examples of allocative rationing is the existence of roughly 37 million people without any health insurance'. We sympathise, and the number of uninsured, net of new people insured, has been rising by about 100,000 a month, every year since that time. But our sympathy rests on the premise that health insurance should be universal, not sold in a voluntary market that is ruled by the 'inverse coverage law' that has spawned a variety of ways to discriminate against those with health needs (Light 1992). Conrad and Brown probably share this assumption; but it is important to be clear that, given the logic of the voluntary health care market, this is not 'rationing'. In the United States, there is no general right to health care. Yet ambivalent feelings lead to Medicare, Medicaid and other public programmes, like food stamps and public housing, as specific interventions to deal with some forms of market failure in the mainstream private market.

Sociologists investigating denied services must take full, proper account of the logic of the market and the way it frames reality. This is central to American-style managed care. Employers and governments have turned health care over to for-profit managed care corporations, to what Uwe Reinhardt (1996) calls in his colourful but insightful account 'bounty hunters'. Employers and governments, after years of failed efforts to get American physicians to help them restrain costs, hired corporate bounty hunters to 'shoot down' costs for rewards in the millions. Was this rationing? They 'shot down' very high fees and bed-day prices by forcing doctors and hospitals to take discounts. Both speak of 'rationing' but what does that mean, except 'less than we're used to having'? Some West Coast surgeons had their fees cut and saw their personal incomes plummet from $500,000 a year to $250,000. Was this rationing? American Medical Association data showed that, overall, physicians' incomes stopped rising and stayed flat. Hospitals claim that discounted payments 'ration' charity care, but even non-profit hospitals have done little charity care, and the percentage of gross revenues devoted to charity care has not dropped substantially. The bounty hunters also cut hospital admissions and shortened lengths of stay. Was this rationing or cutting into the fat of unnecessary hospitalisation?

HMOs (health maintenance organisations) and MCOs (managed care organisa-tions) provide inferior care to patients who have chronic conditions, are elderly or are poor. They deny tests, hospital admissions, or operations, but is this 'rationing'? If we are seeking an authoritative definition of rationing, the answer is not clear. If the corporations use protocols based on effectiveness, even untested ones of their own choosing, or if the procedures are not covered in the particular health insurance policy of that particular patient, those involved may deny that rationing is occurring. The corporations have the same right as any corporation in a voluntary market to provide services according to the contractual terms specified. And yet for those who do not receive care, the results bear a close family resemblance to 'rationing' in other systems. Patients and their doctors often think the denials constitute rationing; but they do not seem to realise that this judgement presumes that health care is a right, when the US system assumes it is a commodity.

Getting inside the 'black box'

Given these definitional uncertainties how should policy makers, economists, researchers and moral philosophers proceed? Rationing takes place in several forms according to the most influential current literature: Diagnosis-related groups (DRGs), cost-sharing or user fees, capitation schemes, denial of services, fixed budgets, waiting lists and requirements for prior authorisation of treatments. We do not doubt that each of these might involve rationing, but they may not.

It depends on how actors conceive of 'rationing', and on actual practice and the details of what happens. Sociologically, what matters are the interactions, power relations, perspectives and agendas of the relevant parties. This is as relevant at the macro level of national political decisions, as it is at the meso level of US HMOs or British Primary Care Trusts, and the clinical micro level. Thus the first research objective is to get inside the 'black box' of organisations at different levels of the health care system to gauge what is happening on the ground.

The need for an up-close look is all too apparent with some of the examples mentioned above. For example, in order to stop the relentless increases in procedures and charges, the US Congress created DRGs by taking the average practices and charges after 25 years of escalation and bundling them into a single payment per diagnostic-related group. As the largest payer, Congress was saying, 'You can live within the totals you have built up, and we will pay no more.' Was this 'rationing'? Hospitals reacted as if it were, by dramatically reducing lengths of stay, nursing staff and the like. Their profit margins soared as they complained about this draconian form of 'rationing' by Congress.

User fees clearly reduce front-end use of services that patients control. Studies show they reduce in about equal proportions both unnecessary and needed services. They are a crude instrument that discriminates by class, but at what point might one say they are 'rationing'? How many of the needed services are effective?

Capitation schemes, like DRGs writ large, are based on historic patterns of utilisation and charges driven up during the decades of fee for service, and the questions are the same. If providers limit access or treatments within capitation contracts, especially US-sized ones, one needs to look more to the providers and their motives than capitation schemes per se.

Across the Atlantic, waiting lists seem to some like an inherent form of rationing, because everyone on them has been seen by a qualified clinician and deemed to need the service or treatment. But what is being rationed, especially if everyone is ultimately treated? The most likely candidates are waiting itself, perhaps suffering, anxiety, the impaired ability to carry out a full life, and the reduced risk of increased morbidity or mortality that early treatment might bring.

Other 'grey areas' in the UK context include prior authorisation of extra contractual referrals (ECRs) in the NHS internal market, and restrictions on the prescribing of 'life-style' drugs such as Viagra (Redwood 2000). In the 'Child B' case, a health authority that had refused to fund a second bone-marrow transplant as an ECR argued that it did so because expert medical opinion suggested that the chance of a successful outcome was minimal. Subsequently, 'Child B' obtained the desired treatment by other means but lived for only a short time. Yet many thought cost had been a factor in the decision and accusations of rationing persisted. Viagra, and more recently the anti-obesity drug Orlistat, were regarded by many British health authorities as medically unnecessary drugs that would not normally be purchased from core budgets. However, some observers argue that these drugs are prescribed for health-damaging conditions, and that a blanket ban which ignores individual patients' circumstances constitutes rationing. The National Institute of Clinical Excellence, the institution set up by the UK Government in 1999 to provide national guidelines on the clinical effectiveness of particular interventions, issued guidance on Orlistat in March 2001, setting out a fairly narrow range of circumstances in which the drug should be prescribed, but has not so far considered Viagra. In all these cases the factors which shape decisions require close empirical examination. Although the presence or absence of rationing is likely to remain a contentious issue, we need to know more about how actors weigh the various factors and whether they perceive that a rationing process is at work.

One test of where rationing begins is to ask: 'under what conditions would you say there is no rationing?' Would this be the case if everyone were seen the same day they were referred, or the same week, or month?' This question can be applied to all the assertions about rationing. At the macro level, how big would the budget have to be before those who claim that the government or programme is rationing would agree that no more rationing is taking place? At the meso level, how many hospitals, how close together, would there have to be before a given stakeholder, or policy analyst, would say that geographical rationing is not taking place? Less than a 60-minute bus ride? Less than 30 minutes? Less than 15? How short would waiting times have to be? Of course, different observers will answer these questions in different ways. They will make a case for drawing the line in one place rather than another, or perhaps talk of grey areas where they acknowledge that it is hard to say. We are brought back once again to the micro-politics of rationing as a struggle over definitions, reflecting different situated interests and perspectives.

Power relations in rationing

Economic concepts of rationing as reasoned choice, or a set of techniques for the rational allocation of resources, tend to obscure the underlying power relationships involved. Whether allocation decisions are made by politicians, managers, doctors or intellectuals, the typical pattern is that a small group of élite actors ration services for others. It is true that decisions about priorities and trade-offs might be made in a more transparent and participatory way (Daniels *et al.* 1996), but in practice such initiatives rarely amount to anything more than short-term experiments. More apparent is an ongoing power struggle in which politicians, policy makers, managers, clinicians and analysts try to justify or challenge allocative decisions. The rhetorics of rationing can be used to support arguments for both less care and more care. Politicians and managers can use it to justify reduced services and budgets, especially for the most vulnerable, in order to advance their own agendas on other fronts. Other managers and clinicians may try to use the 'R' word to mobilise public opposition to service reductions or failure to provide new services. Allegations of rationing can be seen as a particularly powerful form of claims-making activity (Spector and Kitsuse 1977), which at the extreme may lead the public to recognise a new social problem. Thus the use of rationing as political rhetoric is another fit subject for incisive research.

Rationing rests on the belief that those in power have the best interests of their subjects in mind and that one can trust them to allocate scarce resources fairly. Such beliefs are actually empirical questions to be researched. Waiting lists, for example, rest on the public's trust that doctors choose whom to treat next in terms of clinical needs, suffering and life circumstances; but there is little evidence that this is the case. Thus the correlation between long waiting lists and large private practices among surgeons, together with a contract that provides strong incentives to build up one's private practice (perhaps by encouraging long waiters to 'go private'), indicate that power is not always paternalistic (Yates 1996, Light 2000).

These conceptual points pertain directly to a favourite subject of debate, whether rationing should be implicit or explicit. This issue arises, as Mechanic (1995), Hunter (1997), and Griffiths and Hughes (1998) describe, because governments throughout the world have needed to hold down costs on public services and have turned to new modes of purchasing. In a brief history of the origins of managed care (Light 1997a), this is characterised as 'the buyers' revolt' because payers who had passively paid the rising medical bills for years started acting like active buyers. Whatever rationing took place before was implicit, and the argument is that purchasing requires one to be explicit about what services one wants, at what levels of quality and error rates, not unlike Ford purchasing differentials or door handles.

This movement has led, inter alia, to systematic efforts at both the local and national level to compare the outcomes of specified clinical procedures, define standards, collate scientific evidence on the effectiveness of procedures, tests and medicines, and develop guidelines about whether these should be purchased. Nevertheless, some of the best minds in the social sciences, like David Mechanic, Rudolf Klein and David Hunter, have issued warnings about explicit rationing and written in favour of implicit rationing. Many of their warnings are political; explicit rationing of health care will provoke the public and may tie health care policy into knots. They also emphasise the need to consider the highly variable circumstances and clinical conditions of patients who otherwise have the same disorder that would be subjected to the same protocol or explicit rule.

These critics make powerful points about the limitations of formal schemes of rationing. What their arguments can overlook, however, is that implicit rationing by doctors has been rife with evidence of large, unexplained variations, of unnecessary expenditures and of uneven quality because physicians put their autonomy and interests ahead of patients. That is, professional power and autonomy have too often not been exercised in trustworthy ways that manifest the application of medical science to the best interests of patients. Any arguments for the merits of implicit rationing must address these problems. While it is true that 'doctors' specialist knowledge remains irreplaceable, which itself places limits on managers' incursions into medical territory' (Hunter 1997: 56), specialists' knowledge can be – and is – subjected to clinical standards, guidelines and protocols developed by teams of specialists. It is the engineers at Ford who develop the 'specs' for purchasing differentials, not the managers. The key to a solution, we believe, lies in re-conceptualising professionalism around accountability rather than autonomy; so that the uses of power in both explicit and implicit rationing are subject to transparent review. The theoretical point is that rationing of both kinds involves power, but accountability is more effective than trust to keep the best interests of patients in focus . . .

References

Begg, D., Fischer, S. and Dornbusch, R. (1987) *Economics*, 2nd Edition. London and New York: McGraw-Hill.

Conrad, P. and Brown P. (1993) Rationing medical care: a sociological reflection, *Research in the Sociology of Health Care*, 10, 3–22.

Daniels, N. (1994) Meeting the challenges of justice and rationing. *Hastings Center Report*, 24, 4, 27–29.

Daniels, N., Light, D.W. and Caplan, R. (1996) *Benchmarks of Fairness for Health Care Reform*. New York: Oxford University Press.

Donaldson, C. (1996) Economics of priority setting: let's ration rationally! In Smith, R. (ed) *Rationing in Action*. London: BMJ Publishing Group.

Frankford, D.M. (1994) Scientism and economism in the regulation of health care, *Journal of Health Politics, Policy and Law*, 19, 158–9.

Granovetter, M. (1985) Economic action and social structure: the problem of embeddedness, *American Journal of Sociology*, 91, 481–510.

Griffiths, L. and Hughes, D. (1998) Purchasing in the British NHS: does contracting mean explicit rationing? *Health*, 2, 349–71.

Hunter, D.J. (1997) *Desperately Seeking Solutions: Rationing Health Care*. London and New York: Longman.

Katz, M.J. and Rosen, H.S. (1991) *Microeconomics*. New York: Irwin.

LeGrand, J. (1997) Knights, knaves or pawns? Human behaviour and social policy, *Journal of Social Policy*, 26, 149–69.

Light, D.W. (1992) The practice and ethics of risk-rated health insurance, *Journal of the American Medical Association*, 267, 2503–8.

Light, D.W. (1997a) The restructuring of the American health care system. In Litman, T.J. and Robbins, L.S. (eds) *Health Politics and Policy*. Albany, NY: Delmar.

Light, D.W. (1997b) The real ethics of rationing, *British Medical Journal*, 315, 112–15.

Light, D.W. (2000) NHS waiting lists: the hidden agenda, *Consumer Policy Review*, 10, 4, 126–32.

Mechanic, D. (1995) Dilemmas in rationing health care services: the case for implicit rationing, *British Medical Journal*, 310, 1655–9.

Redwood, H. (2000) *Why Ration Health Care?* Trowbridge: The Cromwell Press.

Reinhardt, U. (1996) *A Social Contract for 21st Century American Health Care: Three Tier Health Care with Bounty Hunting*. London: Nuffield Trust.

Roberts, C., Crosby, D., Grundy, P., Lewis, P., Long, J., Shellard, M. and Williams, A. (1996) The wasted millions, *The Health Service Journal*, 106, 5524, 24–7.

Spector, M. and Kitsuse, J.I. (1977) *Constructing Social Problems*. Menlo Park, California: Cummings.

Tanenbaum, S.J. (1994) Knowing and acting in medical practice, *Journal of Health Politics, Policy and Law*, 19, 27–44.

Yates, J. (1996) *Private Eye, Heart and Hip: Surgical Consultants, the National Health Service and Private Medicine*. London: Churchill Livingstone.

Chapter 28

Ray Fitzpatrick and Mary Boulton

QUALITATIVE METHODS FOR ASSESSING HEALTH CARE

From *Quality in Health Care*, 3, 1994: 107–13 (BMJ Publications)

THE EVALUATION OF HEALTH care and efforts to maintain and improve quality in health care have very largely drawn on quantitative methods. Quantification has made possible precise expression of the extent to which interventions are efficient, effective, or appropriate and has allowed the use of statistical techniques to assess the significance of findings. For many questions, however, quantitative methods may be neither feasible nor desirable. Qualitative methods may be more appropriate when investigators are "opening up" a new field of study or are primarily concerned to identify and conceptualise salient issues. Various qualitative methods have been developed which potentially have an enormous role in assessing health care. This paper examines some of the more important forms that have been used in that assessment and outlines principles of good practice in the application of qualitative methodology. It is intended to encourage a wider use of qualitative methods in assessing health care and a greater appreciation of how much such methods have to offer.

The term "qualitative" is sometimes used quite loosely. We will review some of the methods to which the term is properly applied, but first what is *not* a qualitative study should be emphasised. Research based on a small number of patients or respondents should not be considered qualitative just because the sample size is too small to assess statistical significance. This is more likely to prove to be an inadequate quantitative study. Similarly, a study is not qualitative because it is based on answers to a questionnaire about subjective matters nor because data are collected by personal interview. If such data are analysed and reported largely in terms of frequencies and proportions of respondents expressing particular views, that is also a quantitative study. Qualitative research depends upon not numerical but *conceptual* analysis and presentation. It is used where it is important to understand the meaning and interpretation of human social arrangements such as hospitals, clinics, forms of management, or decision making. Qualitative methods are intended to convey to policy makers the experiences of individuals, groups, and organisations who may be affected by policies.

Qualitative methods of data collection

Qualitative methods of collecting data encompass a range of approaches.

In depth interviews

Perhaps the main method of obtaining data for qualitative analysis is by interview. Interviews are a particularly flexible method of gathering data, allowing the investigator to respond to the individual way in which respondents interpret and answer questions. There are various interview formats, but qualitative analysis requires "in depth" interviews so the interviewer can obtain more detailed information than is possible, for example, from an interviewer administered questionnaire, particularly regarding the perceptions and reasons behind respondents' statements. Interviews may be "semistructured," where the interviewer has a fixed set of topics to discuss, or "unstructured," where the interviewer has only very broad objectives in relation to the interview and is largely led by the respondent's priorities and concerns. Unstructured interviews are most appropriate when subject matter is particularly complex or when investigators want to understand reasons for views or are exploring areas which have not previously been extensively described. An interview format increasingly used in health services research is the "critical incident technique," in which respondents are asked to recall the details of a particular experience such as hospitalisation.[1]

Because in depth interviews require the active participation and judgement of the interviewer it is important that they be conducted by interviewers who have been appropriately trained. There is a range of general interviewing skills that are relevant to performance, such as an ability to demonstrate interest in the respondent without excessive involvement that may result in bias and an ability to ask both open ended facilitating questions and specific probes when relevant. The interviewer also needs to understand the general objectives of a study as well as the intentions behind specific questions. Another essential requirement is that interviewers be perceived by respondents as neutral with regard to the subject matter of an interview. For example, hospital staff are inappropriate to conduct interviews about patient satisfaction, and individuals perceived as judgemental are inappropriate for more sensitive topics.

The analysis of in depth interviews normally entails some degree of formal content analysis of what the respondent has said. For this reason investigators usually tape record interviews which can then be transcribed for detailed content analysis. Broad principles of content analysis for qualitative research are discussed below as, to some extent, they are common to all of the methods discussed in this paper.

An illustration of the use of in depth interviews is a study of the neurological management of chronic headache.[2,3] Neurologists were unsure about the appropriateness of their role in this area. The initial purpose of the study was to identify the expectations of patients with chronic headache regarding their neurological referral, and to establish whether those expectations were satisfied. When interviewed before their outpatient appointments, patients proved quite unsure what to expect. Content analysis of these interviews instead disclosed a small number of different concerns felt by patients about their headaches – for example, a need to be reassured about serious disease or a desire to receive advice about how to change lifestyle or diet to avoid headaches. After their neurological consultations a minority of patients did experience serious disappointment with their clinic attendance but for various reasons were very uncomfortable with the language of "satisfaction" or "dissatisfaction" to describe their experiences. Overall the study suggested particular failures of communication in clinics that led to some patients' concerns not being fully addressed.

In this example the primary advantage of in depth interviews was that they allowed the investigator to focus maximally on patients' perceptions of their health problems and responses to health care rather than imposing his own categories. This led to a new and more meaningful typology of patients' concerns. Examples of other qualitative analyses of in depth interviews include studies of dimensions of patients' experiences of care for various chronic health problems,[4] of the role of clinical audit in British medicine,[5] of informal reasons for clinicians' use of echocardiography,[6] and of the concerns of singlehanded GPs in an inner London area.[7]

Focus groups

Groups rather than individuals may be interviewed by means of a technique commonly referred to as a focus group. Typically, eight to ten individuals are recruited to a group discussion about specified topics. The discussion is led by a trained moderator or facilitator and normally lasts for one and a half to two hours. The discussion is tape recorded, transcribed, and subjected to content analysis. Rather like the interviewer conducting in depth interviews, the moderator has a clear agenda of issues on which he or she stimulates discussion but aims to be fairly non-directive in encouraging discussion. Membership of a focus group needs to be reasonably homogeneous; too much heterogeneity in terms of social background or perspective on a topic tends to result in participants feeling inhibited from revealing views. Therefore if the purpose is to identify the range of views of individuals of different social backgrounds the normal practice is to conduct a series of focus groups.

Focus groups are particularly useful where investigators wish to establish quickly the range of perspectives on an issue of importance among different groups – for example, when it is felt necessary to "bridge a gulf" in understanding between providers of a service and the intended users. The dynamics of a well conducted focus group are such that individuals' revelations of their views can "spark off" other participants to reveal broader insights than are possible from individual interviews. However, focus group methods have been compared to "pulling teeth" to stimulate discussion in a group that has no experience or interest in a topic.[8] It is less appropriate in a focus group to probe for elaboration of individuals' statements than is possible in an in depth interview, so that focus groups may be said to be stronger on breadth than depth. The facilitator is less in control of a focus group than is an interviewer with single respondents so it is a method that maximises the expression of perspectives not imposed by the researchers. There are some topics that are sufficiently sensitive that group discussion is inhibiting whereas individual interviews provide a more confidential context for self revelation.

Focus groups are commonly regarded as an exploratory method, so that investigators may conduct them in order to design the questionnaire for a more definitive quantitative survey. Some would argue, however, that focus groups can provide valuable evidence in their own right, provided that investigators are concerned with conceptual rather than numerical analysis.[9]

There are questions still to be addressed with focus group methodology. For example, little is known about how the effects of social desirability and conformity influence expression of views and to what extent heterogeneity of participants influences results. Similarly, though facilitators clearly require substantial inter-personal skills such as ability to listen and to facilitate without becoming so involved as to bias discussion, facilitator effects on the quality of focus groups are not well understood.[9] However, health is a particularly appropriate application for this method,[10] which is being increasingly advocated for use by purchasers in obtaining local views about health and health care.[11,12]

Nominal group techniques

For some purposes a more impersonal and less threatening form of group dynamics may be needed. A somewhat more structured form of gathering data from groups has been developed, called "nominal groups" because exchange and interaction between group members is more controlled than in focus groups. It is considered a technique less prone to the bias arising from vocal individuals influencing a group's views in open discussion.[13]

A nominal group normally is composed of eight members who meet together with a leader who introduces the group's tasks. The leader explains the question or problem on which the group's views are sought. Individuals are asked to list on a paper form their different feelings or experiences in relation to the question (for example, different kinds of disappointments experienced by a group of users of a clinic), without discussion with other group members. Participants are then asked to declare their written comments which are recorded, as closely as possible to the participants' own words, on a blackboard or flipchart. The complete list is then discussed by the group and a preliminary ranking made by the group from most to least important item of the total list. After discussion of this preliminary ranking a second, private ranking of items is performed by individuals on paper. This infor-mation constitutes the researcher's core data. As with focus groups, investigators usually set up several different groups that are needed to represent the different perspectives with interests involved with an issue.

The primary advantages of this form of group research are that individuals may give more carefully considered expression of their views compared with focus groups and are constrained by the tasks to produce more structured and explicit priorities. The structured nature of data gathering means that this is a method particularly appropriate to contexts where technical or complex issues need to be assessed. The primary disadvantage is that individuals are discouraged from "sparking off" each other, so that it is possible that the full range of views and observations are not elicited. Overall, like focus groups, nominal group techniques are a relatively low cost and quick method of exploring the parameters of an issue.

A variant of this methodology has been developed for use in developing professional consensus about appropriate indications for health care interventions. Panels representing relevant clinical expertise are provided with patient vignettes with varying symptoms and other indications. Vignettes are privately rated in terms of degree of appropriateness for the intervention. The group is then actually assembled, it discusses the ratings, and it is given the opportunity to revise prior decisions. A recent example indicates that substantial agreement could be obtained regarding appropriateness for prostatectomy.[14] Most of the steps in data gathering and interpretation of this application of nominal group techniques are actually quantitative, and readers are referred elsewhere for methodological problems associated with such techniques.[15]

Observational studies

When the research question concerns what actually happens in health care settings, rather than participants' perceptions of and responses to it, a more appropriate method of data collection may be direct observation. For this method the investigators attend the events they are concerned with, pay close attention to what goes on, and make a careful record of it for future analysis, using analytical techniques similar to those for other qualitative data.

Careful recording of what occurs is the cornerstone of observational research. Field notes, taken during or immediately after periods of observation, have been the traditional method of recording. The value of field notes depends on the skill and discipline of the investigator in recording as much detail as accurately as possible. Field notes are inevitably selective and so may be subject to observer bias. However, they are a relatively efficient way of recording observations, particularly in sensitive situations, and provide data in a form that is immediately accessible for analysis. Audio recordings and video recordings provide a more detailed and accurate record of events, although the demands of the technology may limit the range of events that can be observed and the tapes themselves present considerable additional demands in terms in transcription before analysis. Tape recordings are attractive in that they allow the investigator to go back and "reobserve" events, which may allow more detailed analysis than is possible with field notes. They also afford a record of the evidence on which interpretations are made which may be inspected by independent observers in establishing the validity of the analysis. However, audio recorders and particularly video recorders have been criticised as being so obtrusive as to change the nature of the events they are recording, thereby invalidating the observation itself. With smaller machines and consulting rooms specifically adapted for recording this is becoming less of a problem, and, in any case, those who have been the subject of audio or video recording have almost always found that the need to deal with the immediate demands of the situation constrain them to carry on in much the same way as they would if they were not being observed.

Investigators may collect data as "participant" or as "non-participant observers." Participant observers participate in the daily life of the organisation over an extended period of time, watching what happens, listening to what is said, and asking questions. It is an exceptionally demanding way of gathering data. The researcher may encounter difficulties in being accepted by the group initially and then in sustaining the role long enough to observe the full range of events. The justification for such efforts is in the way participant observation enables the researcher to see and experience the institutional culture from the point of view of an "insider." Goffman's classic study of asylums illustrates well the unique insights that can be gained by this method of data collection.[16] Goffman joined an American mental hospital as the assistant to the athletic director in order to observe the culture of the institution without drawing attention to himself. The resulting study develops the concept of the "total institution," identifying its core elements and using it as a framework to describe and make sense of the culture of both the patients and the staff. By closely examining what actually went on in the hospital, he was able to get behind official accounts of what the institution did to show the process and strategies that made it work in practice, and the consequences they had for patients' lives.

Participant observation has become less common as a research method, partly because of questions raised about the ethics of covert observation. Non-participant observation allows the researcher to remain as an accepted outsider, watching and recording the interactions as a "fly on the wall." Non-participant observation is particularly useful when the researcher is concerned to describe and conceptualise the "taken for granted" practices of everyday medical life: the routines and strategies that those they are studying develop in carrying out their work which may be so common and familiar as to be outside their conscious awareness. An example is Strong's study described in *The Ceremonial Order of the Clinic* in which he set out to elucidate the rules which govern interactions in medical consultations.[17] On the basis of observations of 1120 paediatric consultations in several medical settings in Scotland and the United States he documented in detail the existence, nature, and scope of the rules which make up the limited number of institutionalised roles universally adopted by patients and doctors.

The main advantage of observation as a method of data collection is in allowing the investigators to "see for themselves," thus avoiding the biases inherent in participants' reports, such as selective perception, poor recall, and the desire to present themselves well. It is particularly appropriate when the investigator is concerned with describing and conceptualising how health services operate – that is, with practices and processes which are directly accessible to an outside observer. Its main drawback is that it limits the number and range of situations that can be studied to those at which the investigator is present. It is the most labour intensive form of data collection and perhaps for this reason is more often used in conjunction with other methods rather than as the main source of data.

Case studies

Case studies are not really a distinctive method of data collection or analysis but warrant separate discussion because they are increasingly used in the study of health care systems. They provide interpretations and analyses that are ultimately qualitative in nature. The most obvious respect in which case studies are qualitative is that typically they involve the study of a single or small number of units where quantitative manipulation of variables associated with units would be inappropriate. However, to a greater extent than the methods discussed so far, case studies often draw on a mixture of quantitative and qualitative data. An example illustrates the point. In 1986 a resource management (RM) inititative was announced for the NHS, the purpose of which was to improve patient care by providing systems whereby managers and clinicians made better informed and more effective use of resources. The initiative was to be piloted in six acute hospitals and the costs and benefits were to be evaluated by a research team.[18] Much quantitative data were gathered by investigators in relation to hospital activities and their costs in the pilot sites over time. However, as a number of other institutional changes to the NHS were simultaneously having effects in both the study hospitals and any potential "control" hospitals outside the pilot it was decided that it would be impossible to isolate quantitative benefits due to the resource management initiative specifically. Moreover, as with most human organisations, NHS defined objectives of the resource management initiative drifted over time. The authors concluded that qualitative evaluation of the initiative based on qualitative and quantitative evidence available was more informative. Qualitative inferences were drawn from the study such as that it was possible to involve clinicians in hospital resource management but that it was not clear that the high administrative and other costs associated with such involvement were matched by benefits to patient care.

Case studies such as the resource management study usually entail a combination of methods. Investigators carry out interviews, conduct participant observation on relevant meetings, and inspect written documents such as minutes or records. A systematic approach to interviews in an organisation can be adopted. For example, in a study of the impact of general management in the NHS, investigators, if confronted with discrepant accounts between different actors, would probe in interviews to obtain possible explanations.[19] Case studies attempt to get an accurate picture by means of "triangulation," whereby the degree of convergence between different sources (for example, interview and documents) is carefully considered.[20] A particular form of checking the plausibility of investigators' explanations is that of 'respondent validation' in which the analysis that has emerged of a setting is presented to participants for their reactions. By means of this technique analysis can be refined and improved by respondents' feedback.[19]

Qualitative analysis of data

If the distinguishing feature of quantitative evidence is the manipulation of numerical data then qualitative analysis is characterised by the development and manipulation of *concepts*. The investigator's primary tasks are the inspection and coding of his or her data in terms of concepts and then the manipulation of such concepts into analyses of underlying patterns. Although there are significant differences of form or emphasis, this crucial role of conceptual analysis is common to all of the qualitative methods outlined above. It is probably the phase of work that is most arcane and mysterious for audiences of qualitative reports and requires some account of how conceptual analysis of qualitative data is actually done.

Whatever method of data collection is used in qualitative methodology, it results in raw material in the form of "text" – written words. The first stage of processing text is to code and classify. The investigator therefore reviews his or her textual material for coding in terms of concepts and categories that may emerge from the material or that inform the investigator's study to begin with. This trans-formed, coded material can then be regrouped or indexed to facilitate further analysis. This stage of grouping and indexing coded material has been considerably eased by the development of computer packages such as Ethnograph, although such technology cannot replace the far more important human interpretation of text before mechanical manipulation.[21]

The next and most difficult stage is the analysis of both the original textual data and the transformed conceptual material. This phase is the most difficult to pre-scribe or indeed describe since it entails a large amount of creative interpretation of evidence. Thought processes include constant comparison of evidence regarding different settings or viewpoints represented in the data and the search for deviant or contrasting observations. One very common feature of this central analytical phase is the development of typologies that convey the range of views, responses, or arrangements under study. Indeed a typology may be one of the central results of a qualitative analysis. Thus in the example cited earlier of a study of patients presenting headaches to neurological clinics a key insight into the strengths and weaknesses of such clinics came from developing a typology of the different major concerns that motivated patients to seek medical help for headache. Patients' views of the benefits of such clinics could be largely understood in terms of these different concerns. A quite contrasting study analysing the role of medical audit advisory groups (MAAGs) identified a typology of three different major models of MAAG.[22] Often it is simply that certain unanticipated themes emerge from content analysis. Elsewhere is described an important study of stroke survivors' views of the benefits of physiotherapy.[23] Several patients regarded physiotherapy as a source of faith and hope for the future. The authors argue that such insights would not emerge from the current batteries of available patient satisfaction instruments used in quantitative analysis, which concentrate on more familiar dimensions of process and outcome.

A variety of intimidating terms have been developed to describe the logic of qualitative analysis including "analytic induction" and "grounded theory".[24] In different ways such accounts emphasise one common feature – namely, that qualita-tive analysis is iterative. The investigator goes back and forth between his developing concepts and ideas and the raw data of texts or, ideally, fresh observations of the field.

Good practice for qualitative research

The accusation is sometimes made that qualitative research is an "easy option." This usually takes the form of an invidious contrast between informally acquired impressions and the systematic rigour of quantitative methodology. In reality the difficulties of obtaining and conveying insights that are convincing to relevant audiences are at least as great for qualitative research. This section outlines some of the general principles of good practice for qualitative methods that have been developed to facilitate analyses that are plausible and relevant to policy. These principles are further developed in a growing number of more detailed guides to qualitative methodology.[25–27]

Sampling

In quantitative studies considerable attention is given to obtaining a sample which is statistically representative of the population of interest so that generalisations may be made from the study. This is generally achieved through random sampling. In qualitative studies numerical generalisations are less important than *conceptual* generalisations. In this case what is important in drawing a sample is to ensure that it contains the full *range* of possible observations so that the concepts and categories developed provide a comprehensive conceptualisation of the subject. The way in which this is done is through "theoretical sampling."[28] On the basis of his or her theoretical understanding the investigator determines what factors might affect variability in the observations and then endeavours to draw the sample in a way which maximises the variability. This may be decided in advance so that, for example, in a study of a clinic the investigator may be careful to interview patients of varying age, sex, social class, and ethnic background or patients seen by different doctors at different times of day. Theoretical sampling may also require adjusting sources of observation in the course of a study to respond to unanticipated patterns or subgroups of experience which may need increased representation in the sample.

Because qualitative data are more cumbersome to manipulate and analyse most qualitative studies are restricted to a small sample size which is unlikely to be statistically representative of the population. Nevertheless, accounts of qualitative research should always provide a clear account of sampling strategies to allow readers to judge the generalisability of the conceptual analyses.

Validity

In the same way every effort is required to establish the validity of analyses based on qualitative material. The two most commonly cited methods of validating qualitative analysis have already been mentioned in relation to case studies – that is, triangulation and respondent validation. In the first method every effort is made to obtain evidence from as diverse and independent a range of sources as possible. This approach is not very different from the process of establishing construct validity for quantitative measures in that one is looking for patterns of convergence between data sources that together corroborate an overall interpretation. Respondent validation requires that investigators obtain subjects' reactions to their analysis and incorporate such reactions into a more complete analysis. However, neither method provides a perfect solution to the problem of validation. Unfortunately, establishing the plausibility of analyses of social settings and organisations such as health care cannot be done by mechanical use of procedures such as triangulation or respondent validation. The world of health care is particularly complex and interpretations of decisions, behaviour, and arrangements will generally vary among participants.

Participants may have various reasons for not agreeing with analyses of their behaviour, and, indeed, such disagreements may provide further revealing evidence of how an organisation works.[26]

It is therefore important that users of qualitative methods adopt a number of principles to convince audiences of the validity of their analyses. Have investigators sampled the diverse range of individuals and settings relevant to their question? How much have they drawn on and collected evidence in terms of interviews, records, field notes, that are in principle capable of independent inspection by others? How much have they drawn on, whenever available or appropriate, quantitative evidence to check or test qualitative statements? To what extent do investigators seem to have sought out observations that might contradict or modify their analyses?[26,29] It remains a matter of judgement for audiences of qualitative studies to determine how systematically investigators have approached such questions in assembling and interpreting their evidence. It is essential that qualitative researchers make more explicit the methods whereby their analyses have emerged so that audiences can make informed judgements about plausibility.

Understanding issues of quality of care

What is the role of qualitative research in understanding issues of quality of care? On the one hand, qualitative methods have enormous potential to illuminate how health care currently operates and the impact of care on patients. Thus puzzling issues such as the persistence of variations in clinical practice should be addressed by qualitative methods. How patients experience and benefit from health services also needs examination by such methods. On the other hand, as more systematic evidence accumulates of effective interventions and appropriate forms of health care, another kind of application of qualitative methods is required. The changes in health services needed to promote quality are organisational and cultural and involve differing perspectives of a diverse range of health professionals, managers, and patients. Mechanisms of change such as clinical audit, quality assurance, and the adoption of clinical guidelines are social processes with meanings to participants that we need to understand. In such a complex environment qualitative methodology will be essential to give us models of how organisations change and innovate to adopt quality in health care.

There is an exciting range of qualitative methods capable of providing basic understanding of the processes and outcomes of health care. Rigorous and transparent attention to methodology is needed to convince audiences of the value of insights into the "black box" of health care. An understanding of these methods will in turn promote a fuller appreciation of the insights they can provide.

References

1   Pryce-Jones M. Critical incident technique as a method of assessing patient satisfaction. In: Fitzpatrick R., Hopkins A., eds. *Measurement of patients' satisfaction with their care*. London: Royal College of Physicians of London, 1993:87–98.

2   Fitzpatrick R., Hopkins A. Illness behaviour and headache, and the sociology of

consultations for headache. In: Hopkins A, ed. *Headache: problems in management.* London: 1988:351–85.

3   Fitzpatrick R., Hopkins A. Patient satisfaction in relation to clinical care: a neglected contribution. In: Fitzpatrick B., Hopkins A., eds. *Measurement of patients' satisfaction with their care.* London: Royal College of Physicians of London, 1993:77–86.

4   Anderson R., Bury M., eds. *Living with chronic illness.* London: Unwin Hyman, 1988.

5   Black N., Thompson E. Obstacles to medical audit: British doctors speak. *Soc Sci Med* 1993;36:849–56.

6   Daly J. Innocent murmurs: echocardiography and the diagnosis of cardiac normality. *Sociology of Health and Illness* 1989;11:99–116.

7   Green J. The views of singlehanded general practitioners: a qualitative study. *BMJ* 1993;307:607–10.

8   Morgan D., Krueger R. When to use focus groups and why. In: Morgan D., ed. *Successful focus groups.* London: Sage, 1993:3–19.

9   Morgan D. Future directions for focus groups. In: Morgan D., ed. *Successful focus groups.* London: Sage, 1993:225–44.

10   de Vries H., Weijts W., Dijkstra M., Kok G. The utilisation of qualitative and quantitative data for health education program planning, implementation and evaluation, a spiral approach. *Health Educ Q* 1992;19:101–15.

11   NHS Management Executive. *Local voices.* London: Department of Health, 1992.

12   Murray S., Tapson J., Turnbull I., McCallum J., Little A. Listening to local voices: adapting rapid appraisal to assess health and social needs in general practice. *BMJ* 1994;308:698–700.

13   Van de Ven A., Delbecq A. The nominal group technique as a research instrument for exploratory health studies. *Am J Public Health* 1972;62:337–42.

14   Hunter D., McKee C., Sanderson C., Black N. Appropriate indications for prostatectomy in the UK – results of a consensus panel. *J Epidemiol Community Health* 1994;48:58–64.

15   Scott E., Black N. When does consensus exist in expert panels? *J Public Health* 1991;13:35–9.

16   Goffman E. *Asylums: essays on the social situation of mental patients and other inmates.* New York: Anchor, 1961.

17   Strong P. *The ceremonial order of the clinic.* London: Routledge, 1979.

18   Packwood P., Keen J., Buxton M. *Hospitals in transition: the resource management experiment.* Milton Keynes: Open University Press, 1991.

19   Pollitt C., Harrison S., Hunter D., Marnoch G. General management in the NHS: the initial impact, 1983–88. *Public Administration* 1991;69:61–83.

20   Bloor M. On the analysis of observational data: a discussion of the worth and use of inductive techniques and respondent validation. *Sociology* 1978;12:545–52.

21   Fielding N., Lee R. eds. *Using computers in qualitative research.* London: Sage, 1991.

22   Humphrey C., Berrow D. Developing role of medical audit advisory groups. *Quality in Health Care* 1993;2:232–38.

23   Pound P., Bury M., Gompertz P., Ebrahim S. Views of survivors of stroke on the benefits of physiotherapy. *Quality in Health Care* 1994;3:69–74.

24   Bryman A., Burgess R. Developments in qualitative data analysis: an introduction. In: Bryman A., Burgess R., eds. *Analysing qualitative data.* London: Routledge, 1993:1–15.

25   Crabtree R., Mitler W. eds. *Doing qualitative research: multiple strategies*. London: Sage, 1993.
26   Silverman D. *Interpreting qualitative data*. London: Sage. 1993.
27   Bryman A., Burgess R., eds. *Analysing qualitative data*. London: Routledge, 1993.
28   Strauss A. *Qualitative analysis for social scientists*. Cambridge: Cambridge University Press, 1987.
29   Dingwall R. Don't mind him – he's from Barcelona: qualitative methods in health studies. In: Daly J. McDonald L., Willis E., eds *Researching health care*. London: Routledge, 1992:161–75.

Chapter 29

Alistair Howitt and David Armstrong

IMPLEMENTING EVIDENCE-BASED MEDICINE IN GENERAL PRACTICE

Audit and qualitative study of antithrombotic treatment for atrial fibrillation

From *British Medical Journal*, 318, 1999: 1324–7

Introduction

DESPITE THE EFFICACY of antithrombotic treatment in preventing stroke in patients with atrial fibrillation,[1] community surveys report a low uptake of such treatment.[2-4] Suggested explanations include general practitioners' reluctance to initiate and monitor treatment,[5] practical difficulties in anticoagulating elderly housebound patients,[6] and lack of authoritative guidelines.[7] Yet a major part of the problem may relate to the proportion of patients eligible for treatment. Clinical trials, from which evidence for effectiveness is derived, usually exclude certain groups of patients, and trial conclusions might not be appropriate for these patients. Patients in clinical trials may also differ from others in their willingness to accept treatment.

The applicability of evidence based medicine to everyday general practice therefore needs to take account of these constraints. The potential scale of any success for an eligible group of patients will be limited by exclusion of those patients for whom treatment would be inappropriate and those who decline after their personal risk is explained. We carried out such an exercise in a general practice, with antithrombotic treatment in atrial fibrillation.

Subjects and methods

Setting and subjects

We conducted our study in a predominantly urban practice in south east England with 13,239 registered patients. We searched the practice's computer database for patients for whom a diagnosis of atrial fibrillation had been recorded and also for all patients who had been prescribed digoxin. We then examined the paper records to confirm the diagnosis.

Measures and procedure

Details of the patients' age, medical history, contraindications to warfarin, housing, and mobility were recorded. Current antithrombotic treatment was recorded as warfarin, aspirin, or no treatment. For patients on warfarin, presence of an additional indication was recorded.

Where records were unclear or incomplete, we invited patients to attend for review. Patients were then categorised by their risk of thromboembolism: currently at risk were patients with chronic or paroxysmal atrial fibrillation; not currently at risk or at low risk were patients with transient atrial fibrillation (only one episode recorded, for example, postoperatively), patients with documented persistent atrial fibrillation, but currently in a regular rhythm (for example, treated thyrotoxicosis and paroxysmal atrial fibrillation not noted in the past 18 months), and patients aged less than 60 years with no additional clinical risk factors.[8]

We stratified patients currently at risk by risk of stroke,[9] and we assessed for eligibility to attend a structured educational interview to discuss antithrombotic treatment. We excluded those who were taking warfarin for an additional indication, those unable to give informed consent (for example, through dementia), or those too ill to participate. We included all other patients with atrial fibrillation, whether taking warfarin or not. Patients were initially approached during consultations or by telephone. We sent a letter with details of the study to those agreeing to participate. Patients unable to attend the surgery were seen at home.

Educational intervention

We asked patients if they were aware that they were at increased risk of stroke and if they were, to give an estimate of that risk.

We used a structured method of giving information about the nature and consequences of having a stroke. Detailed information about aspirin and warfarin treatment was also given. Patients were shown a pictorial representation of their predicted annual risk of stroke (either 4%, 8%, or 12%) and the expected benefits of treatment, amended from the method described by Man-Son-Hing and colleagues,[10] to include risk stratification[9] and aspirin as an alternative treatment to warfarin (Figure 29.1). They were asked which, if any, treatment they would choose, and from this we derived the minimal clinically important difference for warfarin, which is the minimum level of benefit for which they would take warfarin. We recorded this as a percentage reduction in their annual risk of stroke.

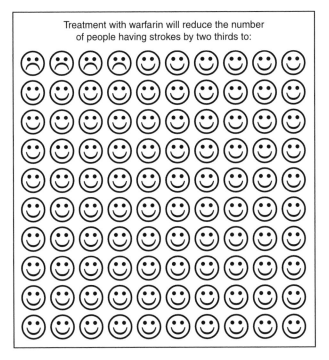

Treatment with warfarin will reduce the number
of people having strokes by two thirds to:

Figure 29.1 Pictorial representation of expected benefit of warfarin treatment shown to patients with predicted annual risk of stroke without any treatment of 12 per cent

During the interviews we made notes of patients' comments and reactions to the information they were given.

We screened patients for conditions associated with atrial fibrillation and other risk factors for stroke. They were all offered echocardiography, which was performed by an experienced echocardiographer within a week of consultation. The report included estimates of left atrial size, left ventricular function, and ejection fraction.

The patients then attended a second interview to decide the antithrombotic treatment they wanted to receive. We recorded the treatment taken after the study.

We analysed data using SPSS for Windows. We performed analyses using χ^2 for cross tabulations, independent samples t test for two group comparisons, and analysis of variance for multiple group comparisons.

Results

We identified 132 patients with a history of atrial fibrillation of whom 100 were judged eligible for warfarin. Of these, we excluded 16 who were unable to consent, eight who were too ill to participate, and 16 who had other clinical indications for taking warfarin. Of the remaining 60 patients, 56 (93%) consented to be interviewed. There was no difference in age or duration of fibrillation between patients attending for interview and the other 44 patients also at risk who were not invited or declined to attend. These 44 patients were more likely to have a history of stroke

(χ^2 5.87, P < 0.05), falls (Fisher's exact test, P < 0.05), and frailty (Fisher's exact test, P < 0.01).

Before the study, 43 patients were taking warfarin, and subsequently 10 patients from the interview group started warfarin. Another seven patients who were taking no treatment started aspirin. One patient who had recently started warfarin to cover an unsuccessful cardioversion decided to switch to aspirin.

None of the clinical sociodemographic variables or the severity measure of predicted annual stroke rate predicted which patients would start warfarin. Twenty-nine patients (52%) agreed to echocardiography, but only one started warfarin because of the test result.

Patients' involvement

Most patients (61%, 34/56) were unaware that they were at risk of stroke, and of those who were aware only two felt able to give an annual estimate of the risk. Of the patients taking warfarin, eight of 17 (47%) were not aware of the risk. Several patients were also unaware that they had an irregular pulse.

Not all patients felt able to make a judgment that could inform derivation of their minimal clinically important difference for warfarin. For those that did, 15 patients already taking warfarin were willing to take it for a lower level of benefit than 20 not taking it, with a mean minimal clinically important difference of 2.4% per annum versus a mean of 4.1% (t test 2.19, P = 0.036). A one way analysis of variance test showed no differences in minimal clinically important difference with differing degrees of risk. The importance of the patients' view of the balance of risk was also evident. Patients' own judgment of their minimal clinically important difference predicted those patients who were going to start warfarin, with a mean minimal clinically important difference at the first interview of 2.56% for those starting warfarin and 4.86% for those not starting warfarin (t test 2.93, P < 0.05).

Although the patients made comparatively few comments about their illness and its treatment at their interview, there were some common themes. For example, many patients who decided not to have warfarin did not see themselves at risk whereas patients choosing warfarin feared the effects of a stroke (Box 29.1).

Box 29.1   Health beliefs

Perceived vulnerability
"I'm not going to have a stroke anyway . . . confident good span of life in front of me." (Patient 12, final treatment aspirin.)

"People who have strokes are overweight, drink and smoke. I don't think it will happen." (Patient 16, final treatment aspirin.)

Perceived seriousness
"If I had a bad stroke, I'd be as good as dead." (Patient 85, started warfarin.)

"I'd rather have a heart attack than a stroke . . . I think stroke is the worst thing out." (Patient 105, started warfarin.)

For others, their advanced age and impending death was an issue. Their response to it was, however, varied and unpredictable. Some seized the chance to prolong their lives whereas others accepted that their lives were limited and did not seem to want them artificially extended (Box 29.2). Many patients included in their responses

---

Box 29.2   Attitudes to death

Seeking to prolong life
"It'll give me a couple of extra years." (Patient 26, aged 82, started warfarin.)

"I want to prolong my life as long as possible." (Patient 120, aged 90, started warfarin.)

Accepting death
"Life's precious, in for a penny, in for a pound. It will eventually happen and I'd rather go as naturally as possible." (Patient 128, aged 90, declined warfarin.)

"Here you are trying to extend the life of an aged person, it's illogical." (Patient 108, aged 86, declined any treatment.)

---

attitudes to change in treatment, which were almost always negative, and many feared the consequences of altering their treatment (Box 29.3).

Box 29.3   Attitudes to change

"I'm feeling a lot better, pity if I've got to change . . . if I change it over. I'll knock it all back again." (Patient 25, decided to continue aspirin.)

"I'd be delighted to come off warfarin . . . [although] I haven't the nerve to give it up." (Patient 81, continued warfarin.)

Discussion

The prevalence rates of atrial fibrillation reported here are similar to those in recent studies from the United Kingdom, suggesting that identification of patients in our study had comparable efficiency.[2–4,11] But out of 132 patients with a recorded history of atrial fibrillation – and 100 in whom it was judged clinically appropriate – only 52 were taking warfarin at the end of the study. Of these, most were already taking it and only 10 started warfarin – that is, even with careful case finding and follow up a large proportion of patients with atrial fibrillation could not be changed to an overtly more effective treatment.

Our study was conducted in only one practice and others might have different background prevalences of atrial fibrillation, concurrent illnesses, and patient responses. The proportion of patients taking warfarin before the intervention was higher than in other studies,[2–4,11] suggesting that the final proportion in our study was not unrepresentatively low. The fact that a half of eligible patients received warfarin after intensive exploration of best management for each patient suggests a major constraint on the uptake of evidence based medicine and a serious dilution of its potential impact.

Why was there such a small effect?

Four groups of patients can be identified out of those judged clinically eligible for warfarin: a small group already taking the drug for other reasons; a group comprising those patients who were taking warfarin solely for their fibrillation after the study; a group, about a quarter of those eligible, who could not be offered treatment because of other factors such as concurrent illness and dementia (as trial protocols often exclude such patients it is clear that trials overestimate the value of treatment in terms of the standard index of number needed to treat): and a group who ultimately declined to be assessed or to start treatment, even though clinically suited. So why did some patients agree to take the drug while others declined?

Sociodemographic factors, including age, did not relate to uptake nor did the presence of additional clinical risk factors. One factor that seemed to make a difference was the measure of patients' willingness to take risks. This finding was further amplified by the patients' comments on treatment. These illustrate the importance of patients' beliefs about the value of treatment, their assessment of personal risk, and their reluctance to change their drugs in the final management decision.

Problems with implementation

Our study also puts into context the view that the problem lies in the difficulty of changing doctors' behaviour to be more in accord with current best evidence. Certainly, changing clinical behaviour may not be easy but this must be seen in the light of other significant barriers to implementing evidence based medicine in general practice.

The first level of implementation, assessing evidence on effectiveness, is essentially population based as it advises on the proportion likely to benefit out of a defined group of patients with the condition. But in applying this evidence to individual patients in routine practice, two further assessments of this evidence need to be made. Firstly, a practitioner based assessment to identify individuals who may benefit from the treatment and secondly, the individual patient has to make the decision as to whether, given the advantages and disadvantages, the treatment is worth taking. Our study has addressed these two, often neglected, stages in the implementation process and illustrates that consent lies at the heart of the third level of implementation – namely, the patient's agreement to take the treatment. Had patients in this study been expressly advised to start warfarin then perhaps the uptake would have been greater. For example, general practitioners overrode a decision to start warfarin in 18 out of 44 patients who were willing to take it after being advised by a doctor involved in a research project.[2] But the approach reported here suggests that a patient centred method, in which as many patients as possible are given an active role in deciding their treatment, produces a less successful outcome regarding warfarin uptake but perhaps a better one regarding the ethics of patient management. It might seem ironic that it is patients who represent an important impediment to implementation of effective treatment given that they apparently have most to benefit, but without their support evidence based medicine is likely to have only limited applicability in general practice.

References

1   Atrial Fibrillation Investigators. Risk factors for stroke and efficacy of antithrombotic therapy in atrial fibrillation. Analysis of pooled data from five randomized controlled trials. *Arch Intern Med* 1994:154:1449–57.

2   Wheeldon NM, Tayler DI, Anagnostou E, Cook D, Wales C. Oakley GDG. Screening for atrial fibrillation in primary care. *Heart* 1998;79:50–5.

3   Sudlow M, Thomson R, Thwaites B, Rodgers H, Kenny RA. Prevalence of atrial fibrillation and eligibility for anticoagulants in the community. *Lancet* 1998;352:1167–71.

4   Lip GYH, Golding DJ, Nazir M, Beevers DG, Child DL, Fletcher RI. A survey of atrial fibrillation in general practice: the West Birmingham atrial fibrillation project. *Br J Gen Pract* 1997;47:285–9.

5   Taylor F, Ramsay M, Voke J, Cohen H. Anticoagulation in patients with atrial fibrillation. GPs not prepared for monitoring anticoagulation. *BMJ* 1993;307:1493.

6   Roderick E, Cox J. Non-valvular atrial fibrillation. *Br J Gen Pract* 1997;47:660–1.

7   Thomson R, McElroy H, Sudlow M. Guidelines on anticoagulant treatment in atrial fibrillation in Great Britain: variation in content and implications for treatment. *BMJ* 1998;316:509–13.

8   Stroke Prevention in Atrial Fibrillation Investigators. Predictors of thromboembolism in atrial fibrillation. I. Clinical features of patients at risk. *Ann Intern Med* 1992;116:1–5.

9   Lip CY, Lowe GD. ABC of atrial fibrillation. Antithrombotic treatment for atrial fibrillation. *BMJ* 1996;312:45–9.

10 Man-Son-Hing M, Laupacis A, O'Connor A, Wells G, Lemelin J, Wood W, *et al.* Warfarin for atrial fibrillation. The patient's perspective. *Arch Interm Med* 1996;156:1811–8.

11 O'Connell JE, Gray CS. Atrial fibrillation and stroke prevention in the community: *Age Ageing* 1996;25:307–9.

Chapter 30

Katie Featherstone and Jenny L. Donovan

RANDOM ALLOCATION OR ALLOCATION AT RANDOM?

Patients' perspectives of participation in a randomised controlled trial

From *British Medical Journal*, 317, 1998: 1177–80

Introduction

THE RANDOMISED CONTROLLED trial is the widely acknowledged design of choice for evaluating medical and surgical treatments.[1,2] Though textbooks and reports of trials in journals focus on issues concerned with design, methods, and results,[1-3] the patient's perspective is relatively neglected. Published research has mostly used questionnaires to examine attitudes towards participation in order to improve accrual. Satisfaction with trial participation is reported by 90–97% of patients.[4-6] Those (75–93% of respondents) who said they would participate in future trials cited altruism[5-7] and personal benefit[5,6,8,9] as reasons. Difficulties with travelling and time taken were the only major criticisms.[4,6,8] Studies of the public or outpatients indicate that 50–75% would probably participate, with 10–20% definitely refusing.[8,10,11-14] Interpretation of these studies is difficult because of their reliance on general issues or hypothetical trials, which do not have direct relevance to actual participation in real trials. Recent research has explored how patients' preferences might be incorporated within trials because of their potential influence on outcome.[15-19]

Two studies have used qualitative research methods to explore more detailed perceptions of methods and terms employed by trials. Roberson et al found that although respondents were familiar with the term "experimental study", two thirds had not heard the term "clinical trial."[20] Snowdon et al, using in-depth interviews with parents of critically ill babies, found that the nature of the trial was often poorly understood and that there were particular problems with the concept of random allocation, and considerable confusion and anger relating to parents' desire for the most suitable treatment for their child.[21]

The existing research record has tended to focus on hypothetical questions, often in trials of rare conditions, or in Snowdon et al's case, parents of critically ill babies.[21] The study reported here uses qualitative research methods to elicit the perspectives of "ordinary" middle aged and elderly men who require elective treatment for a common condition and who have themselves agreed to participate in a pragmatic randomised controlled trial. This paper focuses on the ways in which they make sense of the concept that lies at the heart of the randomised controlled trial: random allocation.

Patients and methods

The study involved patients eligible for the CLasP study. This comprises three linked pragmatic randomised controlled trials to evaluate the effectiveness of a new technology (laser therapy) compared with standard surgery (transurethral resection of the prostate – TURP) for men with acute or chronic urinary retention; and laser surgery, and conservative management (monitoring without active intervention) for men with lower urinary tract symptoms related to benign prostatic disease. The aims of this substudy, to explore the perspectives of patients who agreed or refused to participate in CLasP, meant that qualitative research methods were most appropriate.[22]

Sampling in qualitative research uses non-probability methods, including "purposeful" sampling, in which individuals with particular characteristics are deliberately and systematically selected to explore emerging analytical themes. In this study, 20 participants were interviewed; they came from each of the major clinical centres (11 from A, nine from B), different treatment arms (five conservative management, eight laser therapy, seven TURP), and at different time points (seven within 3 months and five within 5 months of randomisation, and eight after receiving treatment). Men who chose not to participate were also interviewed (these data will be reported elsewhere).

Data were collected by in-depth interviews carried out by KF using a semi-structured checklist of topics,[23-25] covering the same basic issues, including initial symptoms; recall, understanding, and experience of recruitment; feelings about participation; experiences of treatment; and outcome. The aim was to encourage the men to relate stories about their experiences and to explore their understandings of what had happened. Interviews were conducted in the men's homes and recorded on audio tape; they lasted from half an hour to one and a half hours. Each interview was transcribed by KF verbatim, including descriptions of non-verbal factors where appropriate. Analysis of the data proceeded by detailed scrutiny of the transcripts to identify common themes, which were coded; these coded segments of text were included in separate word processing files.[26] These files were expanded with new transcripts and refined, focused, or altered as new themes emerged. Each individual's narrative was examined independently to assess the coherence of each account. Data collection and analysis continued concurrently, according to constant comparison methods of grounded theory, in which data are examined for similarities and differences within themes, retaining the context of the discussion and characteristics of the individuals to aid understanding and allow interpretation and the development of explanations of findings.[27]

Treatment in the CLasP study was allocated to each patient after he had given written informed consent and completed questionnaires and clinical tests, and was done by clinical researchers opening consecutive opaque envelopes. Patients were given an information sheet that described the study as a randomised controlled trial and said that it involved comparing treatments, that one treatment was new (laser therapy), that there was uncertainty about which treatment was best, and that allocation would be by chance and by a clinician opening a sealed envelope.

The results relating to the experience and understanding of randomisation are presented below according to the themes which emerged from the interview data, although space does not permit detailed descriptions of the context surrounding these data. Illustrative quotations are provided, selected for their relevance to the themes and so that the reader can judge the interpretations of the researchers. Names have been changed to protect confidentiality.

Results

Understanding randomisation

Almost all the participants were aware of some aspects of randomisation, and most (14/20) acknowledged the involvement of chance in the allocation of their treatment. Often this was transformed into a description of other (lay) examples of chance, such as a lottery or lucky dip:

> Mr Cooper: But anyway I agreed to have a go at it, a bit of a lucky dip. She has them in envelopes, which operation you are going to get, or which method of treatment you are going to get.

> Mr Symonds: He said, oh yes you've got a swollen prostate, you'll probably have to have an operation but it's a chance you might take, which one of them you take, it comes out the hat, sort of thing you know. It's out of the hat, you cannot pick.

Around half of the men (11) talked about the study in terms of it being a comparison between treatments or an experiment, with the treatment allocation being unknown until the contents of an envelope were revealed:

> Mr Taylor: She told me that I would either have the laser treatment or the operation . . . and at the same time explained that neither she nor the consultant himself knew which I would get until they chose this famous envelope.

A smaller number (four) were also more explicit about clinical equipoise – that the doctor did not know what treatment was best:

Mr Murray: They were unbiased, didn't give you any impression that one was better than the other. But the scheme itself was – I think they wanted to compare, they wanted to do all three and then make a comparison of what the end results were.

Explaining treatment allocation

The majority of men developed detailed narratives to describe and explain their understanding of the method of treatment allocation. While most were able to describe aspects of randomisation, such as the involvement of chance, need for comparison, and concealed allocation, often their narratives contained other lay explanations of what they thought had happened or should have happened. Sometimes this was caused by a clash between experience and expectation – for example, where they had not seen the clinician open the envelope as expected:

Mr Mills: When she first explained it, she said you'll be given an envelope and you take your pick, apparently, and that never happened. . . . I never got offered any envelope. I was just . . . that was the treatment they more or less picked out for me.

Perhaps the most difficult concept for patients to comprehend was clinical equipoise. Lay beliefs and previous experience meant that the men expected clinicians to assign them to treatment based on their specific symptoms, clinical findings, and age:

Mr Symonds: They still let you do the three card trick and they just carry it on because from the very first start it is written in the pamphlets they give you . . . You've got your three choices, your TURPs, your – what do you call it [laser therapy], this one where you're under management, but I think it would be even better if they were to tell you that they prefer, what you're going to get . . . I think that would be better than they let you take your pick when I think, along the lines, that you know you're being conned.

Mr Webster: Well [randomisation] was a bit confusing. It was. They know what's wrong with us. I thought it would just be one operation and that was it. If it was an operation, or if they could have cured it by medication, they would have decided there and then. The other consultant would have decided – you know, this lad needs medication, or, yes, this lad needs the operation.

KF: Did that surprise you?

Mr Webster: Yes it did actually, it did. I could understand it, but I couldn't realise, cope with the idea that whatever the symptoms were, that was the envelope we were going to get . . . I just thought that . . . if it wasn't too bad, I would get the medication . . . but it just seems that they're tossing a coin in the air.

Other common lay views revolved around the influence of fate, luck, and trust:

> Mr Grange: I must say that I was fairly convinced that I was going to get a laser operation. I don't feel at all that those envelopes had anything to do with it.

> Mr Cooper: I preferred the one that I got, so I must have been lucky.

Although the majority of men were able to discuss randomisation, two patients, both from the same centre and randomised to laser therapy, did not believe that their allocation was different from normal clinical practice. Apart from these two, levels of knowledge about randomisation and development of alternative accounts were similar between centres and across treatment arms.

Meanings of trial terms

Another complicating issue was the lay understanding of common terms often used by trialists with specific meanings but which have other meanings outside the confines of randomised controlled trials, such as "trial" and "random." In lay language, the word "trial" means something that is tried out, while "at random" relates to things being done without purpose:

> Mr Bowler: She said there was three options which I had already read about. One was tablets, one was the ordinary operation, and one was laser. I didn't really realise that it was this scheme whereby they were, a trial, you know. Because I didn't think the other one is a trial – TURP. It's longstanding, isn't it?

> Mr Flint: Well, I suppose there's a random system. There isn't a better way really. I mean, if it was just done randomly like that without anybody looking to see how certain results had gone and say, "Oh well, we'll take that one for there, we'll do this one there." If it was done randomly like that, then I suppose it's as good as any.

Discussion

Randomisation and treatment allocation

Most patients were able to describe some aspects of the concept of randomisation, particularly in terms of the involvement of chance, with some having a more detailed understanding of treatment comparison, concealed allocation, and experimental design. In response to a structured questionnaire about randomisation, most would probably have been shown to understand the concept in these basic terms. Qualitative research has shown that individuals routinely attempt to make sense of events by interpreting them in the context of their existing beliefs.[28,29] In attempting to make sense of their participation in this trial, these men produced narratives which on the one hand described their understanding of elements of randomisation, but on the other hand challenged these understandings with, for example, accounts about trusting clinicians to make treatment allocations on the basis of individual clinical characteristics.

The existence of different accounts about treatment allocation could indicate confusion or distortion, as has been suggested elsewhere.[21] The men in this trial acknowledged that randomisation was confusing (see Mr Webster above). Closer examination, however, shows that these apparently contradictory accounts are consistent in their own terms. The men's view that treatment should be determined by clinical and personal characteristics (symptoms or age) is reinforced by the number and complexity of tests and questionnaires they complete during the trial. Any confusion that arises comes from their attempts to make sense of their experience by trying to piece together apparently contradictory accounts – not from a lack of understanding of randomisation.

Information and consent

The terminology used in trials can have different meanings to participants and trialists. The lay definition of "random" (see Mr Flint) implies that treatments are allocated without purpose or control. Similarly, "trial" means that something is being "tried and tested" (see Mr Bowler). Mr Bowler is able to believe that laser therapy is "on trial" but has difficulty with the idea that the standard operation, TURP, is still "on trial." Similar lay definitions have been found elsewhere.[20,21]

Also of importance is consistency between information given to participants and actual practice. In the CLasP study, information given to patients indicated that clinicians would open treatment allocation envelopes in front of patients. In practice, this was not possible. For some, not seeing the envelopes suggested that treatment could have been determined by clinicians. For Mr Symonds, it was the source of distrust about the study. Patient information needs to be clear about procedures to avoid such misinterpretation.

Perhaps more important are the implications for informed consent. Many of these men were struggling to come to terms with different (sometimes competing) views about randomisation. Although all had given written informed consent, it is evident that the majority did not hold a consistent explanation of the scientific method underlying the research. Further research is required to investigate whether these views are found more widely. It is also not clear what impact such beliefs may have on outcome, although some patients were upset by the difficulty of reconciling their views. Some patients doubted the veracity of the trial.

Conclusion

Although this study confirms the importance of providing clear and accurate patient information, it also shows that this in itself is unlikely to ensure consistent interpretation of concepts such as randomisation by participants. The patient information in this study was well received and largely accurately recalled, but patients still struggled with the concepts underlying the design and sometimes developed coexisting contradictory accounts. It may be that participants need to discuss the reasons for particular methods of trial design (such as randomisation) with researchers and reflect on these in order to understand them fully enough to give true informed consent. It is not clear, however, whether this greater understanding would lead to higher or lower levels of accrual to trials, but such an investigation could be linked with research attempting to incorporate patient preferences into randomised controlled trials.[15,16]

References

1   Altman DG. Better reporting of randomised controlled trials: the CONSORT statement. *BMJ* 1996;313:570–1.

2   Pocock SJ. *Clinical trials: a practical approach*. Chichester: Wiley, 1983.

3   Senn S. *Statistical issues in drug development*. Chichester: Wiley, 1997.

4   Henzlova MJ, Blackburn GH, Bradley EJ, Rogers WJ. Patient perception of a long-term clinical trial: Experience using a close-out questionnaire in the studies of left-ventricular dysfunction (SOLVD) trial. *Control Clin Trials* 1994; 15:284–93.

5   Suchanek Hudmon K, Stoltzfus C, Chamberlain RM, Lorimor RJ. Steinbach G, Winn RJ. Participants' perceptions of a phase I colon cancer chemoprevention trial. *Control Clin Trials* 1996;17:494–508.

6   Schron EB, Wassertheil-Smoller S, Pressel S. Clinical trial participant satisfaction: survey of SHEP enrollees. *J Am Geriatr Soc* 1997;45:934–38.

7   Bevan EG, Chee LC, McGhee SM, McInnes GT. Patients' attitudes to participation in clinical trials. *Br J Clin Pharmacol* 1993;35:204–7.

8   Mattson ME, Curb JD, McArdle R, and the AMIS and BHAT Research Groups. Participation in a clinical trial: the patients' point of view. *Control Clin Trials* 1985;6:156–67.

9   Daugherty C, Ratain MJ, Grochowski F, Stocking C, Kodish E, Mick R, *et al.* Perceptions of cancer patients and their physicians involved in phase I trials. *J Clin Oncol* 1995;1:1062–72.

10   Cassileth BR, Lusk EJ, Miller DS, Hurwitz S. Attitudes toward clinical trials among patients and the public. *JAMA* 1982;248:968–70.

11   Slevin M, Mossman J, Bowling A, Leonard R, Steward W, Harper P, *et al.* Volunteers or victims: patients' views of randomised cancer clinical trials. *Br J Cancer* 1995;71:1270–4.

12   Rimer BK, Schildkraut JM, Lerman C, Lin TH, Audrain J. Participation in a women's breast cancer risk counselling trial. Who participates? Who declines? High Risk Breast Cancer Consortium. *Cancer* 1996;77(suppl): 2348–55.

13   Llewellyn-Thomas HA, McGreal MJ, Thiel FC, Fine S, Erlichman C. Patients' willingness to enter clinical trials: measuring the association with perceived benefit and preference for decision participation. *Soc Sci Med* 1991;32:35–41.

14   Bartholow BN, Macqueen KM, Douglas JM Jr, Buchbinder S, McKirnan D, Judson FN. Assessment of the changing willingness to participate in phase III HIV vaccine trials among men who have sex with men. *J AIDs Hum Retrovirol* 1997;16:108–15.

15 Kassirer JP. Incorporating patients' preferences in medical decisions [editorial]. *N Engl J Med* 1994;330:1895–6.

16 Silverman WA. Patients' preferences and randomised trials. *Lancet* 1996;317:1714.

17 Brewin CR, Bradley C. Patient preferences and randomised clinical trials. *BMJ* 1989;299:313–5.

18 McPherson K. The best and the enemy of the good: randomised controlled trials, uncertainty, and assessing the role of patient choice in medical decision making. *J Epidemiol Community Health* 1994;48:6–15.

19 Sutherland HJ. Llewellyn-Thomas HA, Lockwood GA, Trichler DI, Till JE. Cancer patients' desire for participation in treatment. *J R Soc Med* 1980;82:260–3.

20 Roberson NL. Clinical trial participation. Viewpoints from racial/ethnic groups. *Cancer* 1994:74(suppl):2687–91.

21 Snowdon C, Garcia J, Elbourne D. Making sense of randomization: responses of parents of critically ill babies to random allocation of treatment in a clinical trial. *Soc Sci Med* 1997;45:1337–55.

22 Pope C, Mays N. Reaching the parts other methods cannot reach: an introduction to qualitative methods in health and health services research. *BMJ* 1995;311:12–5.

23 Burgess RG. The unstructured interview as a conversation. In: Burgess RG, ed. *Field research: a source book and field mannual.* London: Routledge, 1982:107–10.

24 Hammersley M, Atkinson P. *Ethnography: principles in practice.* London: Tavistock, 1988.

25 Mays N, Pope C, eds. *Qualitative research in health care.* London BMJ publishing Groups, 1996.

26 Miles MB, Huberman EM. *Qualitative data analysis.* 2nd ed. London: Sage, 1994.

27 Glaser BG, Strauss AL. *The discovery of grounded theory.* Chicago: Aldine, 1967.

28 Schutz A. *The phenomenology of the social world.* London: Heinemann Educational, 1972.

29 Williams G. The genesis of chronic illness: narrative reconstruction. *Sociol Health Illness* 1984;6:175–200.

Index